Pharmaceutics and Pharmacology

Pharmaceutics and Pharmacology

Editor: Sean Boyd

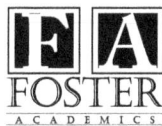

FA
FOSTER
A C A D E M I C S

www.fosteracademics.com

www.fosteracademics.com

FA
FOSTER
ACADEMICS

Cataloging-in-Publication Data

Pharmaceutics and pharmacology / edited by Sean Boyd.
    p. cm.
Includes bibliographical references and index.
ISBN 978-1-63242-511-9
1. Pharmacology. 2. Pharmacy. 3. Drugs. 4. Medical sciences. I. Boyd, Sean.
RM300 .P43 2017
615.1--dc23

Foster Academics,
118-35 Queens Blvd., Suite 400,
Forest Hills, NY 11375, USA

ISBN 978-1-63242-511-9 (Hardback)

Printed and bound in the United States of America.

Contents

Preface IX

Chapter 1   Design and evaluation of Lumefantrine – Oleic acid self nanoemulsifying
             ionic complex for enhanced dissolution...1
             Ketan Patel, Vidur Sarma and Pradeep Vavia

Chapter 2   Silymarin improved 6-OHDA-induced motor impairment in
             hemi-parkisonian rats...11
             Rasool Haddadi, Alireza Mohajjel Nayebi, Safar Farajniya,
             Shahla Eyvari Brooshghalan and Hamdolah Sharifi

Chapter 3   The effect of adipose derived stromal cells on oxidative stress level,
             lung emphysema and white blood cells of guinea pigs model of
             chronic obstructive pulmonary disease...19
             Ahmad Ghorbani, Azadeh Feizpour, Milad Hashemzahi, Lila Gholami,
             Mahmoud Hosseini, Mohammad Soukhtanloo, Farzaneh Vafaee Bagheri,
             Esmaeil Khodaei, Nema Mohammadian Roshan and
             Mohammad Hossein Boskabady

Chapter 4   A comparative study on the physicochemical and biological
             stability of IgG$_1$ and monoclonal antibodies during spray drying
             process...32
             Vahid Ramezani, Alireza Vatanara,
             Abdolhossein Rouholamini Najafabadi, Mohammad Ali Shokrgozar,
             Alireza Khabiri and Mohammad Seyedabadi

Chapter 5   Identifying and prioritizing industry-level competitiveness factors:
             Evidence from pharmaceutical market..39
             Hosein Shabaninejad, Gholamhossein Mehralian, Arash Rashidian,
             Ahmad Baratimarnani and Hamid Reza Rasekh

Chapter 6   Selenium nanoparticle-enriched *Lactobacillus brevis* causes more
             efficient immune responses in vivo and reduces the liver metastasis in
             metastatic form of mouse breast cancer..46
             Mohammad Hossein Yazdi, Mehdi Mahdavi, Neda Setayesh,
             Mohammad Esfandyar and Ahmad Reza Shahverdi

Chapter 7   Tribulus terrestris for treatment of sexual dysfunction in women:
             Randomized double-blind placebo...55
             Elham Akhtari, Firoozeh Raisi, Mansoor Keshavarz, Hamed Hosseini,
             Farnaz Sohrabvand, Soodabeh Bioos, Mohammad Kamalinejad and
             Ali Ghobadi

Chapter 8   Quantification of verbascoside in medicinal species of *Phlomis* and
             their genetic relationships...61
             Parisa Sarkhail, Marjan Nikan, Pantea Sarkheil, Ahmad R Gohari,
             Yousef Ajani, Rohollah Hosseini, Abbass Hadjiakhoondi and
             Soodabeh Saeidnia

Chapter 9   Current approaches of the management of mercury poisoning: need
             of the hour...70
             Mehrdad Rafati-Rahimzadeh, Mehravar Rafati-Rahimzadeh,
             Sohrab Kazemi and Ali Akbar Moghadamnia

Chapter 10   The effects of cichorium intybus extract on the maturation and
             activity of dendritic cells..80
             Mohammad Hossein Karimi, Salimeh Ebrahimnezhad,
             Mandana Namayandeh and Zahra Amirghofran

Chapter 11   Synthesis and cytotoxic properties of novel
             (*E*)-3-benzylidene-7-methoxychroman-4-one derivatives............................87
             Saeedeh Noushini, Eskandar Alipour, Saeed Emami, Maliheh Safavi,
             Sussan Kabudanian Ardestani, Ahmad Reza Gohari, Abbas Shafiee
             and Alireza Foroumadi

Chapter 12   Angiogenic effect of the aqueous extract of *Cynodon dactylon* on
             human umbilical vein endothelial cells and granulation tissue in rat 97
             Hamid Soraya, Milad Moloudizargari, Shahin Aghajanshakeri,
             Soheil Javaherypour, Aram Mokarizadeh, Sanaz Hamedeyazdan,
             Hadi Esmaeli Gouvarchin Ghaleh, Peyman Mikaili and Alireza Garjani

Chapter 13   Doxorubicin-conjugated PLA-PEG-Folate based polymeric micelle
             for tumor-targeted delivery: Synthesis and *in vitro* evaluation.................105
             Zahra Hami, Mohsen Amini, Mahmoud Ghazi-Khansari,
             Seyed Mehdi Rezayat and Kambiz Gilani

Chapter 14   New aspects of *Saccharomyces cerevisiae* as a novel carrier for
             berberine..112
             Roshanak Salari, BiBi Sedigheh Fazly Bazzaz, Omid Rajabi and
             Zahra Khashyarmanesh

Chapter 15   High dose insulin therapy, an evidence based approach to beta
             blocker/calcium channel blocker toxicity..120
             Christina Woodward, Ali Pourmand and Maryann Mazer-Amirshahi

Chapter 16   The cytotoxic activities of 7-isopentenyloxycoumarin on 5637 cells
             via induction of apoptosis and cell cycle arrest in G2/M stage..................125
             Fereshteh Haghighi, Maryam M Matin, Ahmad Reza Bahrami,
             Mehrdad Iranshahi, Fatemeh B Rassouli and Azadeh Haghighitalab

Chapter 17   **Non-addictive opium alkaloids selectively induce apoptosis in cancer cells compared to normal cells**...135
Monireh Afzali, Padideh Ghaeli, Mahnaz Khanavi, Maliheh Parsa,
Hamed Montazeri, Mohammad Hossein Ghahremani and
Seyed Nasser Ostad

Chapter 18   **A new formulation of cannabidiol in cream shows therapeutic effects in a mouse model of experimental autoimmune encephalomyelitis**...143
Sabrina Giacoppo, Maria Galuppo, Federica Pollastro, Gianpaolo Grassi,
Placido Bramanti and Emanuela Mazzon

Chapter 19   *Artemia salina* **as a model organism in toxicity assessment of nanoparticles**...160
Somayeh Rajabi, Ali Ramazani, Mehrdad Hamidi and Tahereh Naji

Chapter 20   **Molecular docking and inhibition studies on the interactions of** *Bacopa monnieri's* **potent phytochemicals against pathogenic** *Staphylococcus aureus*...166
Talha Bin Emran, Md Atiar Rahman, Mir Muhammad Nasir Uddin,
Raju Dash, Md Firoz Hossen, Mohammad Mohiuddin and
Md Rashadul Alam

Chapter 21   **Effect of ethylene glycol dimethacrylate on swelling and on metformin hydrochloride release behavior of chemically crosslinked pH–sensitive acrylic acid–polyvinyl alcohol hydrogel**................................174
Muhammad Faheem Akhtar, Nazar Muhammad Ranjha and
Muhammad Hanif

Chapter 22   **Can donepezil facilitate weaning from mechanical ventilation in difficult to wean patients?**..184
Saeed Abbasi, Shadi Farsaei, Kamran Fazel, Samad EJ Golzari and
Ata Mahmoodpoor

Chapter 23   **Characterization and pharmacological potential of** *Lactobacillus sakei* **1I1 isolated from fresh water fish** *Zacco koreanus*...................................192
Vivek K. Bajpai, Jeong-Ho Han, Gyeong-Jun Nam, Rajib Majumder,
Chanseo Park, Jeongheui Lim, Woon Kee Paek, Irfan A. Rather and
Yong-Ha Park

Chapter 24   **Improved anticancer delivery of paclitaxel by albumin surface modification of PLGA nanoparticles**...204
Mehdi Esfandyari-Manesh, Seyed Hossein Mostafavi, Reza Faridi Majidi,
Mona Noori Koopaei, Nazanin Shabani Ravari, Mohsen Amini,
Behrad Darvishi, Seyed Nasser Ostad, Fatemeh Atyabi and
Rassoul Dinarvand

Chapter 25   **Preliminary investigation of the effects of topical mixture of**
Lawsonia inermis L. and _Ricinus communis_ L. leaves extract in treatment of
osteoarthritis using MIA model in rats.. 212
Atousa Ziaei, Shamim Sahranavard, Mohammad Javad Gharagozlou
and Mehrdad Faizi

Permissions

List of Contributors

Index

Preface

The main aim of this book is to educate learners and enhance their research focus by presenting diverse topics covering this vast field. This is an advanced book which compiles significant studies by distinguished experts. This book addresses successive solutions to the challenges arising in the area of application, along with it; the book provides scope for future developments.

Pharmaceutics is the study of medicine, design and dosage that can be used safely by patients. This book on pharmaceutics and pharmacology discusses topics related to the formulation and manufacturing of pharmaceutical drugs. Drug design and development seek to create drugs from new chemical entities as well as redesign existing drugs. This book contains some path-breaking studies in the field of pharmaceutics and pharmacology. A number of latest researches have been included to keep the readers up-to-date with the global concepts in this area of study. It attempts to understand the multiple branches that fall under this discipline and how such concepts have practical applications. Researchers and students in this field will be assisted by this book.

It was a great honour to edit this book, though there were challenges, as it involved a lot of communication and networking between me and the editorial team. However, the end result was this all-inclusive book covering diverse themes in the field.

Finally, it is important to acknowledge the efforts of the contributors for their excellent chapters, through which a wide variety of issues have been addressed. I would also like to thank my colleagues for their valuable feedback during the making of this book.

Editor

Design and evaluation of Lumefantrine – Oleic acid self nanoemulsifying ionic complex for enhanced dissolution

Ketan Patel, Vidur Sarma and Pradeep Vavia[*]

Abstract

Background: Lumefantrine, an antimalarial molecule has very low and variable bioavailability owing to its extremely poor solubility in water. It is recommended to be taken with milk to enhance its solubility and bioavailability. The aim of present study was to develop a Self Nanoemulsifying Delivery system (SNEDs) of lumefantrine (LF) to achieve rapid and complete dissolution independent of food-fat and surfactant in dissolution media.

Methods: Solubility of LF in oil, co-solvent/co-surfactant and surfactant solution and emulsification efficiency of surfactant were analyzed to optimize the LF loaded self nanoemulsifying preconcentrate. Effect of LF-oleic acid complexation on emulsification, droplet size, zeta potential and dissolution were investigated. Effect of milk concentration and fat content on saturation solubility and dissolution of LF was investigated. Dissolution of marketed formulation and LF-SNEDs was carried out in pH 1.2 and pH 6.8 phosphate buffer.

Results: LF exhibited very high solubility in oleic acid owing to complexation between tertiary amine of LF and carboxyl group of oleic acid (OA). Cremophore EL and medium chain monoglyceride were selected surfactant and co-surfactant, respectively. Significantly smaller droplet size (37 nm), shift in zeta potential from negative to positive value, very high drug loading in lipid based system (> 10%), no precipitation after dissolution are the major distinguish characteristics contributed by LF-OA complex in the SNED system. Saturation solubility and dissolution study in milk containing media pointed the significant increment in solubility of LF in the presence of milk-food fat. LF-SNEDs showed > 90% LF release within 30 min in pH 1.2 while marketed tablet showed almost 0% drug release.

Conclusion: Self nanoemulsification promoting ionic complexation between basic drug and oleic acid hold great promise in enhancing solubility of hydrophobic drugs.

Introduction

Poor aqueous solubility of the existing and New Chemical Entities adversely affects the oral bioavailability. Failure to mimic in vivo performance compare to in vitro potential, variable absorption and so the plasma concentration, requirement of higher dose than actually needed for desired pharmacological activity are some of the major problems associated with poor solubility of drugs. Further, molecules having very poor aqueous solubility with poor oil solubility impose greater formulation challenges for pharmaceutical scientists. Self emulsifying drug delivery system is one the promising strategy to overcome the solubility barrier of drugs, with commercial products in market e.g. Cyclosporin A, Ritonavir, Lopinavir, Fenofibrate etc. Although a versatile approach, it is not suitable for inherently poor oil soluble molecules e.g. Itraconazole, Carbamazepine, Lumefantrine etc. [1-3].

Lumefantrine (LF) is a highly lipophilic flourene derivative and a Biopharmaceutical Classification System (BCS) Class II drug which is an important agent in the treatment of falciparum malaria. Plasmodium Falciparum is an insidious malarial parasite that fatally threatens a major segment of the Sub-Saharan population in Africa. Thus far, existing therapies for treatment of this form of malaria

* Correspondence: vaviapr@yahoo.com
Center for Novel Drug Delivery Systems, Department of Pharmaceutical Sciences and Technology, Institute of Chemical Technology, University under Section 3 of UGC Act – 1956, Elite Status and Center of Excellence – Govt. of Maharashtra, TEQIP Phase II Funded, N. P. Marg, Matunga (E), Mumbai 400 019, India

have been futile due to irregular dosage regimen and insufficient bioavailability afforded by drugs of the quinine class. Lumefantrine is a blood schizonticide, acts by inhibiting detoxification of haem, this toxic haem and free radicals induce parasite death [4,5].

Although a very efficacious molecule, its activity is limited by extremely poor aqueous solubility. Its solubility is far below the critical solubility requirement and so the reported bioavailability is 4–11%. Such vast variability in bioavailability is contributed by the effect of food-fat consumption. Low intrinsic clearance and erratic oral variability and therapeutic levels are more reliably achieved by co-administration with a fatty meal. The oral bioavailability of lumefantrine is highly dependent on food and is consequently poor in acute malaria, showing high degree of variation in different subjects [6]. Poor solubilization leads to incomplete absorption and so inadequate plasma concentrations for antimalarial activity. Due to this chances of treatment failure are higher, which is again associated with increased morbidity, transmissibility and development of resistance. Lumefantrine is an extremely well-tolerated drug, so it is essential to ensure its maximum absorption [6]. Generally milk is recommended to be taken with lumefantrine but availability of milk and its fat content might vary region to region and the variation in antimalarial response to it. This inter-subject variability may gradually induce resistance to artemisinin-based combination therapy, thus making it crucial to increase the dosage regimen. There is only one report on enhancement of dissolution of LF by wet milling technique. However, Nano milling is very high energy consuming process; moreover paper states that nanopowder lumefantrine also requires benzalkonium chloride (BKC) in dissolution media for solubilization [7]. So far there is no report on solubility enhancement of LF by Self nanoemulsifying system. Self nanoemulsifying systems are very well reported in literature for enhancement in solubility of lipophilic drugs. Self emulsifying preconcentrate is made of oil, surfactant, co-surfactant and drug. On dispersion in water it forms < 100 nm sized droplets. Based on oil characteristic it is directly disseminate to systemic circulation or absorb via lymphatic pathway. Oil-surfactant-cosurfactant driven very high solubility, nano-size and permeability results in significantly rise in bioavailability. The spontaneous formation of nanosized emulsion droplets in stomach generates enormously high surface area for drug to diffuse in lumen and absorb rapidly [3,8].

Poor oil solubility of LF has restricted development of lipid based system. In view of this inadequacy, the current study aims at improving the solubility of lumefantrine, especially to eliminate the co administration of milk or any other fatty meal. Considering the basic nature of LF, we have planned to form LF-oleic acid ionic complex and to prepare self emulsifying system of complex by addition

of appropriate surfactant. Such a self emulsifying hydrophobic complex enable rapid dissolution of LF, without need of BKC in dissolution media, hence provide better correlation to in vivo condition. Till date, there is no report on preparation of self emulsification system with drug – oil ionic complex. The main objective of the study was to develop a self nanoemulsifying delivery system of lumefantrine to increase its solubility, which otherwise is dependent on food.

Materials and methods
Materials
Lumefantrine was procured from Mangalam Laboratories Pvt Ltd (India). The following materials were procured from gattefosse India and were used as received: Labrafac CM10 (C 8 -C 10 polyglycolized glycerides), Maisine 35–1 (glyceryl monolinoleate), Lauroglycol FCC (propylene glycol laurate), Labrafil 1944 CS (apricot kernel oil polyethylene glycol [PEG] 6 esters) and Labrafac PG (propylene glycol caprylate/caprate). Cremophor RH 40 (polyoxyl 40 hydrogenated castor oil), Cremophor EL (polyethoxylated castor oil and Solutol HS 15 (polyoxyethylene esters of 12-hydroxystearic acid) were obtained from BASF India Ltd. Gelucire 44/14 (PEG-32 glyceryl laurate) and 50/13 (PEG-32 glyceryl palmistearate) were received from Colorcon Asia (India). Oleic acid, Tween 80 (polyoxyethylene sorbitan monooleate) and PEG 400 were purchased from Merck (India). Deionized water was prepared by a Milli-Q purifi cation system from Millipore (France). Acetonitrile and methanol used in the present study were of high performance liquid chromatography (HPLC) grade. All other chemicals were reagent grade. Empty HPMC capsule shells were procured from ACG Capsules (Mumbai). Milk of different fat content was purchased from Aarey dairy (1.5% fat content) and Gokul dairy (3% fat content) India.

Analytical method
A simple HPLC method was developed for quantitative analysis of lumefantrine in the formulation. The HPLC system was equipped with Jasco PU2080 plus pumps with PDA detector and auto sampler unit. The drug was analyzed using Hypersil C18 column (250 mm × 4.6 mm, 5 μm) with mobile phase composition Methanol – 0.1% TFA in water in the ratio of 80:20 v/v, with 1.5 ml/min flow rate and detector wavelength set to 336 nm.

Methods
Screening of oil
Saturation solubility of Lumefantrine in oil was chosen as the criteria of selection. The solubility of the drug was determined in various natural and derived oils. 1 ml of each of the selected vehicles was added to each cap vial containing an excess of LF. Mixing of the systems was

performed using a vortex mixer. Formed suspensions were then shaken with a shaker at 37°C for 48 hours. After reaching equilibrium, each vial was centrifuged at 15,000 rpm for 5 minutes. The solubility of lumefantrine in oil was then quantified by HPLC method.

Screening of surfactant and co-surfactant

Screening of surfactant was done on the basis of (i) Solubility of LF in surfactant solution and (ii) its emulsification efficiency for LF-oil mixture.

Saturation solubility of the drug was determined in various surfactant solution (1% w/v solutions in water) and co-surfactant. An excess amount of LF was added to 5 ml of the surfactant solution and co-surfactant/co-solvent. Samples were placed in a water shaker bath for 48 hrs. The sample was then centrifuged (15,000) for 10 min followed by analysis of supernatant by HPLC. Oleic acid was selected as oil for lumefantrine solubilization. Various Surfactants, co surfactant and combination thereof were mixed with oleic acid and LF-oleic acid solution in various ratios. The co-solvent/co-surfactant were screened on the basis of emulsification time, droplet size, appearance of final system and its reports on compatibility with capsule shell. 500 mg of each mixture (oleic acid-surfactant or LF-oleic acid-surfactant) was added to 250 ml of water (37°C) with mild stirring (100 rpm on magnetic stirrer). The compositions were evaluated for their emulsifying efficiency for oleic acid and LF-oleic acid mixture. Emulsification time, appearance and type of emulsion, LF precipitation and stability for 24 h etc. parameters were considered to evaluate the emulsification efficiency of surfactant.

LF-SNEDs (Lumefantrine-Self Nanoemulsifying Delivery System) was prepared by dissolving LF in oleic acid (minimal amount require for LF solubilization). Optimized mixture of Surfactant and co-surfacatant were added to LF-oleic acid mixture. Fixed weight of Lumefantrine: Oleic acid (100 mg:325 mg) was mixed with various ratios of Cremophore EL and different co-solvents and co-surfactants. Droplet size and emulsification time was evaluated in order to optimize the quantity of surfactant and co solvent/co surfactant. The prepared LF-SNEDs preconcentrate was filled into HPMC capsules.

Droplet size and zeta potential measurement

One hundred microliters of each LF-SNEDs preconcentrate was added to 100 ml of miliQ water, and gently mixed using a glass rod. The resultant emulsion was analyzed for droplet size (z average diameter) by Dynamic Light Scattering (DLS) using Malvern Zetasizer, USA. The same procedure of dilution used to measure zeta potential by laser dopper microelectrophoresis using same instrument.

Saturation solubility of lumefantrine in milk containing media

Eventhough LF is recommended to be taken with milk, there has been no literature report hitherto on the effect of milk on the solubility of lumefantrine. In an attempt to check the solubility of lumefantrine in milk containing varying amounts of fat, the following two types of milk were chosen: milk containing 1.5% fat (a) and 3.1% fat (b).

Milk of types a and b were added to different test tubes containing water at pH 1.2 buffer USP (Hydrochloric acid) and pH 6.8 phosphate buffer USP at a concentration of 20% v/v under the assumption that an average person consumes 200 ml of milk in a day. Excess amount of drug was added to each test tube and it was kept in a water shaker bath for 24 hours. Thereafter solutions were filtered through 0.45 μm filter to remove the insoluble drugs. Filtrate was diluted suitably distilled water followed by extracted by chloroform. After evaporating chloroform and reconstituting with mobile phase LF was quantified using HPLC. The saturation solubility of lumefantrine with increasing concentrations of milk at different pH was calculated.

In vitro dissolution study

Dissolution of Marketed Formulation was carried out in surfactant free dissolution media with and without milk. Instead of using Fed state dissolution media, a real time method to account for variability in ingested food was used by adding 100 mL and 200 mL of low-fat milk (a) to each dissolution flask respectively. The composition of dissolution media for marketed formulation is mentioned in Table 1. Dissolution of marketed preparation was carried out using USP XXIII apparatus I at 37 ± 0.50°C with a rotating speed of 100 rpm. Samples were taken at every 15 min from each of the flasks and the percentage cumulative release was calculated.

LF-SNEDs preconcentrate was filled in size '0' HPMC capsules. Dissolution Test of LF-SNEDs was carried out in similar dissolution media using sinker. The composition of milk containing dissolution media showed in Table 1.

Table 1 Preparation of dissolution media

Dissolution media	Deionised water	Milk
pH 1.2 buffer USP (HCl)	900	0
	800	100
	700	200
pH 6.8 phosphate buffer USP	900	0
	800	100
	700	200

Results

Screening of oil

The core part of SNEDs is composed of oil, in which drug is solubilized. Hence, it is very much essential to choose the oil having higher solubility for drug. Various types of oil have been screened including fatty acids, medium chain mono/di/tri glycerides, propylene mono/ di glycerides and long chain triglycerides. Castor oil and GMO showed minimal solubility of LF while Medium chain triglycerides, Isopropyl myristate, rice germ oil etc. showed moderate solubility of LF (Table 2). The higher solubility in rice germ oil may be attributed to its high oleic acid content and γ-orizynol [9]. Oleic acid showed significantly higher solubility of lumefantrine – 157 mg of LF/gm of oleic acid. Such a higher solubility is not merely expected form hydrophobic interaction between LF and oleic acid. There must be ionic interaction attributes to this solubility enhancement.

Screening of surfactant

Selection of suitable surfactant is very crucial part for self emulsifying system especially when a fine translucent nanosized emulsion is required. Surfactant was selected on the basis of two criterions: saturation solubility of lumefantrine in 1% w/v surfactant solution (Table 3) and its emulsification efficiency for LF-oleic acid (Table 4).

Table 2 Saturation solubilities of drug in vehicles

Vehicle	Solubility (mg/gm) ± SD (n=3)
Oil	
Castor Oil	5.91± 0.21
Glyceryl Monooleate	7.79 ± 0.29
Sunflower oil	10.57 ± 0.42
Olive oil	11.67 ± 0.37
Acconon CO7	13.22 ± 0.24
Groundnut Oil	14.16 ± 0.43
Corn Oil	19.34 ± 0.61
Captex 300	29.62 ± 0.72
Till oil	33.40 ± 0.8
Isopropyl Myristate	40.85 ± 0.74
Rice germ Oil	59.92 ± 1.19
Oleic Acid	157.20 ± 1.38
Co-surfactant	
Capmul MCM C8	14.99 ± 0.48
Capmul PG8	18.13 ± 0.49
Co-solvent	
Propylene Glycol	0.432 ± 0.11
Ethanol	2.831 ± 0.29
PEG 400	2.852 ± 0.18
Transcutol P	19.267 ± 0.58
Benzyl alcohol	78.024 ± 1.41

Table 3 Saturation solubility of LF in surfactant solution

Surfactant solution (1%)	Solubility (µg/ml) (Mean± SD) (n=3)
Acconon MC8	0.26 ± 0.14
Sodium Deoxytaurocholate	1.33 ± 0.09
Sodium taurocholate	1.42 ± 0.14
Tween 20	9.18 ± 0.13
SLS	10.75 ± 0.28
Lutrol	13.01 ± 0.15
Acconon S 35	13.05 ± 0.17
Gelusire	15.18 ± 0.17
Solutol HS 15	22.49 ± 0.21
TPGS	27.18 ± 0.28
Cremophore EL	44.52 ± 0.29
Cremophore RH40	46.94 ± 0.25
Tween 80	101.63 ± 0.37

Surfactants of chemical diversity – ionic (cholate, SLS) and non ionic (PEG fatty acid esters, PEO-PPO-PEO block co polymers, PEG vitamin E esters etc.) have been screened for solubility of lumefantrine. LF was almost negligible soluble in PEG-medium chain fatty acid ester (Acconon MC8), marginal solubility in ionic surfactant, with highest solubility in Tween 80 (100 ppm). Tween 80 was selected as the surfactant in trials with different co-surfactants to assess the ability of the co-surfactants to improve the clarity of the system. However, Tween 80 does not show good emulsification as the final system remained hazy. Eventhough LF exhibited highest solubility in Tween 80, it was rejected bacause its poor emulsification property for LF-oleic acid (Table 4).

LF-oleic acid-cremophore EL preconcentrate was self nanoemulsify to 50–100 nm sized droplet depending on the amount of cremophore EL (Table 5). However, in all the bathces have shown longer self emulsification time (~ 7 min) on additon into water (Table 6). Reduction in self emulsification time is necessary to release LF immidiately. In order to reduce the emulsification time, addition of co-solvent or co-surfactant facilitating the emulsification process was added. Various co-solvent/ co-surfactant were screened for this purpose. Solubility of LF in Co co-solvent/co-surfactant was not considered as an important criteria for its selection because of very poor solubility of LF in Medium chain monoglycerides, ethanol, PEG and transcutol P. solubiliy of LF was found to be higher in benzyle alcohol compare to other solvents but was rejected in formualtion due to its lower acceptibilty limit and volatile nature.

The emulsification time and appearance of the formulation with different co-surfactants with Cremophore EL were shown in Table 6. Further, droplet size and polydispersity index of various batches of LF-oleic acid mixture with in different ratio of cremophore EL with

Table 4 Emulsification behavior of Oil and Surfactant mixture

Composition	Surfactant	Observation	Emulsification
Oleic Acid	Gelusire 44/14, Tween 80, Solutol HS 15, TPGS, Lutrol F68	Turbid	Poor
LF-Oleic Acid	Gelusire 44/14, Tween 80, Solutol HS 15, TPGS	Turbid	Poor
Oleic Acid	Cremophor RH40	Translucent milky solution	Satisfactory
LF-Oleic acid	Cremophor RH40	Translucent	Good
Oleic Acid	Cremophore EL	Translucent	Good
LF-Oleic Acid	Cremophore EL	Clear and translucent	Excellent

various Co-surfactant/Co-solvent has mentioned in Table 5.

It was found that a oil:surfactant ratio of 1:1.2 yielded the smallest droplet size and a clear translucent system, however, in an attempt to reduce the amount of surfactant in the system the droplet size was compromised slightly and the surfactant concentration was reduced. Thus, a system with an oil:surfactant ratio of 1:1 was chosen. Although transcutol acts as an effective co-solvent in terms of emulsification capacity, it slows down the emulsification time for the system. PEG-400, inspite of being a good candidate for a co-solvent was not chosen due to its hygroscopic tendencies in soft and hard gelatin capsules. Ethanol was not considered as a co-solvent in the final formulation due to its tendency to diffuse out of the shell and it threatens the integrity of the capsule. Capmul MCM-C8, a medium chain monoglyceride was selected as co-surfactant in finally optimized system (LF-SNEDs) since it has given minimal droplet size of 37 nm (Table 5) with comparatively rapid emulsification (Table 6). Moreover there is no report on its any chemical or physical interaction with capsule shell.

Zeta potential

In this study, to account for the electrostatic effects of the drug-lipid interaction, the zeta potential values of self-emulsified formulation were measured at the same drug to lipid ratios as optimized in the above experiments. Zeta potential of SNEDs with and without drug was evaluated to understand effect of LF-oleic acid complex on surface charge. The Zeta Potential of oleic acid self emulsifying system was found to be − 6.73 mv while LF loaded SNEDs exhibited + 4.4 mv zeta potential. The graphical presentation of droplet size, zeta potential and possible orientation of surfactant in LF-SNEDs showed in Figure 1. This indicates the blank formulation has negative zeta potential while addition of drug lead to shift in zeta potential to positive side. The results are in agreement with a study by Nagarsenker et al., suggesting that addition of a basic drug lead to shift in zeta potential from negative to positive [10]. The final composition of LF-SNEDs is mentioned in Table 7.

Saturation solubility of lumefantrine in milk containing media

The saturation solubility of lumefantrine in milk containing media at gastric and intestinal pH was analyzed (Figure 2). Saturation solubility of LF was found to be significantly influenced by pH and presence milk. However, in absence of milk LF showed almost negligible solubility in both pH 1.2 and pH 6.8 buffers. As expected LF has higher solubility at lower pH due to its

Table 5 Particle size analysis of various formulations

Formulation	Co-solvent/Co- surfactant (mg)	Cremophore EL (mg)	Particle size (nm)	PDI
F1	0	250	94.51 ± 7.67	0.329
F2	0	325	65.43 ± 5.49	0.229
F3	0	400	48.4 ± 5.3	0.25
F4	Transcutol P (25)	250	72.25 ± 6.7	0.235
F5	Transcutol P (25)	325	60.5 ± 5.3	0.21
F6	Transcutol P (25)	400	50.25 ± 6.2	0.227
F7	Capmul MCM (25)	250	80.39 ± 8.7	0.254
LF-SNEDs	**Capmul MCM (25)**	**325**	**37.96 ± 4.1**	**0.184**
F9	Capmul MCM (25)	400	53.78 ± 4.81	0.211
F10	Capmul MCM (50)	325	39.49 ± 4.4	0.119
F11	PEG 400 (25)	325	52.98 ± 4.7	0.123
F12	Ethanol (25)	325	41.59 ± 3.5	0.139
F13	Capmul PG8	325	51.71 ± 3.9	0.122

Table 6 Effect of different co-surfactants on emulsification time

Co-surfactant	Emulsification time (min)	Observations
Transcutol P	6.17	Long time to disperse but final system is clear
PEG-400	4.30	Clear system
Capmul PG8	4.70	Translucent nanoemulsion
Capmul MCM-C8	3.16	Translucent nanoemulsion
Without any co-solvent	7.0	Highly viscous clumps take a long time to disperse

basic nature. Saturation solubility of LF increase with increase the fat content of milk, with maximum solubility of 24 ppm was observed in media containing 20% v/v high fat milk at pH 1.2 (Figure 2). Further increase in fat content or milk concentration is expected to proportionally enhance the solubility of LF.

Dissolution profile of marketed formulation in milk containing media

Dissolution profile clearly states that release of LF is highly depend on concenration of milk in dissolution media (Figure 3). The results of dissolution sutdies are complemetaty to saturation solubility study of LF in milk containing media. The dissolution medium without milk showed negligible release and hence it can be predicted that without fat containig food suppliment, bioavailbility and therefore therapeutic response may be very poor. Milk containing dissolution media showed marginal improvement in dissolution of LF. Dissolution of LF is higher at pH 1.2 media compare to pH 6.8, irrespective of milk content. Higher dissolution at pH 1.2 is due to its higher solubility at lower pH. The cumulative

release increases to maximum 12% upon the ingestion of 200 ml of milk in gastric pH.

Dissolution test of lumefantrine self nanoemulsifying system

Comparable dissoluiton profile of marketed formulation and LF-SNEDs at pH 1.2 and pH 6.8 shown in Figure 4. Marketed formulation showed almost negligible release over the period of 60 min, which is by virtue of extemley poor solubility of lumefantrine in aqeous media. LF-SNEDs exhibited significantly enhancement in dissolution compare to marketed preparation. At pH 1.2, more than 90% of LF was found to release within 30 min account of rapid formation of nanoemulasion in contact with aqeuous medium.

Discussion

Oleic acid showed highest solubilizaion capacity of LF owing to complexation between tertiary amine of LF and oleic acid. Complexation of LF and oleic acid was indirectly confirmed by addition of stronger base than lumefantrine. It was assumed that addition of stronger

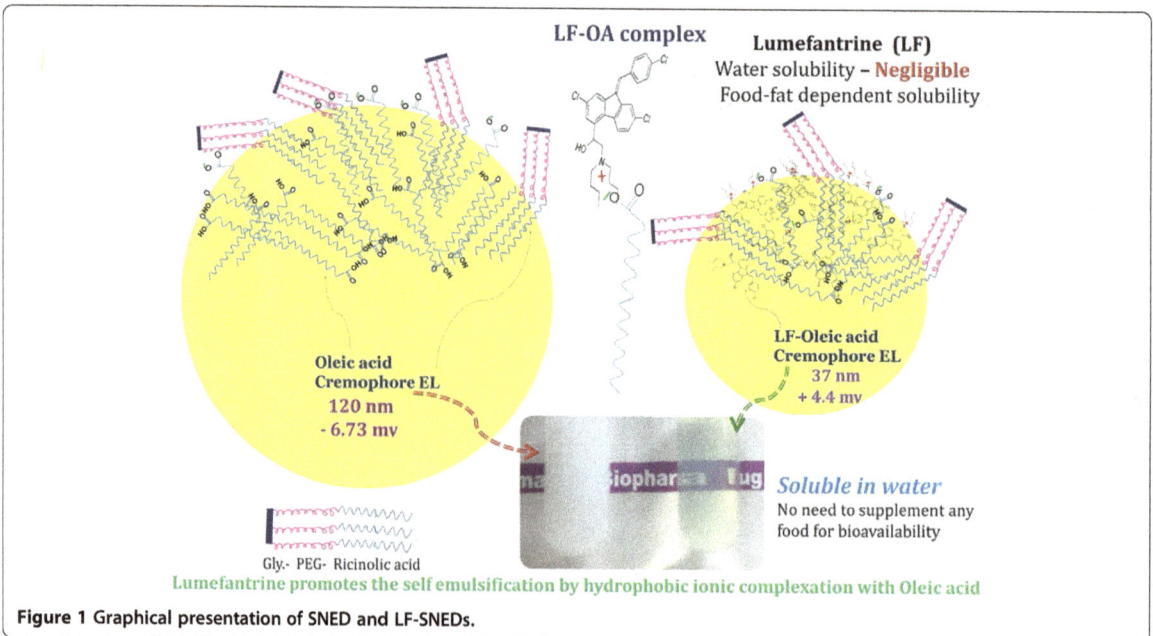

Figure 1 Graphical presentation of SNED and LF-SNEDs.

Table 7 Composition of LF-SNEDs

Lumefantrine	100 mg
Oleic acid	325 mg
Cremophore EL	325 mg
Capmul MCM	25 mg
Total	775 mg

amine containing group in oleic acid will interfere in complexation of amine group of LF with carboxylic acid of oleic acid. The reported pKa value of halofantrine (a similar class of drug) is in the range of 8.2 [11]. So on the basis of structural similarity we assumed that lumefantrine has similar pKa. The pKa of Triethylamine (TEA) is 10.5, which depicts that it is stronger base than lumefantrine. LF was found to be insoluble in oleic acid in the presence of TEA. On this basis it was confirmed that ionic complexation is responsible for significant higher solubility of LF in oleic acid.

Further experimentation on self emulsification property of oleic acid and LF-oleic acid suggested the proof of concept of ionic complexation between LF and oleic acid promote self emulsification (see graphical abstract). It was discovered that a system consisting of only oleic acid (no drug), surfactant and co-solvent is self nanoemulsifying to 120 ± 12 nm while system containing LF-oleic acid, surfactant and consurfactant easily emulsify to nano size translucent dispersion of 37.96 ± 4.1 nm. Addition of LF showed 4 times reduction in droplet size. It means that LF-oleic acid complex is itself promoting the self emulsification, which is otherwise difficult to emulsify oleic acid. We can attribute this to the fact that oleic acid interacts with the amine drug and forms a hydrophobic ion-pairing complex with its carboxylic group. Thus, the functional group of oleic acid which might br interfering in self emulsification, on complexation with drug to it promote the self-emulsifying property. Based on the above results, Oleic acid was selected as the oil. The interaction was reflected in zeta potential study. Shift in Zeta potential of plain oleic acid nanoemulsion – 6.73 mv to + 4.4 mv with LF-oleic acid nanoemulsion also support the ionic interaction between amine of LF and carboxylic acid group of oleic acid. The blank formulation has a negative charge due to the predominance of the anionic oleic acid. The negative charge of blank system is due to presence of carboxylic acid group on surface. Very marginal negative potential of the system is due to poor ionization of oleic acid (pKa – 9.85). Moreover, dense network of PEG of cremophore EL on surface mask zeta potential of the ionized species on surface. Zeta potential of LF-SNEDs was found to be slightly positive, clearly indicating the ionic interaction of LF-oleic acid. The positive charge, in LF-SNEDs can be attributed to masking of anionic charge of oleic acid by complexation with LF and surface orientation of amine group of LF in nanoglobules. This interaction results in significantly higher solubility of LF in oleic acid, further LF-oleic acid complex is expected to be more soluble in oleic acid than lumefantrine itself.

Tween and cremphore both are PEG fatty acid esters but their chemical structures have vast diffence. Cremphore surfactants are more bulky and having higher molecular weight compare to Tween surfactants. Tween 80 has single chian of oleic acid as lipophilic part while cremophore surfactants have three fatty acid chain attahced to PEG-glycerol. This bulkier lipophilic part of cremophore may contributed to better emulsification property of cremophore EL and cremophore RH 40. Hence, further formulations were tested with Cremophore

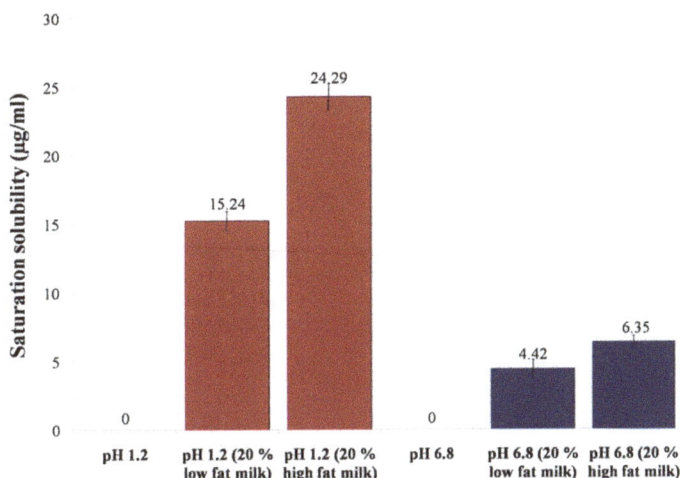

Figure 2 Saturation solubility of lumefantrine in different types of milk at different pH.

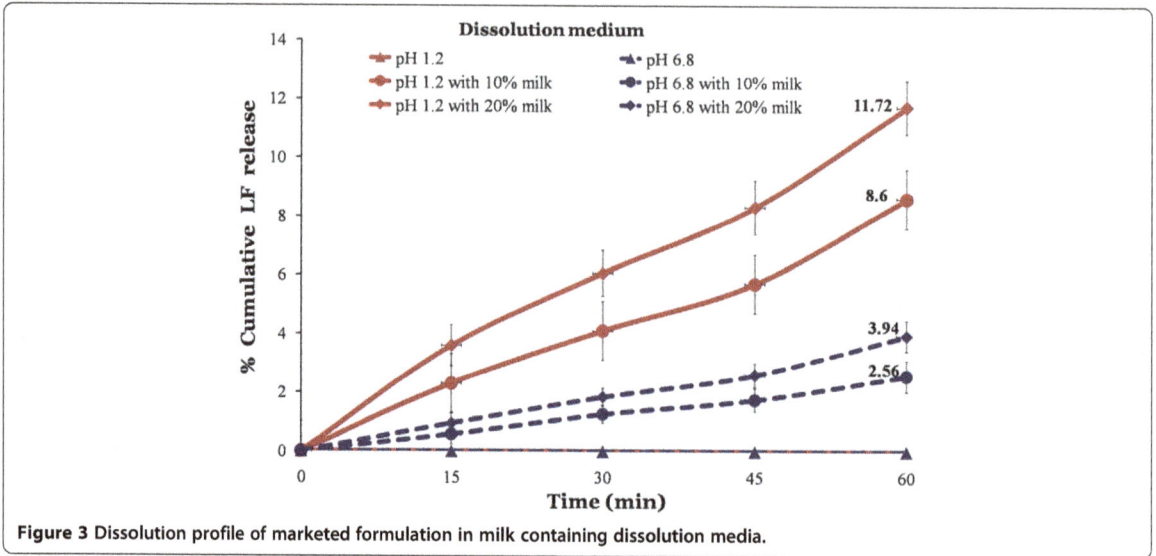

Figure 3 Dissolution profile of marketed formulation in milk containing dissolution media.

EL and Cremophore RH 40. We have observed that free fatty acid e.g. oleic acid is difficult to emulsify in comparision to its glyceryl esters. Though Cremophore RH 40 showed a slightly better solubilising capacity, it was dismissed in favour of Cremophore EL as the latter portrayed a clearer and more transparent emulsion on redispersion. Also, Cremophor RH40 (polyoxyl 40 hydrogenated castor oil) appeared to be less readily digested than Cremophor EL (polyoxyl 35 castor oil). An explanation for differences in the digestability of the structurally similar Cremophor surfactants is not very clear in literature but may reflect differences in the reactivity of the saturated (hydrogenated) castor oil glyceride backbone in Cremophor RH40 leading to the generation of slightly different reaction products with polyethylene oxide, when

compared with Cremophor EL (which is generated by polyethoxylation of unsaturated castor oil) [12]. Alternatively the slightly larger polyethylene oxide content of Cremophor RH 40 may have more effectively masked the approach and binding of pancreatic enzymes (and therefore hydrolysis) when compared with Cremophor EL. Cremophore EL has an IIG limit of 599 mg making it a feasible and non-toxic component in the system.

Self-emulsification of oil-surfacatant preconcentrate proceeds through formation of Liquid Crystalline phase (LC) at oil–water interface. The rate and extent of water penetration into LC phase determines the rate of emulsification. Rapidity of self emulsification is governed by weakness and viscosity of intermediate LC [13,14]. Medium chain monoglyceride (MCM) has ability to

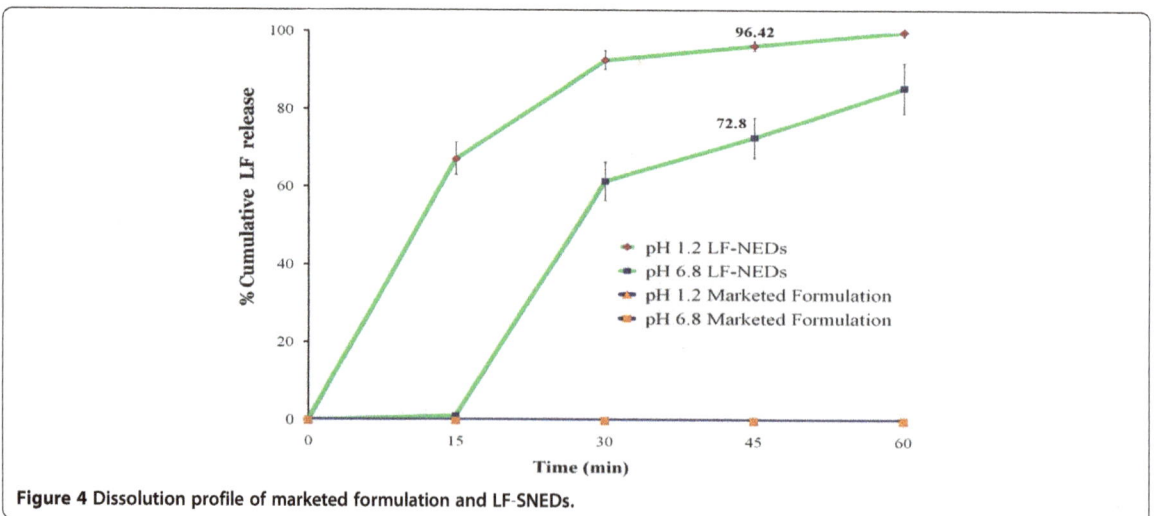

Figure 4 Dissolution profile of marketed formulation and LF-SNEDs.

form such LC phase especially when mixed with hydrophilic surfactant [14].

It was observed that increasing concentrations of fat in milk brought about an increase in saturation solubility of lumefantrine whereas no solubility was observed at the gastric and intestinal pH in the absence of milk. Triglycerides are the major component of milk fat. These medium to long chain triglycerides of milk contributing to marginal solubility of lumefantrine in milk. Higher the fat content of milk, higher will be the solubility of LF in it.

This indicates the extreme necessity of fat containing diet for its solublilization and therefore absoption. Possibility of failure in therapeutic response can not be denied with such a poorly soluble drug as discussed in introduction part.

Increase in solubility with increase in milk content is prime reason for enhacement in bioavailability of LF when given with milk. The results are in agreement with a bioavailability study carried out on healthy human volunteer to evaluate the effect of food/fat on bioavailability of LF. Bindschedle et al. have reported 16 fold enhancement in bioavailability in the presence of food [15]. Ashley et al. have reported 90% of maximum AUC was achieved with 36 ml of soya milk [6]. Ensuring that volunteer receives milk or fat with given medicine is feasible under study conditions but difficult to guarantee during routine treatment in malaria patients. However, the availability of milk, composition of fat and the amount of milk consumed varies from person to person and thus there is no conclusive prediction of the bioavailability in the LF.

LF-oleic acid ionic hydrophobic complex emulsify to nanosize by cremophore EL, generating an enormously high surface area. Accroding to noyes-whitney equation reduction in droplet size lead to significant enhancement in dissolution while Prandlt equation suggests the significant reduction in diffusion layer thickness with nanosizing of particle [16].

One more important thing to take into consideration is dissolution media does not contain any surfactant. Generally, in dissolutin studies of hydrophobic drug, surfactant is added to maintain sink condition and to prevent precipitaion of drug-in dissolution media. USP recommends use of 1% w/v Benzalkonium chloride (BKC) in dissoultion media. The saturation solubilty of LF in 0.1 M HCl with 1% w/v BKC is 119 ± 3 ppm, sufficient to solubilize 120 mg of LF in dissolution media [16]. The most important advantage of LF-SNEDs system is complete dissolution of LF without use of such surfactant in dissoltion media. Both the dissolution media pH 1.2 and pH 6.8, do not contain BKC or other surfactant, still LF-SNEDs capable enough to solubilize drug without precipiatation. Amount of cremophore EL in dosage form is just 325 mg, leading to 0.36% w/v in 900 ml of dissolution media. This concentration is much below to maitain sink condition for LF in dissolution media (Table 3). Hence, we can predict that LF remains in solubilized state in dissolution media because of its comlexation with oleic acid. The complex formation promote the faster self emulsification and dissolution and further inhibit the precipitaion of drug once solubilized. In phosphate buffer 6.8, slow dissolution of capsule shell resulted in 10 min lag period for solubilitzation. After opening of capsule dissolution profile is similar to that of pH 1.2.

Conclusion

Hydrophobic ionic complexation based self nanoemulsifying delivery system of LF showed remarkabley higher dissolution profile, eliminating the requirement of food/fat for LF solubilization. Lumefantrine has very high solubility in oleic acid due to complexation between tertiary amine of LF and oleic acid. Higher the solubiilty of drug in oil, higher the drug loading capacity of formulation. For drug having higher dose, ionic complexation with oleic acid would be effective strategy to enhance solibilty by self nanoemulisfying formulation. Selection of an ideal surfactant and co-surfactant is very much essential to emulsify the complex to nano sized globule within short period of time. Sponteneous formation of nanoemulsion lead to rapid dissolution of a hydrophobic drug, which may offer food/fat independent bioavailability. Ionic complexation with self emulsifying delivery offer an easy, cost effective and industry feasible approach for solubilization of basic hydrophobic drugs.

Competing interest

The authors declare that they have no competing interest.

Authors' contributions

KP and VS have carried out studies mentioned in article. PV has guided this project and made substantial contributions for data interpretation and involved in drafting the manuscript and revising it critically. All authors read and approved the final manuscript.

Acknowledgment

Authors are thankful to University Grant Commission, Govt. of India for research fellowship awarded and All India Council for Technical Education (AICTE-NAFETIC) for research facilities provided.

References
1. Thomas VH, Bhattachar S, Hitchingham L, Zocharski P, Naath M, Surendran N: The road map to oral bioavailability: an industrial perspective. *Expert Opin Drug Metab Toxicol* 2006, 2:591–608.
2. Stegemann S, Leveiller F, Franchi D, de Jong H, Lindén H: When poor solubility becomes an issue: from early stage to proof of concept. Eur J Pharma Sci 2007, 31:249–61. Patel AR, Vavia PR: Preparation and in vivo evaluation of SMEDDS (self-microemulsifying drug delivery system) containing fenofibrate. *AAPS J* 2007, 9:E344–E345.
3. Singh SP, Raju KSR, Nafis A, Puri SK, Jain GK: Intravenous pharmacokinetics, oral bioavailability, dose proportionality and in situ permeability of antimalarial lumefantrine in rats. *Malar J* 2011, 10:293.

4.   Ezzet F, Mull R, Karbwang J: The population pharmacokinetics of CGP 56697 and its effects on the therapeutic response in malaria patients. *Br J Clin Pharmacol* 1998, **46**:553–561.

5.   Ashley EA, Annerberg A, Kham A, Brockman A, Singhasivanon P, White NJ: How much fat is necessary to optimize lumefantrine oral bioavailability? *Trop Med Int Health* 2007, **12**:195–200.

6.   Gahoi S, Jain GK, Tripathi R, Pandey SK, Anwar M, Warsi MH: Enhanced antimalarialactivity of lumefantrine nanopowder prepared by wet-milling DYNO MILL technique. *Colloids Surf B: Biointerf* 2012, **95**:16–22.

7.   Date AA, Nagarsenker MS: Design and evaluation of self-nanoemulsifying drug delivery systems (SNEDDS) for cefpodoxime proxetil. *Int J Pharm* 2007, **329**:166–172.

8.   Pawar SK, Vavia PR: Rice Germ Oil as Multifunctional Excipient in Preparation of Self- Microemulsifying Drug Delivery System (SMEDDS) of Tacrolimus. *AAPS PharmSciTech* 2012, **13**:254–261.

9.   Patel KD, Padhye SG, Nagarsenker MS: Duloxetine HCl lipid nanoparticles: preparation, characterization, and dosage form design. *AAPS Pharm Sci Tech* 2012, **13**:125–133.

10. Babalola CP, Adegoke AO, Ogunjinmi MA, Osimosu MO: Determination of physicochemical properties of halofantrine. *Afr J Med Med Sci* 2003, **32**:357–359.

11. Cuiné JF, McEvoy CL, Charman WN, Pouton CW, Edwards GA, Benameur H, Porter CJ: Evaluation of the impact of surfactant digestion on the bioavailability of danazol after oral administration of lipidic self-emulsifying formulations to dogs. *J Pharm Sci* 2008, **97**:995–1012.

12. Lopez-Montilla JC, Herrera-Morales PE, Pandey S, Shah D: Spontaneous emulsification:mechanisms, physicochemical aspects, modeling and applications. *J Disp Sci Techn* 2002, **23**:219–268.

13. Biradar SV, Dhumal RS, Paradkar AR: Rheological investigation of self-emulsification process: effect of co-surfactant. *J Pharm Pharm Sci* 2009, **12**:164–174.

14. Bindschedler M, Degen P, Lu ZL, Jiao XQ, Liu GY, Fan F: Comparative biovailability of benflumetol after administration of single oral doses of co-artemether under fed and fasted conditions to healthy subjects (abstract P-01-96). *Proceedings of the Xivth International Congress for Tropical Medicine and Malaria, Nagasaki, Japan* 1996:17–22.

15. Müller RH, Jacobs C, Kayser O: Nanosuspensions as particulate drug formulations in therapy. *Rationale for development and what we can expect for the future. Adv drug deliv rev* 2001, **23**:3–19.

16. Umapathi P, Ayyappan J, Quine SD: Development and Validation of a Dissolution Test Method for Artemether and Lumefantrine in Tablets. *Trop J Pharm Res* 2011, **10**:643–653.

Silymarin improved 6-OHDA-induced motor impairment in hemi-parkisonian rats: behavioral and molecular study

Rasool Haddadi[1,3], Alireza Mohajjel Nayebi[2,3*], Safar Farajniya[2], Shahla Eyvari Brooshghalan[2] and Hamdolah Sharifi[4]

Abstract

Background: Neuroinflammation and oxidative stress has been shown to be associated with the development of Parkinson disease (PD). In the present study, we investigated the effect of intraperitoneal (i.p.) administration of silymarin, on 6-OHDA-induced motor-impairment, brain lipid per-oxidation and cerebrospinal fluid (CSF) levels of inflammatory cytokine in the rats.

Results: The results showed that silymarin is able to improve motor coordination significantly ($p < 0.001$) in a dose dependent manner. There was a significant ($p < 0.001$) increase in MDA levels of 6-OHDA-lesioned rats whereas; in silymarin (100, 200 and 300 mg/kg, i.p. for 5 days) pre-treated hemi-parkinsonian rats MDA levels was decreased markedly ($p < 0.001$). Furthermore the CSF levels of IL-1β was decreased ($p < 0.001$) in silymarin (100, 200 and 300 mg/kg) pre-treated rats up to the range of normal non-parkinsonian animals.

Conclusion: We found that pre-treatment with silymarin could improve 6-OHDA-induced motor imbalance by attenuating brain lipid per-oxidation as well as CSF level of IL-1β as a pro-inflammatory cytokine. We suggest a potential prophylactic effect for silymarin in PD. However, further clinical trial studies should be carried out to prove this hypothesis.

Keywords: Silymarin, Catalepsy, MDA, IL-1β, 6-OHDA, Rotarod, Rat

Introduction

Parkinson's disease (PD) is the second most common and progressive neurodegenerative disorder worldwide with a prevalence of approximately 1% in people over age 60. Clinically, the disease is characterized by resting tremor, rigidity, bradykinesia and postural instability [1-3]. Progression of these symptoms is secondary to the selective loss of dopaminergic (DA) neurons in the substantia nigra pars compacta (SNpc) [4]. The primary cause of PD is still unknown although aging appears to be a major risk factor. Indeed, mitochondrial impairment and elevated oxidative stress have been linked to the PD pathogenesis [5]. It is well agreed that chronic neuro-inflammation has part in the pathogenesis of the disease

* Correspondence: nayebia@tbzmed.ac.ir
[2]Drug Applied Research Center, Tabriz University of Medical Sciences, Tabriz, Iran
[3]Department of Pharmacology and Toxicology, Faculty of Pharmacy, Tabriz University of Medical Sciences, Tabriz, Iran
Full list of author information is available at the end of the article

[6,7]. For the first time in 1988, McGeer et al. reported increase of activated microglia in the SNc of parkinsonian patients, which was showed the involving of neuroinflammation in PD [8]. Chronic neuro-inflammation causes to damage of neural cells through generation of reactive oxygen species (ROS). In the brain, activated microglia are a major origin of cytokines and oxidizing radicals which are produced subsequent to activation of intracellular peroxidases and oxidative processes [9]. ROS can activate pro-inflammatory pathways and subsequently cause to damage of vulnerable neurons. Several studies showed that both oxidative stress and neuro-inflammation play a role in the neurodegeneration of SNc observed in PD [10,11]. The dopaminergic neurons (DA-neurons) of SNc are highly vulnerable to oxidative stress due to the high oxygen demand of this brain region together with the low levels of antioxidant enzymes [12]. Previous studies have demonstrated increase of activated microglia in the SNc of parkinsonian patients [8]. It has been found that microglial activation result in the

decrease of DA-neurons in patients suffering from PD [13,14]. Furthermore, the levels of proinflammatory cytokines such as tumor necrosis factor alpha (TNF-α), interleukin-1beta (IL-1β) and IL-6 that expressed by glial cells, increased markedly in the serum, brain and cerebrospinal fluid (CSF) of patients with PD [8,15,16]. To present, no effective therapies have been developed to treat PD; however, modulation of neuroinflammation is important to modify disease progression.

Silymarin (SM), is a polyphenolic flavonoid derived from the seeds and fruits of the milk thistle plant (*Silybum marianum*), routinely used to treat liver diseases and have antioxidative [17], anti-apoptotic [18], anti-inflammatory [19,20], and neuroprotective properties [21]. The anti-oxidative activity of SM is due to the scavenging of free radicals and activation of superoxide dismutase [22]. SM inhibits microglia activation and decreases inflammatory mediators; the mechanisms by which it protects dopaminergic neurons from lipopolysaccharide induced neurotoxicity [23]. Furthermore, several studies demonstrated protective effects of SM in several experimental models of neuronal injury, particularly in focal cerebral ischemia and cerebral ischemia−reperfusion-induced brain injury in rats [24,25]. However, less information is available about its effect on motor deficits associated with Parkinson disease. Therefore, the present study aims to investigate the effect of SM on 6-hydroxydopamine (6-OHDA)-induced motor imbalance and modification of cerebral levels of IL-1β and MDA as indicators of neuro-inflammation and oxidative damage.

Material and methods
Chemicals
All chemicals were purchased from Sigma Chemical Co. (USA). Solutions were made freshly on the days of experimentation by dissolving drugs in physiological saline (0.9% NaCl) except for silymarin which was dissolved in 50% polyethylene glycol (PEG). The drugs were injected intraperitoneally (i.p.) except for 6-hydroxydopamine (6-OHDA) which was injected into right substantia nigra pars compacta (SNc).

Animals
Male Wistar rats (220 ± 20 g) were used in this study. The animals were given food and water ad libitum and were housed in standard polypropylene cages, four per cage at a ambient temperature of 25 ± 2°C under a 12-h light/12-h dark cycle. Animals were habituated to the testing conditions including being transferred to the experimental environment, handled, weighed, and trained on the test platform for 10 min 2 days before the behavioral investigations were conducted. The present study was carried out in accordance with the ethical guidelines for the Care and Use of Laboratory Animals of Tabriz

University of Medical Sciences, Tabriz, Iran (National Institutes of Health Publication No. 85–23, revised 1985).

Experimental protocol
In the beginning of study only the rats that showed normal walking on rotarod (700 ± 20 sec) were subjected to further experimentation. The healthy animals were randomized into 8 groups each consisting of eight rats. Rats in group 1 (control or intact) received no injection and were left untreated for the entire period of the experiment. Rats in group 2 (sham operated) were injected with saline containing 0.2% (w/v) ascorbic acid into SNc. Rats in group 3 received only 6-OHDA (8 µg/2 µl/rat; intra-SNc). Rats in group 4 pre-treated with vehicle PEG (i.p.) daily for 5 consecutive days and then were received intra-SNc injection of 6-OHDA in the same way as group 3. Rats in group 5 (positive control) pre-treated with i.p. administration of silymarin 200 mg/kg once daily (9 a.m.). Rats in groups 6 to 8 pre-treated with i.p. administration of silymarin (100, 200 and 300 mg/kg) once daily (9 a.m.) for 5 days and then were received intra-SNc injection of 6-OHDA in the same way as group 3 and then, after 3 weeks as recovery period, all animals were tested by rotarod.

At the end of experiments, the animals were anesthetized by i.p. injection of ketamine (80 mg/kg) and xylazine (10 mg/kg) and their cerebro-spinal fluid (CSF) were collected (as described below) and prepared for further analysis of IL-1β. Then animals were euthanized by an overdose of ether and the striatal tissue samples prepared for MDA assay.

Surgical procedures
The animals were anesthetized by i.p. injection of ketamine (80 mg/kg) and xylazine (10 mg/kg). After the rats were deeply anaesthetized (loss of corneal and toe pad reflexes), they were fixed in a stereotaxic frame (Stoelting, Wood Lane, IL, USA) in the flat position. The scalp hairs were completely shaved, swabbed with povidone iodine 10% and a central incision made to reveal skull. The coordinates for this position were determined according to the rat brain in stereotaxic coordinates [26] anteroposterior from bregma (AP) = −5.0 mm, mediolateral from the midline (ML) = 2.1 mm and dorsoventral from the skull (DV) = −7.7 mm. Desipramine (25 mg/kg, i.p.) was injected 30 min before intra-nigral injection of 6-OHDA to avoid degeneration of noradrenergic neurons. Then 6-OHDA (8 µg/per rat in 2 µl saline with 0.2% ascorbic acid) was infused by infusion pump at the flow rate of 0.2 µl/min into the right substantia nigra. At the end of injection, cannula was kept for an additional 2 min and then slowly was withdrawn. Sham-operated animals were submitted to the same procedure except 2 µl vehicle of 6-OHDA

(0.9% saline containing 0.2% (w/v) ascorbic acid) was infused into the SNc.

Cannula verification

For confirmation of placement of the cannula in the SNc of the brain, at the end of experiments all rats with guide cannula were euthanized by a high dose of ether and decapitated. The brains were removed and placed in a formaldehyde (10%) solution. After 1 week, the tissues were then embedded in paraffin. Then serial sections (3 μm) were cut with a microtome (Leitz, Germany), and as shown in (Figure 1), the placement of the tip of the cannula in the SNc, AP from bregma = −5.0 mm, was microscopically controlled (Figure 1). Data from rats with an incorrect placement of injecting cannula were excluded from the analysis.

Rotarod assay test

Animals were transferred to the experimental room at least 1 h before the test in order to let them habituate to the test environment. Assessment of motor coordination and balance was done by a commercially available rat rotarod apparatus on the day of 21 after 6-OHDA injection (Figure 2). Rat was mounted on the rotarod (18 RPM) and the time latency to fall from the rod was automatically recorded. All observations were made between 9 AM and 4 PM by an observer who was blind to the entity of treatments. All rats were pre-trained for 2 days in order to reach a stable performance. The latency to fall from the apparatus was recorded. Motor

balance was assessed three weeks after neurotoxin injection in four consecutive times, each lasting 720 s (with one hour interval). Values were expressed as retention time on the rotarod in the four test trails.

CSF sampling

At the end of experiments, the anesthetized rats were mounted in a stereotaxic frame. The surface of the neck region were shaved and swabbed with ethanol (70%). The position of the animal's head was sustained downward at almost 45°. A needle (scalp vein-23) which connected to a draw syringe was put horizontally and centrally into the cisterna magna for CSF collection with no incision at this region. The colorless CSF sample was slowly drawn into the syringe in a volume of 100 μl. The CSF samples were kept frozen at −70°C until assessment by enzyme-linked immunosorbent assay (ELISA) method.

Malondialdehyde (MDA) assay

For MDA assessment, rats (n = 8) were euthanized, and selected brain regions (midbrain) were rapidly removed, cleaned, and immediately frozen in liquid nitrogen. Subsequently, tissue samples were weighed and homogenized (IKA Homogenizer, Staufen, Germany) in ice-cold buffer phosphate (50 mM, pH 6.0 at 4-8°C) and then were centrifuged at 10000 rpm for 20 min at 4°C. The supernatant was aliquot and stored at −80°C for further analysis. The MDA concentration in the supernatant was measured as described before [27]. Briefly, trichloroacetic acid and TBARS reagent were added to

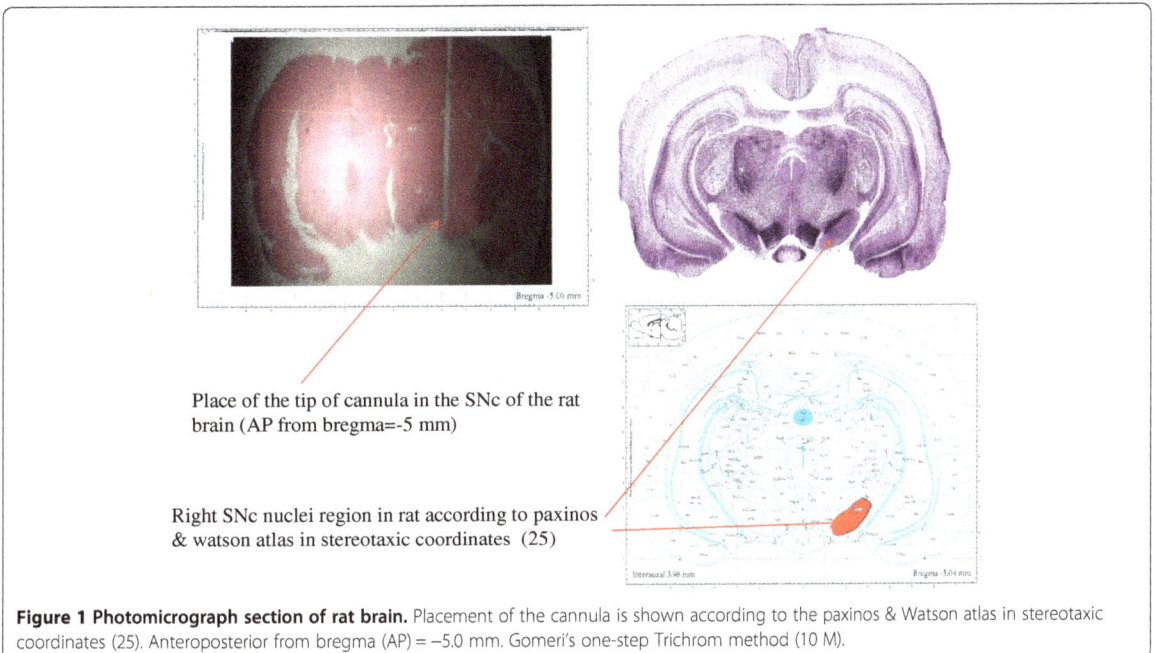

Place of the tip of cannula in the SNc of the rat brain (AP from bregma=-5 mm)

Right SNc nuclei region in rat according to paxinos & watson atlas in stereotaxic coordinates (25)

Figure 1 Photomicrograph section of rat brain. Placement of the cannula is shown according to the paxinos & Watson atlas in stereotaxic coordinates (25). Anteroposterior from bregma (AP) = −5.0 mm. Gomeri's one-step Trichrom method (10 M).

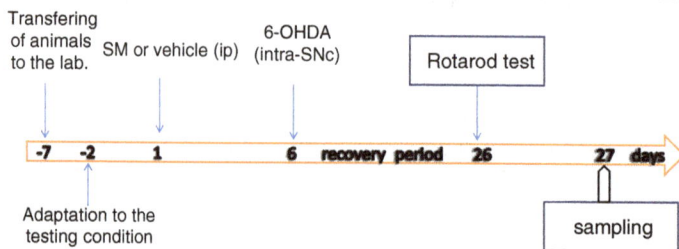

Figure 2 Schematic representation of the experimental procedure; see text for details.

supernatant, then mixed and incubated at 100°C for 80 min. After cooling on ice, samples were centrifuged at 1000 × g for 20 min and the absorbance of the supernatant was read at 532 nm. TBARS results were expressed as MDA equivalents using tetraethoxypropane as standard. The protein content of the supernatant was measured using Bradford Protein Assay kit (Sigma Chemical, St. Louis, MO).

IL-1β assay

The CSF level of IL-1β was determined by using commercial ELISA kits (Rat IL-1β kits, IBL, Hamburg, Germany) according to the manufacture's instruction. Conditions were the same for all assays. Briefly, the frozen CSF samples were diluted, added into the wells and incubated at room temperature for 120 min on a microplate shaker. After washing, diluted Streptavidin-Horseradish peroxidase-conjugated anti-mouse IL-1β was reacted for 60 min at room temperature (on microplate shaker set at 200 rpm). After washing again, the wells were developed with tetramethyl benzidine (TMB) for 10 min and the optical densities were read at 450 nm with an ELISA reader.

The concentration of the IL-1β was expressed as pg/ml of CSF.

Statistical analysis

Data were expressed as the mean ± SEM, and were analyzed by one-way ANOVA in each experiment. In the case of significant variation ($p < 0.05$), the values were compared by Tukey test.

Results

The effect of intra-SNc-injection of 6-OHDA on motor- balance

The effect of intra-SNc injection of 6-OHDA on motor-coordination was evaluated by rotarod test. The duration of time to fall from rotating rod was evaluated in three groups of rats: normal, sham operated and 6-OHDA (8 μg/2 μl/rat)-lesioned rats. Drugs and vehicle were injected into the SNc through the implanted guide cannula. As shown in Figure 3, 6-OHDA was able to induce significant ($p < 0.001$) motor imbalance in comparison with both normal and sham-operated rats so that 6-OHDA- lesioned rats fail to maintain their equilibrium

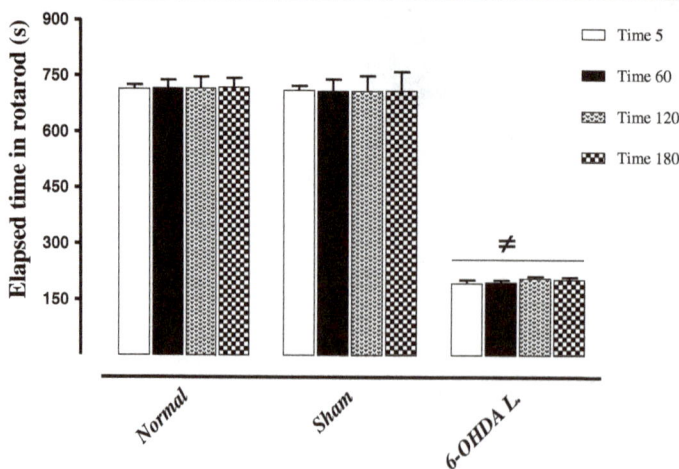

Figure 3 The rotarod results of normal, sham-operated and 6-OHDA-lesioned (8 μg/2 μl/rat) rats. Each bar represents the mean ± SEM of elapsed time on the rod (s); n = 8 rats for each group; [*]$p < 0.001$ as compared with normal and sham-operated groups. (L = .Lesioned).

on rotarod and a significant decrease (367% in compare with normal group) in retention time on rotarod was observed in these animals (Figure 3).

Effect of silymarin on 6-OHDA induced motor-incoordination

The effect of pre-treatment with silymarin (100, 200 and 300 mg/kg, i.p.) and its vehicle for 5 days, on 6-OHDA induced motor-incoordination was assessed 3 weeks after injection of 6-OHDA. In these groups motor balance was tested on 21 days after surgery for 4 repeated times (5, 60, 120 and 180 min). The results indicated that silymarin (in all 3 doses) significantly ($p < 0.001$)

improved motor balance in 6-OHDA lesioned rats in a dose dependent manner (Figure 4A) so that the latency time to fall off increased (198%, 287% and 304%) in lesioned rats pre-treated with 100, 200 and 300 mg/kg of SM with respect to rats treated with vehicle, respectively. No alteration was observed on rotarod elapsed time in vehicle pre-treated rats (Figure 4B).

Effects of 6-OHDA and silymarin on the brain level of MDA

To investigate the possible involvement of MDA as a marker of the oxidative stress in PD we appraised the level of MDA in the ventral midbrain (brain region

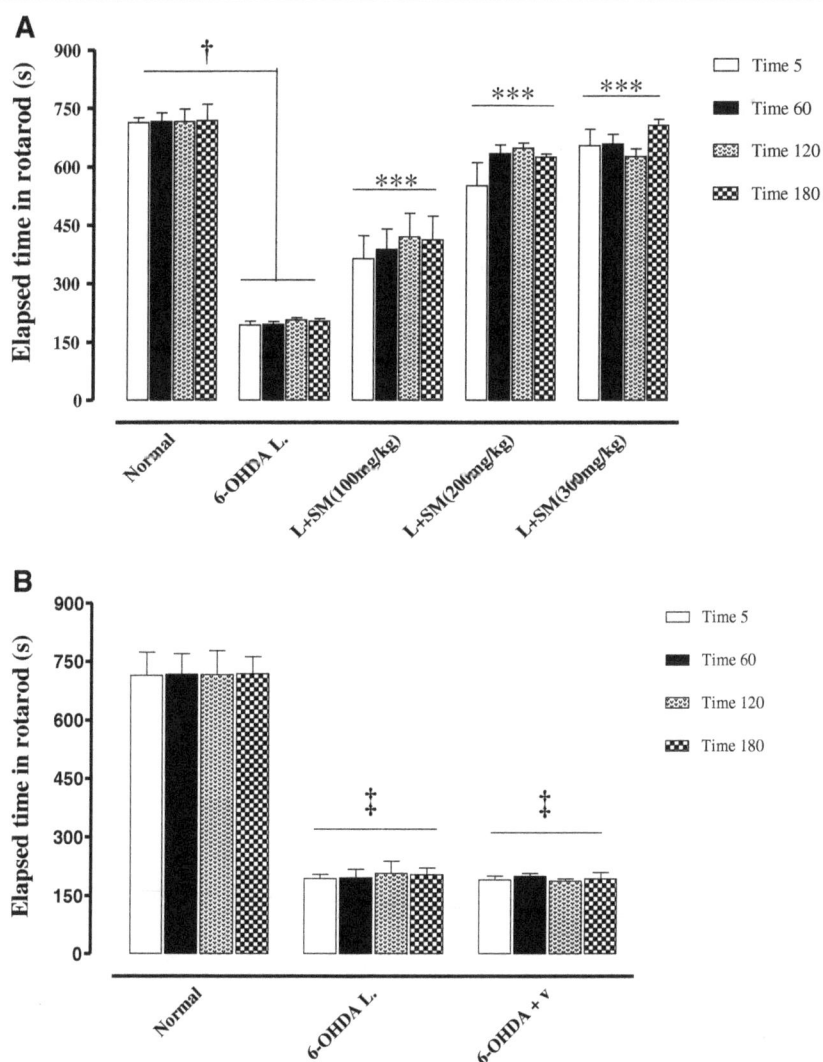

Figure 4 The rotarod test results of 6-OHDA (8 μg/2 μl/rat)-lesioned rats that pre-treated with silymarin (100, 200 and 300 mg/kg, i.p. for 5 days) (A) and silymarin vehicle (B). Each bar represents the mean ± SEM of elapsed time (s) on the rod; n = 8 rats for each group; [†]p <0.001 between normal and 6-OHDA groups; ***p < 0.001 when compared with 6-OHDA lesioned rats; [‡]p < 0.001 when compared with normal rats. (SM = Silymarin); (V = Vehicle of silymarin); (L = .Lesioned).

containing the SNc dopaminergic neurons). In the present study 6-OHDA injection given to the rats resulted in a significant (p < 0.001 vs. control) increase in lipid peroxidation in brain tissue, as measured by an increase in the level of MDA in the brain (Figure 5). The MDA level in the brain was found to reduce from 11.4 ± 1.1 nm/mg protein in 6-OHDA group to 6.62 ± 0.51, 6.25 ± 0.48 and 5.6 ± 0.63 (p < 0.001) nm/mg pr., in SM (100, 200, and 300 mg/kg/day) pre-treated groups, in a dose dependent manner, respectively (Figure 5).

Effect of silymarin on the CSF level of IL-1β

To further explore on the protection against 6-OHDA induced Parkinson disease by silymarin, the potential effect of silymarin on the level of IL-1β, which is a key pro-inflammatory cytokine released following microglia activation, was investigated in the present study. The results showed that 6-OHDA markedly increased the IL-1β level by 286.5% (P < 0.001 vs. control) (Figure 6). Pre-treatment with silymarin with all three doses (100, 200, and 300 mg/kg/day) significantly attenuated the level of IL-1β from 332.8 ± 52 pg/ml of CSF in the 6-OHDA group to 129.5 ± 26 (P < 0.001), 113.2 ± 11 (P < 0.001), and 86.16 ± 7 (P < 0.001) pg/ml respectively, in a dose-dependent manner (Figure 6).

Discussion

We have previously reported that short-term administration of silymarin at induction of PD by 6-OHDA prevents from catalepsy and reduces myeloperoxidase activity and inflammatory cytokines [28]. In the present study it has been indicated that SM improves motor impairment following intra-SNc injection of 6-OHDA in rats and amends the neuroinflammation and oxidative stress factors.

Different beneficial effects of silymarin have been reported in several in vitro and in vivo studies. Recently, the beneficial effect of silymarin has been reported in an Alzheimer's disease rat model [29]. However, less information is available about its effect on motor impairment in experimental models of PD. Behavioral assessment is a strong hallmark in evaluation of neuroprotection. Particularly, in rodents, motor-incoordination which is a reliable marker of the nigrostriatal neurodegeneration, is one symptoms of PD that can be created by unilateral intra-SNc injection of 6-OHDA and assessed by rotarod as a common standard motor-balance test [30]. In the 6-OHDA-induced PD model used in the present study, 6-OHDA caused a significant motor-imbalance, so that walking of rats on the rotating drum was lesser in 6-OHDA lesioned group compared to the control group. This is in accordance to previous studies reported that 6-OHDA (8-12 μg/2 μl/rat) induces motor-imbalance as an early symptom of PD by decreasing number of SNc neurons [30,31]. Indeed unilateral lesion of SNc compels a rat to put its weight abnormally on the both sides of its body for movement and equilibrium; hence this cause to motor disorders and motor asymmetry [31,32].

According to the results, silymarin (in all three doses) improved motor-incoordination induced by 6-OHDA. Baluchnejadmojarad et al. reported that silymarin attenuates the rotational behavior in 6-OHDA-lesioned rats and protects nigrostriatal neurons against 6-OHDA-induced neurodegenerative process [21]. 6-OHDA has pro-oxidant activity which causes to neurotoxicity. This toxin subsequent of auto-oxidation in the extracellular space, produce reactive oxygen species (ROS) [33]. Furthermore, it has been reported that 6-OHDA induce DA cells degeneration selectively by generation of free radicals and subsequently induction of oxidative stress and

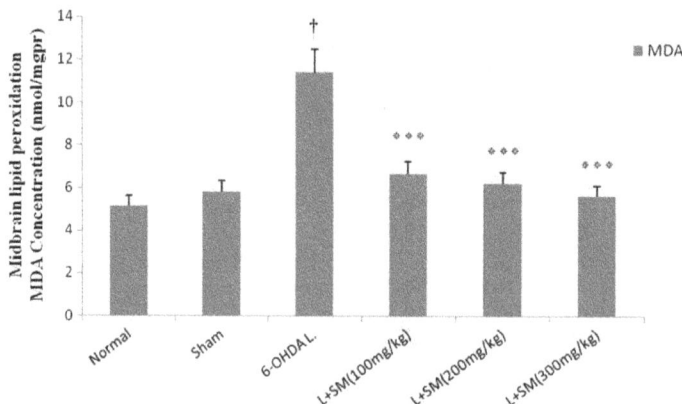

Figure 5 The effect of i.p. administration of silymarin (SM) at the doses of 100, 200, and 300 mg/kg/day (for 5 days) on lipid peroxidation in midbrain as measured by MDA concentration. Values are mean ± SEM (n = 8). †P < 0.001 from respective normal value; ***P < 0.001 as compared with 6-OHDA injected group using one way ANOVA with Tukey post hoc test. (L = .Lesioned).

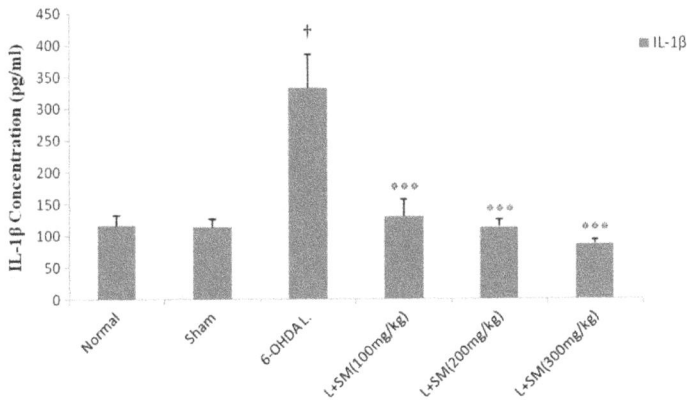

Figure 6 The effect of i.p. administration of silymarin (SM) at the doses of 100, 200, and 300 mg/kg/day (for 5 days) on IL-1β concentration in CSF (Figure 6). Values are mean ± SEM (n = 8). †P < 0.001 from respective normal value; ***P < 0.001 as compared with 6-OHDA injected group using one way ANOVA with Tukey post hoc test. (L = .Lesioned).

mitochondrial respiration dysfunction [34]. Additionally, oxidative stress result in microglia activation which leads to neurotoxicity of DA-neuron [14]. We suggest that the observed enhancement of motor balance in silymarin pre-treated hemi-parkinsonian rats in this study may be due to its possible neuroprotective effect. This effect may be exerted through counteracting oxidative stress process [35] maybe through regulating antioxidant defense system as well as inhibition of free radical generation [35].

To investigation of this issue, we also evaluated brain levels of MDA as lipid peroxidation marker in silymarin pre-treated hemi-parkinsonian rats. Malondialdehyde, a thiobarbiturate reactive substance, which formed as an end product of the peroxidation of lipids, served as an index of the intensity of oxidative stress. Our result showed a marked increase in midbrain lipid peroxidation as evidenced by elevation of MDA concentration in 6-OHDA-lesioned rats whereas, silymarin prevented dose-dependently from increase of MDA levels and restored it to the range of intact animals. According to these finding, we thought that silymarin attenuates the severity of oxidative stress through inhibition of lipid peroxidation. Also, it has been reported that the level of brain superoxide dismutase (SOD) and glutathione reductase (GR) as antioxidant enzymes decreased in parkinsonian rats and SM restored their levels in parkinsonian animals [21,36], which are totally in agreement with our findings.

Another key finding of the present study was that the reduction of brain MDA levels in silymarin pre-treated parkinsonian rats was associated with a significant decrease in pro-inflammatory cytokine. Our results showed that hemi-parkinsonian rats have a significant increase in CSF level of IL-1β, whereas its level was restored up to the normal range of intact animals by silymarin. This

is in accordance with other previous studies which show that 6-OHDA- neurotoxicity induced by microglia activation and subsequent increase of TNF-α, IL-6 and IL-1β levels in both substantia nigra (SN) and striatum [8,37-39]. DA neurons in SNc are vulnerable to inflammatory affront as a major exciter of neurodegenerative disease because of high density of microglia in SNc [40]. Pro-inflammatory cytokines such as TNF-α, IL-6 and IL-1β are released by activated microglia in striatum and SN [41], which have an important role in neurotoxicity [42]. It was noted that SM reduced the levels of IL-6 and TNF-α as well as suppression of MPO activity in hemi-parkinsonian rats [28]. Furthermore silymarin inhibit nuclear factor kappa B (NF-kB) activation in DA neurons [23], and down-regulate cyclooxygenase-2 (COX-2) in brain [25], which could subsequently decrease release of IL-1β.

The anti-oxidant activity can be considered as a possible neuroprotective mechanism of silymarin in PD. It can be postulated that neuroprotective and anti-neuroinflammatory effects of silymarin, in 6-OHDA induced hemi-parkinsonian rats, are almost due to reduction of pro-inflammatory cytokines and suppression of oxidative stress.

Conclusion

In conclusion, we found that short-term pre-treatment with silymarin improved 6-OHDA-induced motor-imbalance and protected animals against neurotoxicity of 6-OHDA. Furthermore silymarin decreased CSF levels of IL-1β and decreased lipid peroxidation as evidenced by striatal level of MDA in 6-OHDA-lesioned rats. We suggest a possible protective role for SM against neuro-inflammation and oxidative damages induced in PD. More clinical investigations should be done to prove its therapeutic application in PD.

Competing interest
The authors declare that they have no competing interest.

Authors' contributions
RH involved in doing behavioral experiments and drafting. MNA the supervisor of the study participated and involved in concept, design, support of study, interpretation of data and final check of the draft. SF has made contribution in study as an advisor. SEB and HS involved in doing behavioral experiments. All authors read and approved the final manuscript.

Acknowledgement
We wish to thank the Director of Drug Applied Research Center, Tabriz University of Medical Sciences for supporting this study.

Author details
[1]Student Research Committee, Tabriz University of Medical Sciences, Tabriz, Iran. [2]Drug Applied Research Center, Tabriz University of Medical Sciences, Tabriz, Iran. [3]Department of Pharmacology and Toxicology, Faculty of Pharmacy, Tabriz University of Medical Sciences, Tabriz, Iran. [4]Urmia University of Medical Science, Urmia, Iran.

References
1. Jankovic J, Stacy M: **Medical management of levodopa-associated motor complications in patients with Parkinson's disease.** *CNS Drugs* 2007, **21:**677–692.
2. Smeyne RJ, Jackson-Lewis V: **The MPTP model of Parkinson's disease.** *Mol Brain Res* 2005, **134:**57–66.
3. Warner TT, Schapira AHV: **Genetic and environmental factors in the cause of Parkinson's disease.** *Ann Neurol* 2003, **53:**S16–S25.
4. Rodriguez-Oroz MC, Jahanshahi M, Krack P, Litvan I, Macias R, Bezard E, Obeso JA: **Initial clinical manifestations of Parkinson's disease: features and pathophysiological mechanisms.** *Lancet Neurol* 2009, **8:**1128–1139.
5. Obeso JA, Rodriguez-Oroz MC, Goetz CG, Marin C, Kordower JH, Rodriguez M, Hirsch EC, Farrer M, Schapira AH, Halliday G: **Missing pieces in the Parkinson's disease puzzle.** *Nat Med* 2010, **16:**653–661.
6. Hirsch EC, Hunot S: **Neuroinflammation in Parkinson's disease: a target for neuroprotection?** *Lancet Neurol* 2009, **8:**382–397.
7. Lee J-K, Tran T, Tansey MG: **Neuroinflammation in Parkinson's disease.** *J Neuroimmune Pharmacol* 2009, **4:**419–429.
8. McGeer P, Itagaki S, Boyes B, McGeer E: **Reactive microglia are positive for HLA-DR in the substantia nigra of Parkinson's and Alzheimer's disease brains.** *Neurology* 1988, **38:**1285–1285.
9. Block M, Hong J: **Chronic microglial activation and progressive dopaminergic neurotoxicity.** *Biochem Soc Trans* 2007, **35:**1127–1132.
10. Hirsch EC, Vyas S, Hunot S: **Neuroinflammation in Parkinson's disease.** *Parkinsonism Relat Disord* 2012, **18:**S210–S212.
11. Varçin M, Bentea E, Michotte Y, Sarre S: **Oxidative stress in genetic mouse models of Parkinson's disease.** *Oxid Med Cell Longev* 2012, **2010:**624925. doi:10.1155/2012/624925.
12. Floyd RA: **Antioxidants, oxidative stress, and degenerative neurological disorders.** *Exp Biol Med* 1999, **222:**236–245.
13. Kim WG, Mohney RP, Wilson B, Jeohn GH, Liu B, Hong JS: **Regional difference in susceptibility to lipopolysaccharide-induced neurotoxicity in the rat brain: role of microglia.** *J Neurosci* 2000, **20:**6309–6316.
14. Cicchetti F, Brownell A, Williams K, Chen Y, Livni E, Isacson O: **Neuroinflammation of the nigrostriatal pathway during progressive 6-OHDA dopamine degeneration in rats monitored by immunohistochemistry and PET imaging.** *Eur J Neurosci* 2002, **15:**991–998.
15. Mogi M, Harada M, Riederer P, Narabayashi H, Fujita K, Nagatsu T: **Tumor necrosis factor-α (TNF-α) increases both in the brain and in the cerebrospinal fluid from parkinsonian patients.** *Neurosci Lett* 1994, **165:**208–210.
16. Brodacki B, Staszewski J, Toczyłowska B, Kozłowska E, Drela N, Chalimoniuk M, Stępien A: **Serum interleukin (IL-2, IL-10, IL-6, IL-4), TNFα, and INFγ concentrations are elevated in patients with atypical and idiopathic parkinsonism.** *Neurosci Lett* 2008, **441:**158–162.
17. Mandegary A, Saeedi A, Eftekhari A, Montazeri V, Sharif E: **Hepatoprotective effect of silymarin in individuals chronically exposed to hydrogen sulfide; modulating influence of TNF-α cytokine genetic polymorphism.** *Daru* 2013, **21:**28.
18. Manna SK, Mukhopadhyay A, Van NT, Aggarwal BB: **Silymarin suppresses TNF-induced activation of NF-κB, c-Jun N-terminal kinase, and apoptosis.** *J Immunol* 1999, **163:**6800–6809.
19. Gupta O, Sing S, Bani S, Sharma N, Malhotra S, Gupta B, Banerjee S, Handa S: **Anti-inflammatory and anti-arthritic activities of silymarin acting through inhibition of 5-lipoxygenase.** *Phytomedicine* 2000, **7:**21–24.
20. Esmaily H, Vaziri-Bami A, Miroliaee AE, Baeeri M, Abdollahi M: **The correlation between NF-κB inhibition and disease activity by coadministration of silibinin and ursodeoxycholic acid in experimental colitis.** *Fundam Clin Pharmacol* 2011, **25:**723–733.
21. Baluchnejadmojarad T, Roghani M, Mafakheri M: **Neuroprotective effect of silymarin in 6-hydroxydopamine hemi-parkinsonian rat: involvement of estrogen receptors and oxidative stress.** *Neurosci Lett* 2010, **480:**206–210.
22. Muzes G, Deak G, Lang I, Nekam K, Gergely P, Feher J: **Effect of the bioflavonoid silymarin on the in vitro activity and expression of superoxide dismutase (SOD) enzyme.** *Acta Physiol Hung* 1991, **78:**3–9.
23. Wang MJ, Lin WW, Chen HL, Chang YH, Ou HC, Kuo JS, Hong JS, Jeng KCG: **Silymarin protects dopaminergic neurons against lipopolysaccharide-induced neurotoxicity by inhibiting microglia activation.** *Eur J Neurosci* 2002, **16:**2103–2112.
24. Raza SS, Khan MM, Ashafaq M, Ahmad A, Khuwaja G, Khan A, Siddiqui MS, Safhi MM, Islam F: **Silymarin protects neurons from oxidative stress associated damages in focal cerebral ischemia: A behavioral, biochemical and immunohistological study in Wistar rats.** *J Neurol Sci* 2011, **309:**45–54.
25. Hou Y-C, Liou K-T, Chern C-M, Wang Y-H, Liao J-F, Chang S, Chou Y-H, Shen Y-C: **Preventive effect of silymarin in cerebral ischemia–reperfusion-induced brain injury in rats possibly through impairing NF-κB and STAT-1 activation.** *Phytomedicine* 2010, **17:**963–973.
26. Paxinos G, Watson C: *The rat brain in stereotaxic coordinates.* UK: Academic press, Elsevier Inc.; 2007.
27. Kaya H, Sezik M, Ozkaya O, Dittrich R, Siebzehnrubl E, Wildt L: **Lipid peroxidation at various estradiol concentrations in human circulation during ovarian stimulation with exogenous gonadotropins.** *Horm Metab Res* 2004, **36:**693–695.
28. Haddadi R, Mohajjel Nayebi A, Brooshghalan SE: **Pre-treatment with silymarin reduces brain myeloperoxidase activity and inflammatory cytokines in 6-OHDA hemi-parkinsonian rats.** *Neurosci Lett* 2013, **555:**106–111.
29. Yaghmaei P, Azarfar K, Dezfulian M, Ebrahim-Habibi A: **Silymarin effect on amyloid-β plaque accumulation and gene expression of APP in an Alzheimer's disease rat model.** *Daru* 2014, **22:**24.
30. Nayebi AM, Rad SR, Saberian M, Azimzadeh S, Samini M: **Buspirone improves 6-hydroxydopamine-induced catalepsy through stimulation of nigral 5-HT (1A) receptors in rats.** *Pharmacol Rep* 2010, **62:**258–264.
31. Carvalho MM, Campos FL, Coimbra B, Pêgo JM, Rodrigues C, Lima R, Rodrigues AJ, Sousa N, Salgado AJ: **Behavioral characterization of the 6-hydroxidopamine model of Parkinson's disease and pharmacological rescuing of non-motor deficits.** *Mol Neurodegene* 2013, **8:**14.
32. Meredith GE, Sonsalla PK, Chesselet M-F: **Animal models of Parkinson's disease progression.** *Acta Neuropathol* 2008, **115:**385–398.
33. Hanrott K, Gudmunsen L, O'Neill MJ, Wonnacott S: **6-hydroxydopamine-induced apoptosis is mediated via extracellular auto-oxidation and caspase 3-dependent activation of protein kinase Cδ.** *J Biol Chem* 2006, **281:**5373–5382.
34. Barnum CJ, Tansey MG: **Modeling neuroinflammatory pathogenesis of Parkinson's disease.** *Prog Brain Res* 2010, **184:**113–132.
35. Nencini C, Giorgi G, Micheli L: **Protective effect of silymarin on oxidative stress in rat brain.** *Phytomedicine* 2007, **14:**129–135.
36. Fabiana M, Andrea T, Giulia S, Cecilia B, Manuel ZMJ, Giorgio C-F, Patrizia H: **Neuroprotective effect of sulforaphane in 6-hydroxydopamine-lesioned mouse model of Parkinson's disease.** *Neurotoxicology* 2013, **36:**63–71.
37. Mogi M, Togari A, Tanaka K, Ogawa N, Ichinose H, Nagatsu T: **Increase in level of tumor necrosis factor (TNF)-α in 6-hydroxydopamine-lesioned striatum in rats without influence of systemic L-DOPA on the TNF-α induction.** *Neurosci Lett* 1999, **268:**101–104.
38. Nagatsu T, Mogi M, Ichinose H, Togari A: **Changes in cytokines and neurotrophins in Parkinson's disease.** *J Neural Transm Suppl* 2000, **36:**277–290.

39. Mogi M, Harada M, Kondo T, Riederer P, Inagaki H, Minami M, Nagatsu T: Interleukin-1β, interleukin-6, epidermal growth factor and transforming growth factor-α are elevated in the brain from parkinsonian patients. *Neurosci Lett* 1994, **180**:147–150.

40. Qin L, Wu X, Block ML, Liu Y, Breese GR, Hong JS, Knapp DJ, Crews FT: Systemic LPS causes chronic neuroinflammation and progressive neurodegeneration. *Glia* 2007, **55**:453–462.

41. Shadrina M, Slominsky P, Limborska S: Molecular mechanisms of pathogenesis of Parkinson's disease. *Int Rev Cell Mol Biol* 2010, **281**:229–266.

42. Sawada M, Imamura K, Nagatsu T: Role of cytokines in inflammatory process in Parkinson's disease. *J Neural Transm Suppl* 2006, **70**:373–381.

The effect of adipose derived stromal cells on oxidative stress level, lung emphysema and white blood cells of guinea pigs model of chronic obstructive pulmonary disease

Ahmad Ghorbani[2], Azadeh Feizpour[1], Milad Hashemzahi[1], Lila Gholami[1], Mahmoud Hosseini[3], Mohammad Soukhtanloo[4], Farzaneh Vafaee Bagheri[1], Esmaeil Khodaei[1], Nema Mohammadian Roshan[5] and Mohammad Hossein Boskabady[1*]

Abstract

Background: Chronic obstructive pulmonary disease (COPD) is a worldwide epidemic disease and a major cause of death and disability. The present study aimed to elucidate pharmacological effects of adipose derived stromal cells (ASCs) on pathological and biochemical factors in a guinea pig model of COPD. Guinea pigs were randomized into 5 groups including: Control, COPD, COPD + intratracheal delivery of PBS as a vehicle (COPD-PBS), COPD + intratracheal delivery of ASCs (COPD-ITASC) and COPD + intravenous injection of ASCs (COPD-IVASC). COPD was induced by exposing animals to cigarette smoke for 3 months. Cell therapy was performed immediately after the end of animal exposure to cigarette smoke and 14 days after that, white blood cells, oxidative stress indices and pathological changes of the lung were measured.

Results: Compared with control group, emphysema was clearly observed in the COPD and COPD-PBS groups ($p < 0.001$). Lung histopathologic changes of COPD-ITASC and COPD-IVASC groups showed non-significant improvement compared to COPD-PBS group. The COPD-ITASC group showed a significant increase in total WBC compared to COPD-PBS group but there was not a significant increase in this regard in COPD-IVASC group. The differential WBC showed no significant change in number of different types of leukocytes. The serum level of malondialdehyde (MDA) significantly decreased but thiol groups of broncho-alveolar lavage fluid (BALF) increased in both cell treated groups ($p < 0.05$ for all cases). Weight of animals decreased during smoke exposure and improved after PBS or cell therapy. However, no significant change was observed between the groups receiving PBS and the ones receiving ASCs.

Conclusion: Cell therapy with ASCs can help in reducing oxidative damage during smoking which may collectively hold promise in attenuation of the severity of COPD although the lung structural changes couldn't be ameliorated with these pharmacological therapeutic methods.

Keywords: COPD, Stromal cells, Malondialdehyde, Thiol, Emphysema, WBC, Guinea pigs

* Correspondence: boskabadymh@mums.ac.ir
[1]Neurogenic Inflammation Research Centre and Department of Physiology, School of Medicine, Mashhad University of Medical Sciences, Mashhad 9177948564, Iran
Full list of author information is available at the end of the article

Background

Chronic obstructive pulmonary disease (COPD) is a progressive lung disease. Its three most common pathological changes are chronic bronchitis, chronic obstructive bronchiolitis and emphysematous destruction of the lung parenchyma [1]. Emphysema, the main histopathologic feature of COPD, leads to a decrease in elastic recoil and therefore continuation of decrease in small airway patency during expiration causing a not fully reversible airflow limitation and increase in the lung residual volume [2]. This airway obstruction may contribute to respiratory failure and weight loss leading to cachexia [3] and eventually death. Thus, finding a fundamental and curative approach for this disease is of vital importance.

The other characteristic feature of COPD, as well as other respiratory diseases, is the oxidant-antioxidant imbalances. This imbalance is reported to be developed by the increased lipid peroxidation which is known as an index of oxidative stress and a reduction of antioxidant capacity. Decrease in plasma protein sulfhydryl concentrations in COPD patients is well documented [4]. There are also other evidences suggesting the role of reactive oxygen species in lung inflammation of COPD patients which can be a direct effect or through lipid peroxidation products [5]. Therefore, increasing the antioxidant capacity is one of the main concerns in the pharmacological treatment of COPD.

For treatment of such respiratory diseases as asthma, bronchodilating agents are helpful but the airflow limitation and accelerated loss of lung function caused by COPD cannot be reversed by this type of treatments [4,6]. The existing treatments for COPD only change the symptoms, quality of life and exacerbation frequency, while a fundamental or effective therapy is yet to be achieved. Recent advances in regenerative medicine and cell therapy have led to successful attempts to restore damaged tissues. Therefore, cell-based therapy might be a more promising therapeutic option for COPD.

Adipose tissue derived stromal cells (ASCs) and mesenchymal stem cells (MSCs), derived from ASCs or bone marrow, are readily available sources of stromal/stem cells required for cell therapy [5-10]. Many researchers such as Schweitzer et al. [5], Ahmed et al. [6], Gupta et al. [7], Baber et al. [8], Shigemura et al. [9] and Ishiazwa et al. [10] have contributed to cell therapy of lung diseases by local or systemic administration of ASCs/MSCs to the animal model of different lung injuries induced by elastase, monocrotaline or endotoxin and have observed promising pharmacological effects.

The MSCs are reported to interfere with oxidative stress and induce lung parenchymal regeneration [5,11]. Mesenchymal stem cells can ameliorate the pulmonary damages by two mechanisms. One is protecting the vascular bed endothelial cells from apoptosis by paracrine effects of several growth factors such as Hepatocyte growth factor (HGF) and Vascular endothelial growth factor (VEGF). The other mechanism is acquiring the phenotype or markers of airway or alveolar epithelial cells and vascular endothelial cells. In addition, it has been shown that transplantation of ASCs into elastase-treated emphysema models augments alveolar and vascular regeneration by enhancement of epithelial cell proliferation, inhibition of alveolar cell apoptosis and promotion of angiogenesis in lung vasculature [9,12]. Lung emphysematous destruction induced by COPD is well studied by different studies. However, MSCs ameliorative effect on COPD in guinea pigs, the main model of respiratory diseases, induced by cigarette smoking, the main cause of COPD in human was not investigated. On the other hand, some researches documented a pharmacological protective effect on the epithelial cells during oxidative damage by involvement of such cytokines as insulin-like growth factor (IGF) [7,8], HGF [9], and IL-6 [13] which raise the question if the MSCs may exert their therapeutic effect by an antioxidant function through secreting cytokines. There are few studies on the topic of antioxidant function of stem cells such as the one documenting that MSC protection of the kidneys against ischemia/reperfusion injury may be at least in part due to their antioxidant effects [14]. Another study also confirms an antioxidant along with a neuroprotective function for MSCs which have been previously approved in an *in vitro* study on neuroblastoma cells exposed to an oxidative stress [15]. However, such studies aren't formerly performed on the oxidative damage induced in the lungs of COPD model guinea pigs.

Considering the pathological changes occurring during COPD, at least three targets exist for intervention including inflammation, emphysematous destruction, and oxidative stress [5,14,15] among which the two latter ones are the focus of this study.

As far as we know, there is no study to investigate the ameliorative effect of ASCs on cigarette smoking-induced lung injury in guinea pigs, the main animal model of COPD. Therefore, the present study aimed to elucidate the pharmacological effects of local and systemic injection of ASCs on oxidative factors, lung pathology and white blood cells in cigarette smoke induced COPD in guinea pigs.

Methods
Animals and groups

Thirty one guinea pigs (600–800 g) were kept in a temperature controlled room while a 12-h on/12-h off light cycle was maintained. All animal experiments were carried out according to the ethical guidelines of the animal care of the Mashhad University of Medical Sciences. They were categorized to 5 groups as follows:

a) Control group, the animals were exposed to ambient air rather than smoke (n = 6).
b) COPD group, the animals were exposed to cigarette smoke for 3 consecutive months (n = 9).
c) COPD + PBS, the animals were exposed to cigarette smoke and then received PBS as vehicle via intratracheal injection (n = 5).
d) COPD + intratracheal delivery of ASCs (COPD-ITASC), the animals were exposed to cigarette smoke and then received 10^6 ASCs via intratracheal injection (n = 6).
e) COPD + intravenous injection of ASCs (COPD-IVASC): the animals were exposed to cigarette smoke and then received 10^6 ASCs via intravenous injection (n = 5).

Biochemical assays and lung pathological examination were done 14 days after treatment with cell or vehicle.

Exposure of animals to cigarette smoke

Exposure of guinea pigs to cigarette smoke was performed according to the method designed by Boskabady and Kiani with some modifications [16]. Briefly, the animals were placed in a special box which was divided into two parts: one held the body of the animal and the other one held its head (dimensions: 15×12×7 cm). Twenty millilitre puffs of cigarette smoke were drawn out of the cigarettes using a syringe and then exhausted at a rate of two puffs per minute into the animals' head chamber (every 30 seconds, one puff of cigarette smoke was dragged into the head chamber). Exposure of animals to each cigarette lasted for 8–9 minutes, with a 10 minutes resting period between two cigarettes. The animals were exposed initially to one cigarette per day and gradually increasing to a maximum of 5 cigarettes per day over a period of 20 days. In short, the animals were exposed to cigarette smoke (Magna: Nicotine = 5, tar = 6) for totally 3 consecutive months, 5 days per week, and 5 cigarettes per day (the cigarettes' filters weren't removed).

Preparation of stromal cells

Adipose tissues were obtained from healthy guinea pigs weighing 600–800 g. They were anesthetized by intra peritoneal injection of ketamine (150 mg/kg) and xylazine (6 mg/kg). Subcutaneous inguinal fat deposits were resected and under laminar hood, the fat tissue was minced into 1–2 mm pieces by means of a sterile scalpel [17]. The tissue pieces were incubated at 37°C for 60 minutes in PBS containing 2 mg/ml collagenase meanwhile being shaken (60 cycles/min) [18,19]. After centrifugation (300 g for 8 minutes), the floated lipid layer was

discarded and the stroma-vascular fraction was collected, washed and re-suspended in DMEM medium supplemented with 10% FBS, 100 units/ml penicillin and 100 µg/ml streptomycin [19,20]. The cells were seeded into tissue culture flask and passaged when 60–80% confluent and used at passages three to six.

Differentiation of stromal cell

For differentiation to adipocyte, the stromal cells were seeded in 12-well culture plate and then incubated in DMEM supplemented with 3% FBS, 66 µM biotin, 250 µM IBMX, 1 µM dexamethasone, 34 µM d-panthothenate, 5 µM indomethacin and 0.2 µM insulin. The cells were maintained in differentiation medium for 3 days and then exposed to the adipocyte maintenance medium consisting of DMEM, supplemented with 3% FBS, 66 µM biotin, 1 µM dexamethasone, 34 µM d-panthothenate and 0.2 µM insulin. After additional 9 days of incubation, adipogenesis was confirmed by Oil Red O which stains intracellular triglyceride droplets. For staining, the cells were fixed with 10% formalin and then incubated with Oil Red O solution. Thereafter, the cells were washed three times with distilled water and photographed using inverted microscope [19].

For osteocyte differentiation, the stromal cells were incubated in DMEM supplemented with 10% FBS, 10 µg/ml ascorbic acid, 5 mM β-glycerol phosphate and 0.1 µM dexamethasone. The cells were maintained in the differentiation medium for two weeks and the culture medium was replaced every 3 days [21]. For Alizarin red staining, the cells were fixed with 10% formalin and then incubated with 2% Alizarin red solution. Thereafter, the cells were washed three times with distilled water and photographed using inverted microscope [22].

Stromal cell labeling and tracing

The cells were harvested, suspended in PBS and incubated with 2 µM cell tracker CM DiI (Invitrogen) for 5 min in 37°C and 15 min in 4°C in the absence of light. After 20 min of staining, it was centrifuged at 1500 for 5 min, washed with PBS, centrifuged again and suspended in 0.3 ml PBS. It was finally dragged to a 27 gauge insulin syringe and was prepared for injection to the animals' jugular vein or trachea. After 2 weeks of ASCs administration (either intratracheal or intravenous), the animals were euthanized and 4 µm sections were provided from different regions of their lung. Existence of the CM-DiI labeled stromal cells was detected under fluorescent microscope.

Intratracheal and systemic delivery of stromal cells

The guinea pigs of COPD-ITASC group were anesthetized and after exposing the trachea, 0.3 ml PBS containing 10^6 cells was injected under direct vision to the trachea using a 27 gauge insulin syringe. Viability of injected cells was found to be more than 90% as assessed with trypan blue staining.

In COPD-IVASC group, the animals were anesthetized and the jugular vein was exposed. Then, a volume of 0.3 ml PBS containing 10^6 cells was injected into the vein using a 27 gauge insulin syringe.

Total WBC and differential WBC measurement

Total WBC was counted in duplicate in a hemocytometer (in a Burker chamber) in blood stained with Turk solution (1:10 dilution, consisted of 1 ml of glacial acetic acid, 1 ml of gentiac vialet solution 1% and 100 ml distilled). Differential WBC was determined in blood samples stained with Turk solution and Wright-Giemsa, respectively. Briefly, differential cell counts were done on thin slide, prepared with smearing blood sample, using Wright-Giemsa stain. According to staining and morphological criteria, differential cell analysis was carried out under a light microscope by counting 100 cells, and the percentage of each cell type was calculated.

Biochemical assays

After sacrificing the guinea pigs, broncho-alveolar lavage fluid (BALF) was prepared from the lung by locating a cannula into trachea and lavage of the lungs with 2 mL of saline for 5 times (total: 10 mL). BALF was then centrifuged at $2500 \times g$ for 10 min and the supernatant was collected for measurement of thiol groups' concentration.

Total thiol groups were measured using 2,2'-dinitro-5,5'-dithiodibenzoic acid (DTNB) which reacts with the SH groups to produce a yellow colored complex with peak absorbance at 412 nm [23,24]. In summary, 1 mL Tris-EDTA buffer was added to 50 µL of BALF and sample absorbance was read at 412 nm against Tris-EDTA buffer alone (A1). Then, 20 µL of DTNB reagent (10 mM in methanol) was added to the mixture and after 15 min, the sample absorbance was again read (A2). Total thiol concentration was calculated using this equation: Total thiol (mM) = (A2-A1-blank) × 1.07/0.05 × 13.6.

Five ml blood sample was collected gently from the left ventricle and placed in a citrate containing blood collection tube not to be coagulated. The blood was centrifuged and the serum was separated and kept in $-70°C$ for further measurement of MDA concentrations. MDA level, as an index of lipid peroxidation, was measured. MDA reacts with thiobarbituric acid (TBA) as a thiobarbituric acid reactive substance (TBARS) to produce a red colored complex which has peak absorbance at 535 nm. Two mL from reagent of TBA/trichloroacetic acid (TCA)/ hydrochloric acid (HCL) was added to 1 mL of serum, and the solution was heated in a water bath for 40 minutes. After cooling, the whole solutions were centrifuged at 1000 g for 10 minutes. The absorbance was measured at 535 nm [25]. The MDA concentration was calculated as follows: C (m) = Absorbance/(1.56 × 10^5).

Lung pathology

After fixation of the lung specimen in formalin and staining with H&E, the tissue sections were evaluated under a light microscope by a pathologist. The pathologic changes in the lung of COPD, COPD-PBS, COPD-ITASC and COPD-IVASC groups were evaluated according to the intensity of emphysema. Three intensities of parenchymal destruction were considered for scoring the emphysema observed in the lungs. Scoring of pathological changes was performed as previously described [16]. For this purpose, the percent of the area containing mild, moderate or severe emphysema was multiplied by the number 1, 2 or 3, respectively and the total score for each section was calculated.

Animals weight measurement

The weight of the animals of all groups was measured at the beginning of the study (week 0) and after 3 months (at the end of exposure period); but in COPD-PBS, COPD-ITASC and COPD-IVASC groups, the weight of animals was also measured after a further 2 weeks (at the end of treatment with PBS or ASC cells).

Statistical analysis

All the data were quoted as mean ± SEM and compared by means of Instat software. The data of COPD animals were compared to the control ones using unpaired "t" test. The same test was used for the comparison between PBS and either COPD + ITASC or COPD + IVASC as well as between COPD + PBS and COPD. In addition, the comparison between the weights of animals at three time points during the procedure was performed using ANOVA. Significance was accepted at p < 0.05.

Results

Stromal cell characterization

Figure 1A and C shows the morphology of stromal cells isolated from adipose tissue of guinea pig. The cells were adherent and showed significant expansion in the cultures (Figure 1A). After passage 3, they had a spindled, fibroblast appearance in culture that is consistent with MSCs morphology.

To determine whether the cells have pluripotent capacity, before intratracheal or intravenous injection, a number of them were cultured in differentiating media specific for adipocyte and osteocyte. Oil Red O staining showed the accumulated triglyceride droplets in the cells cytoplasm which confirms adipogenic differentiation capacity of the isolated stromal cells (Figure 1B). In addition, Alizarin Red staining revealed extracellular matrix mineralization which confirms osteogenic differentiation capacity of the stromal cells (Figure 1D).

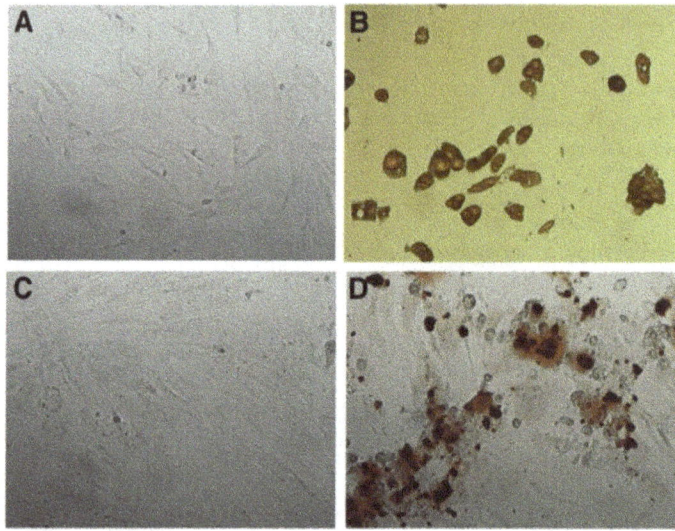

Figure 1 Differentiation of adipose derived stromal cells to adipocyte and osteocyte lineages. The stromal cells were cultured in adipogenic or osteogenic differentiating media for 12 and 14 days, respectively. **A**: Oil Red O staining of cells cultured in control media; **B**: Oil Red O staining of cultured cells in adipogenic differentiating media; **C**: Alizarin Red staining of cells cultured in control media; **D**: Alizarin Red staining of cells cultured in osteogenic differentiating media. Magnification × 100.

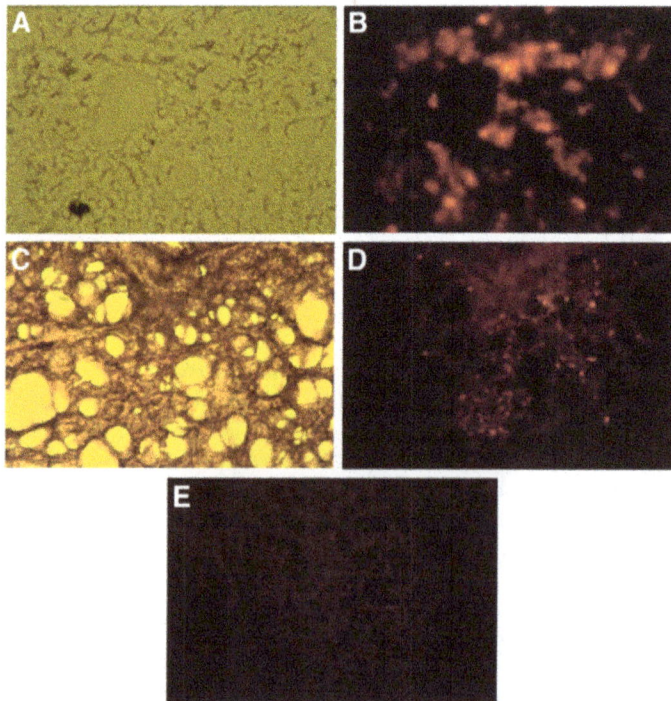

Figure 2 Fluorescence microscopic photographs of lungs after intratracheal delivery of CMDiI-labeled stromal cells. A: Phase-contrast microscopic image of lung from normal animal harvested 2 days after injection of labeled stromal cells into trachea (Magnification × 200); **B**: The same field under fluorescent microscope. **C**: Phase-contrast microscopic image of formalin fixed lung from COPD animal harvested 14 days after injection of labeled stromal cells into trachea (Magnification × 100); **D**: The same field under fluorescent microscope; **E**: Fluorescence microscopic image of lung from COPD animal harvested 14 days after injection of PBS as vehicle (Magnification × 100).

Stromal cell detection in the lung

To detect stromal cells in airway structures, the CM-DiI labeled cells were injected to trachea. Figure 2 shows fluorescence microscopy of stromal cells after 2 or 14 days of intratracheal delivery. Two days after intratracheal injection, microscopic image of lung from normal guinea pig (guinea pig experiencing no treatment) confirmed the delivery of stromal cells into both large and small airway structures (Figure 2A and B). The CM-DiI-labeled stromal cells were also detected in the lung from COPD guinea pig 14 days after intratracheal administration (Figure 2C and D). There was no fluorescence signal in the lung harvested from COPD animal 14 days after injection of PBS as vehicle (Figure 2E).

To ensure pulmonary delivery of stromal cells after intravenous injection, fluorescence microscopy was also done on lung sections two days after cell injection. The labeled cells were detected in the lung alongside resident cells in airways and alveolar structures (Figure 3A and B). In separate homing experiments, the labeled cells were administered systemically via intravenous injection to a COPD guinea pig. Fourteen days after administration of the cells, fluorescence signals of labeled cells were still detected in the lung (Figure 3C, D and E).

Lung histopathological results

Three consecutive months of exposing animals to the cigarette smoke caused a considerable destruction of alveolar walls and consequently widespread emphysema as H&E stained sections show. The same changes were observed in the COPD-PBS group and there was no significant difference between the emphysema score in COPD-PBS and COPD groups. The change in emphysema score of COPD-ITASC and COPD-IVASC animals was non-significant compared to the COPD-PBS group (Figure 4).

Biochemical results

BALF thiol concentration had a significant decrease in COPD compared with control group ($P < 0.001$). There was also a significant reduction in this factor in COPD-PBS group compared to the COPD animals ($P < 0.05$). The thiol concentration increased in both treated groups with stromal cells, but it was only significant in COPD-IVASC compared to COPD-PBS group ($P < 0.05$), (Figure 5).

Concentration of MDA had a significant increase in the COPD group compared with the control animals ($P < 0.01$) which was not significantly different with COPD-PBS groups (Figure 6). The concentration of MDA

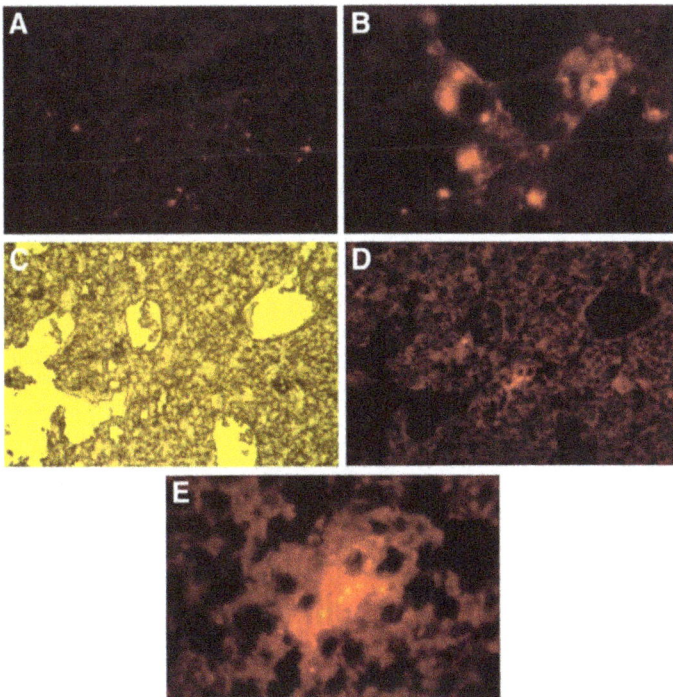

Figure 3 Fluorescence microscopic photographs of lungs after systemic delivery of CMDiI-labeled stromal cells. A and **B**: Lung homing of labeled stromal cells two days after injection of cells into jugular vein of normal guinea pig (Magnification: A = ×100, B = ×400); **C**: Phase-contrast microscopic image of formalin fixed lung from COPD animal harvested 14 days after injection of labeled stromal cells into jugular vein (Magnification × 100); **D**: The same field under fluorescent microscope (Magnification × 100); **E**: The same field under fluorescent microscope with magnification of × 400.

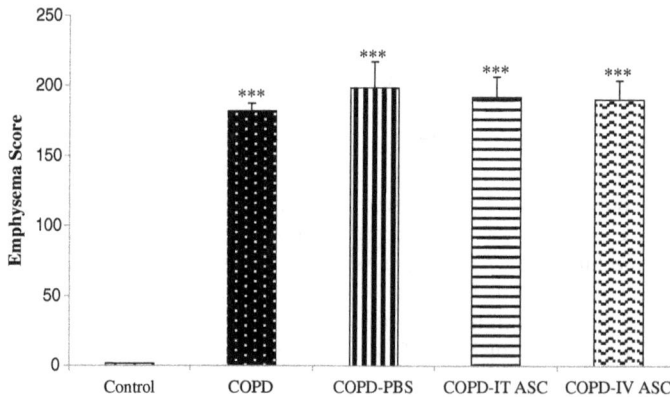

Figure 4 Effect of adipose derived stromal cells (ASCs) therapy on pathological changes of the lung according to the scoring method mentioned in the text. Data are shown as mean ± SEM. ***$P < 0.001$ as compared with control group. The animals in COPD-PBS, COPD-ITASC and COPD-IVASC groups were exposed to cigarette smoke for 3 months and then received PBS, intratracheal injection of ASCs and intravenous injection of ASCs, respectively. For scoring, the percent of the area containing mild, moderate or severe emphysema was multiplied by the number 1, 2 or 3, respectively.

in both treated groups with the stromal cells showed a significant reduction compared to the COPD-PBS animals ($P < 0.05$).

Total and differential WBC counts

There was a significant increase in total WBC in the COPD compared to the control group ($P < 0.01$). No significant difference was observed between the total WBC counts in COPD-PBS and COPD group (Figure 7A). There was a significant increase in this parameter in the COPD-ITASC group compared to COPD-PBS animals but no significant difference was observed between COPD-IVASC and COPD-PBS groups. There was no significant difference in the number of eosinophil, neutrophils, lymphocytes and monocytes between various groups (Figure 7B).

Animals weight changes

There was an increase in the weight of the animals of control group after 3 months of ambient air exposure but all the other groups showed a significant reduction in this parameter after 3 months of cigarette smoking except for COPD-IVASC group in which this increase wasn't significant (Figure 8). After the surgery and injection of stromal cells or PBS, all the three groups showed a significant increase in animals' weight during the two weeks before being euthanized.

Discussion

In many studies pertaining to asthma and COPD, the most widespread small animal species used are the mice or rats while guinea pigs are the most susceptible species and a significant airspace enlargement happens in their

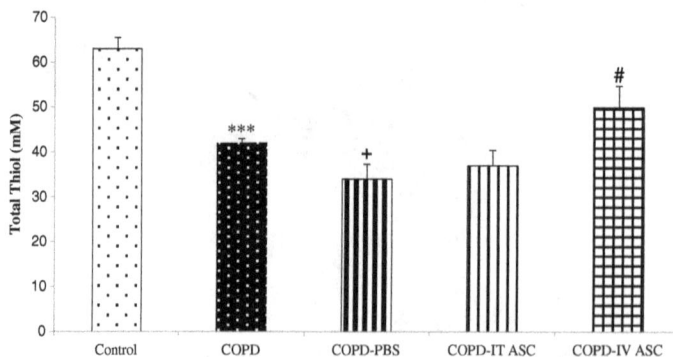

Figure 5 Thiol total concentration in broncho-alveolar lavage fluid in different groups. Data are shown as mean ± SEM. ***$P < 0.001$ as compared with control group. #$P < 0.05$ as compared with COPD-PBS group. +$P < 0.05$ as compared with COPD group. The animals in COPD-PBS, COPD-ITASC and COPD-IVASC groups were exposed to cigarette smoke for 3 months and then received PBS, intratracheal injection of ASCs and intravenous injection of ASCs, respectively.

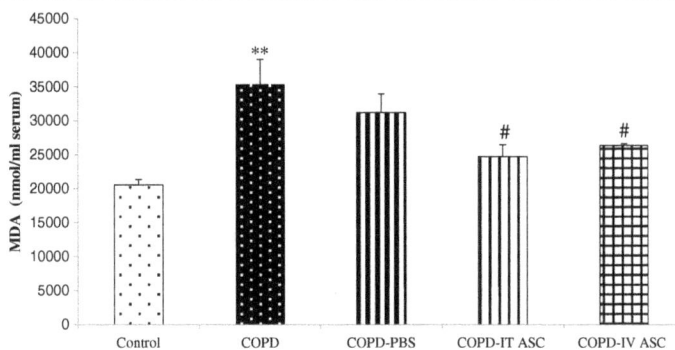

Figure 6 Serum concentration of malondialdehyde (MDA) in different groups. Data are shown as mean ± SEM. **$P < 0.01$ as compared with control; #$P < 0.05$ as compared with COPD-PBS. The animals in COPD-PBS, COPD-ITASC and COPD-IVASC groups were exposed to cigarette smoke for 3 months and then received PBS, intratracheal injection of ASCs and intravenous injection of ASCs, respectively.

lungs after a few months of cigarette smoke exposure [26]. Besides, the most considerable advantage of guinea pigs, as a respiratory disease model, its airway pharmacology and physiological processes of these animals are similar to human such as the airway autonomic system, allergic reaction and responses to agonists and antagonists. The other side of the coin is that using guinea pigs in animal studies has some disadvantages too, including absence of transgenic animals, a lack of variety in guinea pig strains, and a noticeable axon reflex that is questionable whether it is present in human airways or not [27]. Therefore, despite the easier procedures and lower expenses in working with rats or mice, guinea pig was chosen as an animal model of COPD in the present study.

It is documented that the structural changes considered important in COPD are as follows: destruction of alveolar wall and existence of emphysema, alveolar space enlargement due to emphysema, increase in alveolar septum due to infiltration of leukocytes and penetration of smoke particles, elastolysis and collagen fiber deposition in alveolar septa and pulmonary vessel wall [16]. The major reasons for these changes caused by cigarette smoking are inflammatory responses, oxidative damage and changes in protease-anti protease balance. According to the results of the present study, emphysema was observed in the lungs of the smoke-exposed group of animals, so that the adjacent alveolar spaces were joined to each other due to the parenchymal destructions and air space enlargements were clearly observed. This is consistent with other studies demonstrating physiological and morphological changes induced by cigarette smoke in lung of guinea pigs [16,27,28]. In the present study, treatment of smoke exposed animals by stromal cells showed no significant improvement in the intensity of the smoke-induced emphysema. As all the procedure of familiarizing animals to the new habitat, smoke exposure and cell administrations took several months, it was assumed that higher age

of the animals at the end of the study might be interfering with cell therapy. Therefore, the inconvenient histopathology result might be due to the lack of regenerative mechanisms or decreased numbers of progenitor cells in the lung parenchyma or a stromal vascular fraction of the older subjects [10]. Kasper et al. also worked on MSC properties in bone marrow; they documented that not only these cells' potential regeneration decreases with age but also their migration capability and number in bone marrow decreases as an individual grows older [29]. Furthermore, the number of systemically or locally injected cells varies from 1×10^6 to 5×10^7 in different studies on the effect of MSCs on lung injuries [9,10,30]. Accordingly, another reason of the observed result in this part of our study might be due to the inevitable low number of injected cells. The number of stromal cells was intentionally chosen to be low in this experiment because in a study, carried out by Lee et al., it was demonstrated that intravenous injection of high number of MSC into mice contributed in embolism in the lung which may be fatal [31]. Consistently, Furlani et al. documented that some of their animals died of pulmonary embolism after abdominal aorta injection of high and low doses of MSCs (1×10^6 MSCs or 0.2×10^6), while no death was observed in the present study [32]. In addition, one of the most probable reasons for the absence of improving pharmacological effects of cell therapy on structural changes of the lung is that these changes take place during a long period of development of COPD which is well known to be rarely reversible. For this reason, in further studies, the effect of cell therapy is recommended to be examined during different stages of development of COPD not at the end of the disease development.

The results of this study also showed increased total WBC in the blood of smoke exposed animal and COPD-PBS group. However, cell therapy did not affect changes in blood total WBC. The probable reasons for the absence of improving effects of cell therapy on this parameter

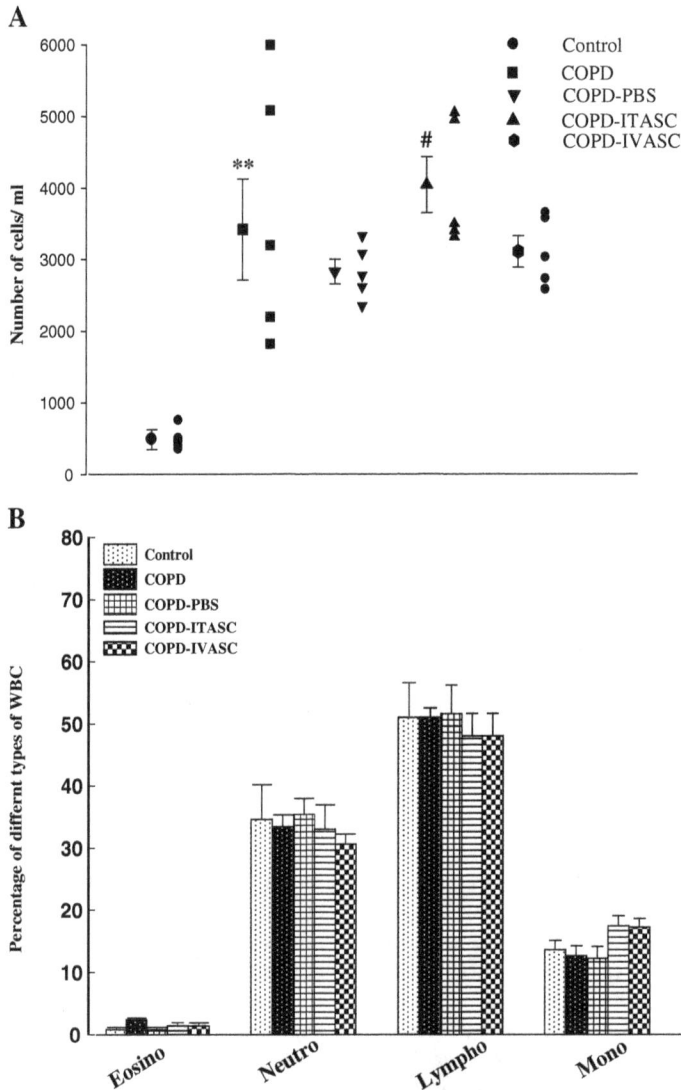

Figure 7 Effects of adipose derived stromal cells therapy on white blood cell counts in blood of different groups. Effects of adipose derived stromal cells (ASCs) on total white blood cell (WBC), **(A)** and its effect on differential WBC **(B)** counts. Data are shown as mean ± SEM. The animals in COPD-PBS, COPD-ITASC and COPD-IVASC groups were exposed to cigarette smoke for 3 months and then received PBS, intratracheal injection of ASCs and intravenous injection of ASCs, respectively.

could also be due to taking place of this change during a long period of development of COPD which is difficult to be affected by this method of therapy. However, further studies regarding the effect of cell therapy during different stages of development of COPD could be of great value. The ranges of differential WBC counts reported in this study may seem inconsistent with normal values. However, the ranges for lymphocyte, neutrophil and eosino-phil number are 30-80%, 20-60% and 0-7% respectively in guinea pig which is different from human [33]. Our

previous studies also showed similar range of differen-tial WBC counts in guinea pigs [34,35].

In the present study, the cells injected into the trachea or the jugular vein of the animals were traced to confirm that they have reached the injured lung. As described be-fore, the labeled stromal cells were detectable in the tissue even 2 weeks after cell therapy. It is consistent with an-other study reporting the persistence of MSCs 21 days fol-lowing their injection into the trachea [8]. Schweitzer et al. also documented that systemically delivered adipose

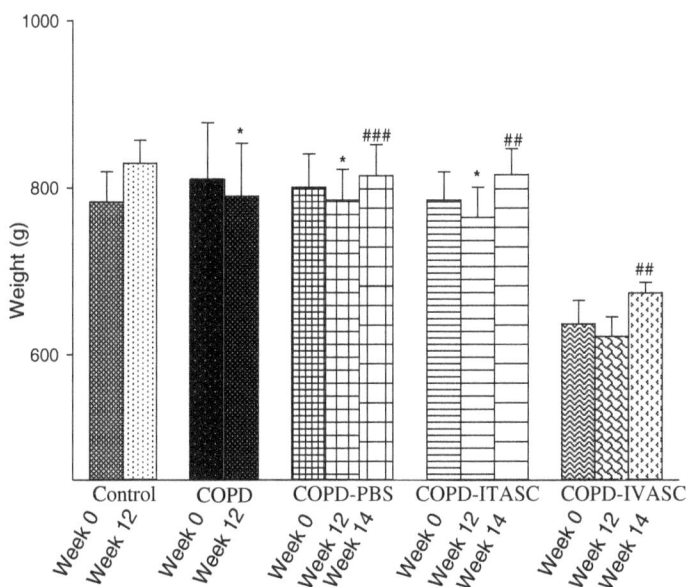

Figure 8 Body weight in guinea pigs of different groups. Data are shown as mean ± SEM values of body weight at three time points: at the first of the 3 months of inhalation (Week 0), on the last day of the 3 months of inhalation (Week 12) and 2 weeks after surgery (Week 14). *$P < 0.01$ as compared with week 0; ##$P < 0.01$ and ###$P < 0.001$ as compared with week 12. The animals in COPD-PBS, COPD-ITASC and COPD-IVASC groups were exposed to cigarette smoke for 3 months and then received PBS, intratracheal injection of ASCs and intravenous injection of ASCs, respectively.

stem cells were detectable in the parenchyma and large airways of the lungs up to 21 days after injection [5]. It seems that two weeks recovery, given to the animals after administration of the cells, is a proper time for the stromal cells to exert their impact either by regeneration in the damaged tissue or by paracrine effects.

The results of the present study showed that the oxidative stress was increased in the smoke exposed group both in their BALF and serum measured by an increase in the concentration of MDA in serum and a decrease in the thiol groups in BALF. It is well documented that cigarette smoke contains stable compounds that undergo redox-cycle to form reactive oxygen species such as superoxide radicals, hydrogen peroxide, hydroxyl radicals etc. [36]. Our results are in accordance with the study carried out by Qamar et al., who reported the debility in antioxidant defenses after intratracheal instillation of cigarette smoke extract in rats [36]. Since there was no significant difference in the MDA and thiol concentration between COPD and COPD-PBS groups, it can be concluded that the PBS injection had no pharmacological effect on the parameter under investigation. BALF thiol concentration of the treated groups with intratracheal and intravenous administration of stromal cells increased significantly in COPD-IVASC group. However, both treated groups showed significant decrease in serum MDA concentration. These findings confirmed the ameliorative effect of stromal cells

on the oxidative damage caused by cigarette smoke. Consistently, the antioxidant effect of mesenchymal stem cells within the stromal-vascular fraction of subcutaneous adipose tissue has been previously shown by Kim et al. documenting that these cells have potent antioxidant activity and protect HDFs from oxidative injury by decreasing apoptotic cells [11].

Considering the results, although the animals were kept in boxes with low possibility of movement and high probability of gaining weight during three months, being exposed to cigarette smoke during these months caused a considerable decrease in body weight of almost all the animals. Complied with these results, Schweitzer et al. documented that patients affected by emphysema often exhibit progressive respiratory symptoms and loss of lung function culminating in respiratory failure and systemic weight loss [5]. There are plenty of other studies demonstrating the effect of cigarette smoking on body weight loss [37,38]. In the present study, after finishing the three months of smoke exposure, the surgery and administration of the cells or PBS to the animals led to a significant increase in body weight. As Schweitzer et al. documented, therapeutic effects of adipose stem cells aren't restricted to the lung but also contains restoring the weight loss sustained by guinea pigs during cigarette smoke exposure [5]. However, the weight gain after the surgery, in the present study, can't be associated with the treatment with stromal cells because this improvement was observed in the PBS receiving groups too. Therefore, it can be concluded that smoke cessation and lower mobility of the animals due to the surgery might be the initial source of gaining weight.

In the present study, the applied method of exposing the animals to cigarette smoke resulted in exposure of all the animals to the same concentration of cigarette smoke as follows; every 30 second a twenty ml puff of smoke was dragged into the head chamber using a 20 ml syringes and duration of exposure of the animals to each cigarette was about 8 minutes with the same duration of rest between each two successive cigarettes. This protocol was maintained during the whole procedure and the smoke concentration in the head chamber was maintained the same for all the groups. This obviously leads to the similar levels of plasma nicotine and its metabolite as well as similar levels of plasma carboxyhemoglobin. Therefore, the variations observed in the results of different groups are just due to the variations in treatment protocol between them.

Conclusions
In conclusion, both intratracheal and intravenous cell therapy lead to pharmacological effect on reduction of oxidative damage and restoring the weight loss during smoking which may collectively hold promise in attenuation of the severity of the disease in the patients experiencing COPD although the lung structural changes couldn't be ameliorated with these therapeutic methods. However, more investigations are needed to further assess the pharmacological effects of adipose derived stromal cells on the microscopic structure of the damaged lung induced by cigarette smoke.

Competing interest
The authors declare that they have no competing interest.

Authors' contributions
AG: help in study design, supervision of experiments, statistical analysis and preparation of manuscript, AF: performance of experiment, help in statistical analysis and manuscript preparation, MH: help in performance of experiment, LG: help in performance of experiment, MH: help in study design and supervision of experiments, MS: Bichemichal analysis, FVB: help in performance of experiment, EK: help in performance of experiment, NMR: Patholofical evaluations, MHB: study design, supervision of experiments, help in statistical analysis and preparation of manuscript. All authors read and approved the final manuscript.

Acknowledgments
This study was financially supported by the Research Council of Mashhad University of Medical Sciences. This paper is a part of M.Sc. thesis.

Author details
[1]Neurogenic Inflammation Research Centre and Department of Physiology, School of Medicine, Mashhad University of Medical Sciences, Mashhad 9177948564, Iran. [2]Pharmacological Research Center of Medicinal Plants, School of Medicine, Mashhad University of Medical Sciences, Mashhad, Iran. [3]Neurocognitive Research Center and Department of Physiology, School of Medicine, Mashhad University of Medical Sciences, Mashhad, Iran.

[4]Department of Clinical Biochemistry, School of Medicine, Mashhad University of Medical Sciences, Mashhad, Iran. [5]Department of Pathology, School of Medicine, Mashhad University of Medical Sciences, Mashhad, Iran.

References
1. Pauwels RA, Buist AS, Ma P, Jenkins CR, Hurd SS: Global strategy for the diagnosis, management, and prevention of chronic obstructive pulmonary disease: National Heart, Lung, and Blood Institute and World Health Organization Global Initiative for Chronic Obstructive Lung Disease (GOLD): executive summary. Resp Care 2001, 46:798–825.
2. Saetta M, Ghezzo H, Kim W, King M, Angus G, Wang N, et al: Loss of alveolar attachments in smokers. A morphometric correlate of lung function impairment. Am Rev Respir Dis 1985, 132:894–900.
3. Jeffery PK: Structural and inflammatory changes in COPD: a comparison with asthma. Thorax 1998, 53:129–136.
4. Celli B, MacNee W, Agusti A, Anzueto A, Berg B, Buist A, et al: Standards for the diagnosis and treatment of patients with COPD: a summary of the ATS/ERS position paper. Eur Respir J 2004, 23:932–946.
5. Schweitzer KS, Johnstone BH, Garrison J, Rush NI, Cooper S, Traktuev DO, et al: Adipose stem cell treatment in mice attenuates lung and systemic injury induced by cigarette smoking. Am J Respir Crit Care Med 2011, 183:215–225.
6. Gladysheva ES, Malhotra A, Owens RL: Influencing the decline of lung function in COPD: use of pharmacotherapy. Int J COPD 2010, 5:153–164.
7. Gupta N, Su X, Popov B, Lee JW, Serikov V, Matthay MA: Intrapulmonary delivery of bone marrow-derived mesenchymal stem cells improves survival and attenuates endotoxin-induced acute lung injury in mice. J Immunol 2007, 179:1855–1863.
8. Baber SR, Deng W, Master RG, Bunnell BA, Taylor BK, Murthy SN, et al: Intratracheal mesenchymal stem cell administration attenuates monocrotaline-induced pulmonary hypertension and endothelial dysfunction. Am J Physiol-Heart C 2007, 292:1120.
9. Shigemura N, Okumura M, Mizuno S, Imanishi Y, Nakamura T, Sawa Y: Autologous transplantation of adipose tissue-derived stromal cells ameliorates pulmonary emphysema. Am J Transplant 2006, 6:2592–2600.
10. Ishizawa K, Kubo H, Yamada M, Kobayashi S, Numasaki M, Ueda S, et al: Bone marrow-derived cells contribute to lung regeneration after elastase-induced pulmonary emphysema. FEBS Lett 2004, 556:249–252.
11. Kim W-S, Park B-S, Kim H-K, Park J-S, Kim K-J, Choi J-S, et al: Evidence supporting antioxidant action of adipose-derived stem cells: protection of human dermal fibroblasts from oxidative stress. J Dermatol Sci 2008, 49:133–142.
12. Ahmed S, Katsha SO, Xin H, Kanehira M, Sun R, TNaY S: Paracrine factors of multipotent stromal cells ameliorate lung injury in an elastase-induced emphysema model. ASGCT 2010, 19:196–203.
13. Yamamoto C, Yoneda T, Yoshikawa M, Fu A, Tokuyama T, Tsukaguchi K, et al: Airway inflammation in COPD assessed by sputum levels of interleukin-8. CHEST J 1997, 112:505–510.
14. Drost E, Skwarski K, Sauleda J, Soler N, Roca J, Agusti A, et al: Oxidative stress and airway inflammation in severe exacerbations of COPD. Thorax 2005, 60:293–300.
15. MacNee W: Oxidative stress and lung inflammation in airways disease. Eur J Pharmacol 2001, 429:195–207.
16. Boskabady MH, Kiani S: The effect of exposure of guinea pig to cigarette smoke and their sensitization in tracheal responsiveness to histamine and histamine receptor (h1) blockade by chlorpheniramine. Pathophysiol 2007, 14:97–104.
17. Ghorbani A, Varedi M, Hadjzadeh MR, Omrani GH: Type-1 diabetes induces depot-specific alterations in adipocyte diameter and mass of adipose tissues in the rat. Exp Clin Endocrinol Diabetes 2010, 118:442–448.
18. Ghorbani A, Hadjzadeh MR, Rajaei Z, Zendehbad SB: Effects of fenugreek seeds on adipogenesis and lipolysis in normal and diabetic rat. Pak J Biol Sci 2014, 17:523–528.
19. Ghorbani A, Jalali SA, Varedi M: Isolation of adipose tissue mesenchymal stem cells without tissue destruction: a non-enzymatic method. Tissue Cell 2014, 46:54–58.
20. Ghorbani A, Abedinzade M: Comparison of in vitro and in situ methods for studying lipolysis. ISRN Endocrinol 2013, 2013:205385.

The effect of adipose derived stromal cells on oxidative stress level, lung emphysema and white...

31

21. Hsu LW, Goto S, Nakano T, Chen KD, Wang CC, Lai CY, et al: The effect of exogenous histone H1 on rat adipose-derived stem cell proliferation, migration, and osteogenic differentiation in vitro. J Cell Physiol 2012, 227:3417–3425.

22. Raynaud C, Maleki M, Lis R, Ahmed B, Al-Azwani I, Malek J, et al: Comprehensive characterization of mesenchymal stem cells from human placenta and fetal membrane and their response to osteoactivin stimulation. Stem Cells Int 2012, 2012:658356.

23. Sadeghnia HR, Yousefsani BS, Rashidfar M, Boroushaki MT, Assadpour E, Ghorbani A: Protective effect of rutin on hexachlorobutadiene-induced nephrotoxicity. Ren Fail 2013, 35:1151–1155.

24. Sadeghnia HR, Kamkar M, Assadpour E, Boroushaki MT, Ghorbani A: Protective effect of safranal, a constituent of Crocus sativus, on quinolinic acid-induced oxidative damage in rat hippocampus. Iran J Basic MedSci 2013, 16:73–82.

25. Khodabandehloo F, Hosseini M, Rajaei Z, Soukhtanloo M, Farrokhi E, Rezaeipour M: Brain tissue oxidative damage as a possible mechanism for the deleterious effect of a chronic high dose of estradiol on learning and memory in ovariectomized rats. Arq Neuro-Psiquiat 2013, 71:313–319.

26. Wright JL, Churg A: Cigarette smoke causes physiologic and morphologic changes of emphysema in the guinea pig. Am J Res Crit Care Med 1990, 142:1422–1428.

27. Boskabady MH, Kiani S, Aslani MR: Tracheal responsiveness to both isoprenaline and beta-adrenoreceptor blockade by propranolol in cigarette smoke exposed and sensitized guinea pigs. Respirol 2006, 11:572–578.

28. Canning BJ, Chou Y: Using guinea pigs in studies relevant to asthma and COPD. Pulm Pharmacol Ther 2008, 21:702–720.

29. Kasper G, Mao L, Geissler S, Draycheva A, Trippens J, Kühnisch J, et al: Insights into mesenchymal stem cell aging: Involvement of antioxidant defense and actin cytoskeleton. Stem cells 2009, 27:1288–1297.

30. Yun Luan XZ, Kong F, Cheng G-H, Qi T-G, Zhang Z-H: Mesenchymal stem cell prevention of vascular remodeling in high flow-induced pulmonary hypertension through a paracrine mechanism. Int Immunopharmacol 2012, 14:432–437.

31. Lee RH, Pulin AA, Seo MJ, Kota DJ, Ylostalo J, Larson BL, et al: Intravenous hMSCs improve myocardial infarction in mice because cells embolized in lung are activated to secrete the anti-inflammatory protein TSG-6. Cell Stem Cell 2009, 5:54–63.

32. Furlani D, Ugurlucan M, Ong L, Bieback K, Pittermann E, Westien I, et al: Is the intravascular administration of mesenchymal stem cells safe?: Mesenchymal stem cells and intravital microscopy. Microvas Res 2009, 77:370–376.

33. Suckow MA, Stevens KA, Wilson RP: The laboratory rabbit, guinea pig, hamster, and other rodents. San Diego: Access Online via Elsevier; 2012.

34. Boskabady MH, Keyhanmanesh R, Khamneh S, Ebrahimi MA: The effect of Nigella sativa extract on tracheal responsiveness and lung inflammation in ovalbuminsensitizedguinea pigs. Clinics 2011, 66:879–887.

35. Boskabady MH, Bayrami G, Tabatabaee A: The effect of the extract of Crocus sativus and its constituent safranal, on lung pathology and lung inflammation of ovalbumin sensitized guinea-pigs. Phyto Med 2012, 19:904–911.

36. Qamar W, Sultana S: Farnesol ameliorates massive inflammation, oxidative stress and lung injury induced by intratracheal instillation of cigarette smoke extract in rats: an initial step in lung chemoprevention. Chem-BiolInteract 2008, 176:79–87.

37. Chen H, Hansen MJ, Jones JE, Vlahos R, Bozinovski S, Anderson GP, et al: Cigarette smoke exposure reprograms the hypothalamic neuropeptide Y axis to promote weight loss. Am J Resp Critic Care Med 2006, 173:1248–1254.

38. Kubo S, Kobayashi M, Masunaga Y, Ishii H, Hirano Y, Takahashi K, et al: Cytokine and chemokine expression in cigarette smoke-induced lung injury in guinea pigs. Eur Resp J 2005, 26:993–1001.

A comparative study on the physicochemical and biological stability of IgG$_1$ and monoclonal antibodies during spray drying process

Vahid Ramezani[1,2], Alireza Vatanara[1*], Abdolhossein Rouholamini Najafabadi[1], Mohammad Ali Shokrgozar[3], Alireza Khabiri[4] and Mohammad Seyedabadi[5]

Abstract

Background: The main concern in formulation of antibodies is the intrinsic instability of these labile compounds. To evaluate the physicochemical stability of antibody in dry powder formulations, physical stability of IgG$_1$ and a monoclonal antibody (trastuzumab) during the spray drying process was studied in a parallel study and the efficacy of some sugar based excipients in protection of antibodies was studied.

Results: The SDS-PAGE analysis showed no fragmentation of antibodies after spray drying in all formulations. The secondary structure of antibodies contained 40.13 to 70.19% of β structure in dry state. Also, CD spectroscopy showed the similar secondary structure for trastuzumab after reconstitution in water. ELISA analysis and cell culture studies were conducted in order to evaluate bioactivity of monoclonal antibody. Formulations containing combination of excipients provided maximum tendency of trastuzumab to attach to the ELISA antigen (86.46% ± 2.3) and maximum bioactivity when incubated with SKBr$_3$ cell line (the cell viability was decreased to 65.99% ± 4.6). Incubation of formulations with L929 cell line proved the biocompatibility of the excipients and non-toxic composition of formulations.

Conclusion: The IgG$_1$ and trastuzumab demonstrated similar behavior in spray drying process. The combination of excipients containing trahalose, hydroxypropyl beta cyclodextrin and beta cyclodextrin with proper ratio improved the physical and chemical stability of both IgG$_1$ and monoclonal antibody.

Keywords: Antibody, Trastuzumab, Spray drying, Trehalose, Hydroxypropyl beta cyclodextrin, Beta cyclodextrin

Background

Monoclonal antibodies as an important part of therapeutic proteins are approved for treatment of various chronic and life threatening diseases. Their specific action and relatively low side effects have contributed to vast application of antibodies in many diseases [1]. The majority of antibodies are administrated by injection ordinarily; however, new antibodies and new administration routes such as inhalation [2], transdermal [3], vaginal [4], oral [5] and nasal [6] are investigated broadly as new delivery systems.

The main concern in formulation of antibodies is the intrinsic instability of these labile compounds. Generally,

proteins are sensitive molecules to various physical instabilities like denaturation, aggregation, fragmentation and chemical reactions such as deamination, oxidation and isomerization [7,8]. Embedding of protein in dry matrix improves the stability versus physical and chemical degradation by various mechanisms [9-11].

Spray drying as a one-step process has been widely studied in production of dry powders containing proteins [12]. As a limitation, proteins as like as antibodies could be destabilized due to the high temperature and pressures in this process. In this way, the effects of various excipients [9,12] and process variables [12,13] have been investigated in lots of studies [9,10,12,13]. In our previous study, D-optimal design was conducted to optimize IgG$_1$ formulation in the presence of sugars and cyclodextrins in order to understand how the spray drying affects the antibody. But as like as many other

* Correspondence: vatanara@tums.ac.ir
[1]Department of Pharmaceutics, Faculty of Pharmacy, Tehran University of Medical Sciences, Tehran, Iran
Full list of author information is available at the end of the article

researches, these efforts have been focused on the processing of IgG as a model antibody and extension of the results of a general antibody to the monoclonal antibodies remains as a challenge. To the extent of our knowledge, no systematic study has been reported as a comparison between these two categories of antibodies. In the present work, trastuzumab as a monoclonal antibody was formulated parallel to the IgG_1 in the presence of sugar based excipients and the physical stability were compared. Trastuzumab is an important humanized monoclonal antibody that is approved in treatment of breast cancer with over-expressed HER2 receptor [14,15]. So, assessment of the biological activity of trastuzumab is supportive to evaluate the conformational stability of protein during the process.

Material and methods

Materials

Hydroxypropyl beta cyclodextrin (HPβCD) was obtained from Acros (Belgium) and Beta cyclodextrin (βCD) was purchased from Sigma (USA). Trehalose dehydrate, potassium phosphate dibasic and disodium sulfate were acquired from Merck (Germany). Trastuzumab (Herceptin®) was purchased from Roche Ltd (Hungary) and the chemicals were from sigma (USA). Human IgG_1 (with molecular weight of about 150 KD) was supplied by Kedrion (Italy). Prior to each investigation, low molecular weight additive of antibody solution was removed by dialysis with deionized water (cut off: 15 kDa).

Spray drying of antibody formulations

Spray drying was performed on various aqueous solutions of antibody with different excipients according to Table 1. The design of study was in accordance with the findings of previous studies on IgG_1. A lab scale Buchi-191 spray dryer (Buchi, Switzerland) was employed to obtain the dry antibody powder. The inlet temperature of 100°C, air flow rate of 700 L/h, liquid feed rate of

1.7 mL/min, and aspiration rate of 100% were selected. The resulted dry powders were collected in dry and well closed glass vials and stored at 4°C.

Size exclusion chromatography

Size exclusion chromatography (SEC) was conducted to evaluate the percentage of soluble IgG aggregations as one of the most important physical instabilities. In order to separate the monomer from aggregated antibody, a 300 mm TSK 3000 SWXL column (Tosoh Biosep, Germany) was employed. Approximately, 20 μL of each sample containing 2.5 mg/mL was injected. The mobile phase consisted of 0.1 M disodium hydrogen phosphate and 0.1 M sodium sulfate (pH 6.8) with flow rate of 0.5 mL/min. The antibody concentration was measured by a UV detector (Waters, USA) at 280 nm. All experiments were performed in triplicate.

Sodium dodecyl sulfate polyacrylamide gel electrophoresis (SDS-PAGE)

In order to determine the antibody fragmentation, non-reducing sodium dodecyl sulphate-poly (acrylamide) gel electrophoresis (SDS-PAGE) was performed. Polyacrylamide gel 10% was prepared and diluted sample with concentration of 100 μg/mL was loaded. The samples were mixed with equal volumes of sample buffer before loading. Protein molecular weight marker of Fermentas® (Germany) was used to estimate the sample molecular weight.

Fourier transformation infrared spectroscopy (FT-IR)

Nicolet Magna spectrometer (USA) was applied to record the infrared spectra. Briefly, 2 mg of each sample was pressed with 200 mg KBr to make a clear tablet. The Jasco Spectra Manager® software (Japan) was used to deconvolution the spectra and detect the changes in secondary structure of antibody. Second derivative spectrum of amide I region (1600–1700 cm^{-1}) is a useful indicator to

Table 1 Composition of various formulations of IgG_1 and trastuzumab

Formulation	IgG_1	Trastuzumab	HPβCD	βCD	Trehalose
F_1	-	1	-	-	-
F_2	-	1	1	-	-
F_3	-	1	-	1	-
F_4	-	1	-	-	1
F_5	-	1	1	1	0.26
F_6	1	-	-	-	-
F_7	1	-	1	-	-
F_8	1	-	-	1	-
F_9	1	-	-	-	1
F_{10}	1	-	1	1	0.26

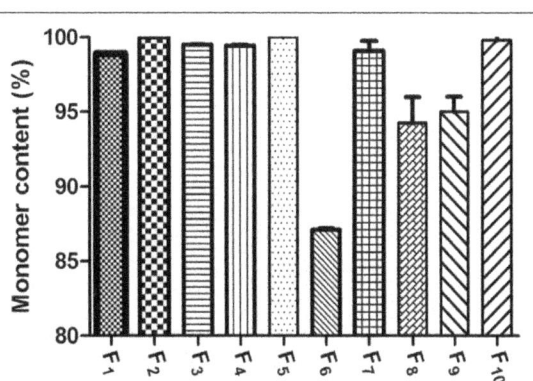

Figure 1 The percent of antibody monomer in microparticles immediately after spray drying analyzed by size exclusion chromatography (SEC).

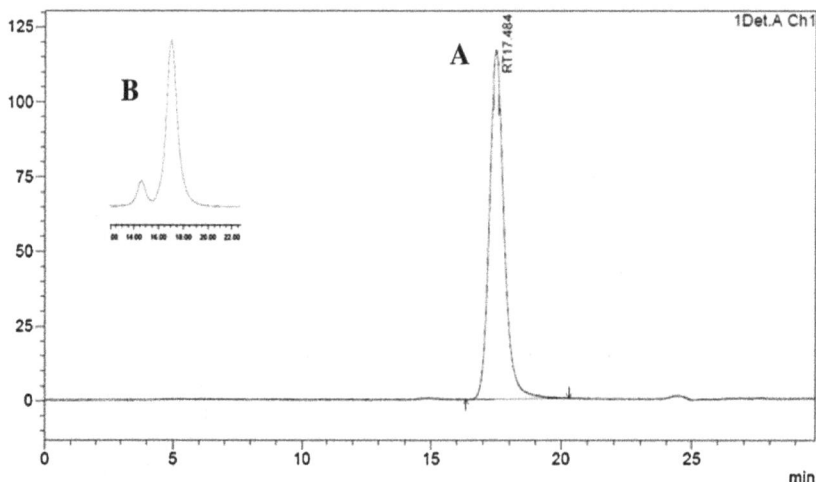

Figure 2 Size exclusion chromatography of F_5 (A); as shown, the aggregation related pick (B) has been disappeared in this formulation.

understand the protein structure. The percent of β sheet, α helix and turn was calculated by mixed Gaussian/ Lorentzian function considering β sheet structure absorption in 1640 cm^{-1} and 1695–1690 cm^{-1}, α helix in 1660–1650 cm^{-1} and turns from 1690 to1665 cm^{-1}.

Circular dichroism (CD)

Circular dichroism spectroscopy (AVIV, USA) was applied to analysis the secondary structure of monoclonal antibody after reconstitution. Proper amounts of processed powder were dissolved in purified water to make 250 µg/mL solutions. Measurement of buffer and antibody samples were performed in far-UV spectrophotometer at 20°C from 195 to 260 nm with the interval of 1 nm. Buffer spectra were substracted from the relevant protein solutions and converted to mean residual ellipticity. Deconvolution was performed to estimate the secondary structure of trastuzumab spectra. The secondary structure was calculated considering the molecular weight of 148 kDa for trastuzumab and a total number of 1328 amino acids.

Enzyme-linked Immunosorbent Assay (ELISA)

Direct ELISA was performed in order to determine the in-vitro activity of spray dried trastuzumab. Briefly, a 96 wells plate from Nunc (USA) was coated with 6 µg/mL of recombinant human HER_2 protein in carbonate/bicarbonate buffer over-night. The plate was blocked with 2% w/v BSA for 1 h at 37°C after three times of washing. About 100 µL of samples were added and incubated for 2 h at 37°C. After washing, 100 µL of the goat anti human antibody conjugated with horse radish peroxidase (HRP) was added and incubated at room temperature for 1 h. The bounded antibody was determined with tetramethyl benzemidine (TMB) as the proxidase substrate for 15 min and the concentration was determined at 650 nm by a STAT FAX 4700 ELISA reader (USA).

Cell culture studies

The human breast cancer cell line $SKBr_3$ and human fibroblast L929 were obtained from cell culture collection of Pasteur institute of Iran. $SKBr_3$ was cultured in RPMI medium supplemented with 10% of fetal bovine albumins

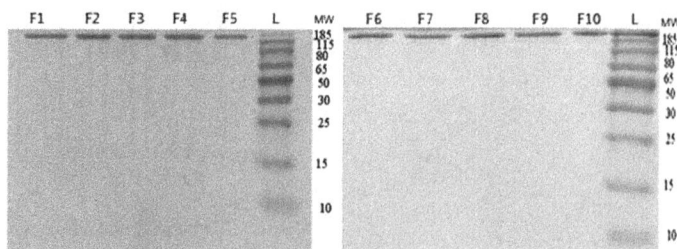

Figure 3 SDS-PAGE of formulations contained trastuzumab and IgG_1. The standard molecular weights were run in the left of gel.

and the L929 cell line was cultured in Dulbecco's modified Eagle's medium with 5% of fetal bovine albumin. Both culture mediums contained 1% of L-glutamine, 100 UI/mL of penicillin G and 100 mg/mL of streptomycin and maintained at 37°C in a humid atmosphere of 5% CO_2. For the experiment, the cells were harvested after brief incubation with trypsin (0.05%, w/v) and EDTA (0.02%, w/v).

Primarily, the cells were incubated with various concentrations of trastuzumab in the range of 10^1 to 10^6 ng/mL and the dose–response of trastuzumab on SKBr3 cells was determined. Further examinations were performed on the samples in concentrations of 10^5 ng/mL. To evaluate the biological activity of monoclonal antibody in various spray dried samples, the proper amount of each sample were dissolved in 100 mL of medium and added to 96-well plates in triplicate with 2×10^2 cells/well. Cell viability was assayed with mono tetrazolium 3-[4,5-dimethylthiazol-2-yl]-2,5-diphenyl tetrazolium bromide (MTT) colorimetric method. Briefly, the cells were exposed to tetrazolium after 48 h incubation with trastuzumab samples. Living cells were able to metabolized tetrazolium to non-soluble formazan, the formazan salts was dissolved and quantified using spectrophotometer plate reader (BioTek, USA) at 540 nm. The negative control was medium without trastuzumab and the positive control included unprocessed standard trastuzumab with determined concentration.

Statistical analysis

Data are presented as means ± SD and LSD-test was performed to evaluate the differences between groups. The statistical significance of results is considered with a P value less than 0.05. The graphs have been drawn by GraphPad® Prism 5and Microsoft® Excel 2007.

Results and discussion

Similar to other proteins, antibodies can undergo degradation pathways during the spray drying process. Protein degradation can reduce the efficient binding of protein to the receptors and decrease the bioactivity. So it is very impotent to ensure the physical stability as well as biological activity of monoclonal antibodies after spray drying or other processes. In our previous study, optimization and characterization of IgG_1formulations led to use a combination of trehalose, HPβCD and βCD which resulted in protection of antibody structure up to 99.81 ± 0.7%. In the present study, as shown in Table 1, these excipients were employed in order to evaluate the stability of trastuzumab as a monoclonal antibody in comparison with IgG_1.

Physical stability of antibody

The percent of antibody aggregates after spray drying are presented in Figure 1. The pattern of aggregation in IgG_1 and trastuzumab was similar; however, the percent

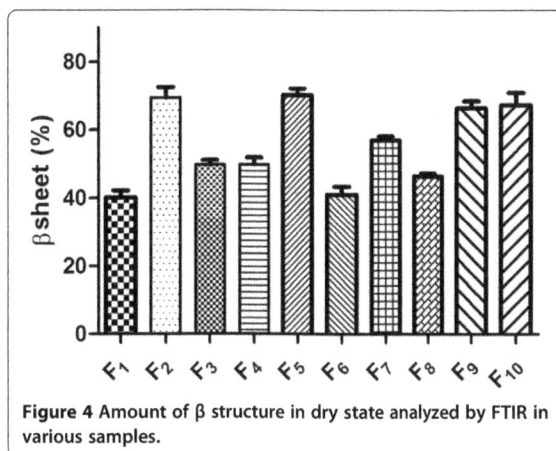

Figure 4 Amount of β structure in dry state analyzed by FTIR in various samples.

of aggregations were different. As seen, the pure IgG_1 contained 87.1% monomer and pure trastuzumab contained 98.9% monomer after process. Application of excipients successfully decreased the aggregation in both of antibodies. In this way, the efficacy of HPβCD was greater than βCD and trehalose. Combination of trehalose, HPβCD and βCD in the F_5 showed the highest effectiveness in protection of the trastuzumab monomer. As seen in Figure 2, the pick related to the trastuzumab dimmer in SEC chromatogram has been disappeared. This point implicates the synergistic effect of sugars in protection of antibody monomer. Similar observations have demonstrated the synergism effect of various sugars in preservation of proteins by water substitution mechanism [10].

Non reducing SDS-PAGE was performed in order to reveal fragmentation of antibodies during the spray drying. In this type of SDS-PAGE, reducing agents are not used and consequently, evaluation of protein structure is possible without reduction of di-sulfide bounds. Therefore,

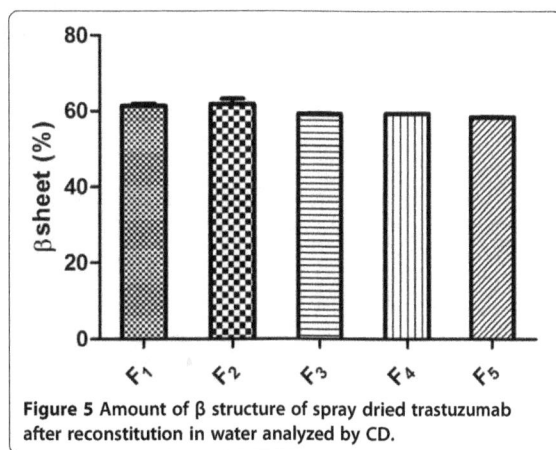

Figure 5 Amount of β structure of spray dried trastuzumab after reconstitution in water analyzed by CD.

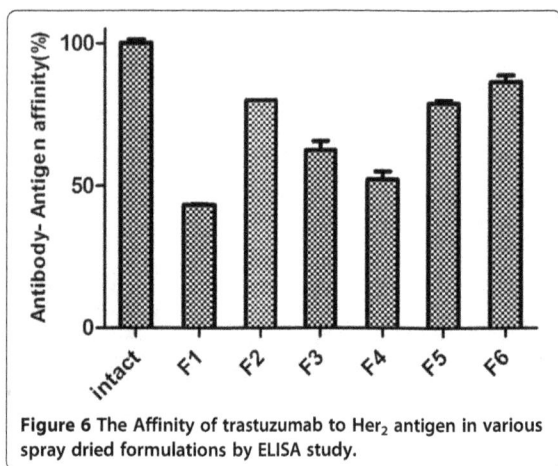

Figure 6 The Affinity of trastuzumab to Her$_2$ antigen in various spray dried formulations by ELISA study.

detection and quantification of process-related fragmentation would be possible. As shown in Figure 3, all formulations of both trastuzumab and IgG$_1$ present bonds just in 150 kDa and there is no distinct bond in lower molecular weight regions. Amphlett G et al. (1996) showed that the bonds such as Asp-Gly and Asp-Pro are more sensitive to cleavage in proteins backbone. So the proteins are prone to cleavage and fragmentation in these places [16]. Moreover, disulfide bonds cleavage lead to formation of antibody fragments of 25 and 50 kDa. If fragmentation took place during the spray drying process, we expected to observe the distinct bonds in SDS-PAGE gel, but the results suggested that process stresses did not affect the trastuzumab backbone. So the data implicated that the short time exposure of antibodies to harsh conditions of spray drying did not induce antibody fragmentation.

The secondary structure of antibody samples was evaluated by FTIR spectroscopy in dry state. As presented in Figure 4, the lowest ratio of β structures (40.13 ± 2.1%) was perceived when pure antibodies were processed by spray drying and presence of excipients in the formulations of antibody increased the β structures content; Where, F$_2$ provided 69.35% and F$_5$ contained 70.19% of

β structure. Processing of pure IgG$_1$ lead similarly to 41.01% of β structures and F$_{10}$ as the formulation containing the composition of excipients, preserved the high amounts of β structure after spray drying (67.21%).

The secondary structure of monoclonal antibody, after reconstitution in water, was assessed using far-UV CD spectrophotometer. The amounts of β sheet and β turns in the processed trastuzumab were about 60%. Comparison of FTIR and CD data revealed that dehydration of trastuzumab resulted in substantial and measurable conformational changes and it emphasize that protein structure is highly depended on protein type and formulation conditions, but these changes can be reversible or irreversible. According to the Figure 5, results indicated that trastuzumab reforms to the native structure after reconstitution in water. In agreement, similar studies showed that selection of proper stabilizers minimize the structural changes of proteins such as poly-L-lysine [17], acetate dehydrogenase and phosphor fructokinase [18].

Biological activity

The biological activity of trastuzumab depends on its ability to target the extracellular domain of human epidermal growth factor receptor protein in tumor cells. Trastuzumab therapy reduces the tumor cells proliferation by several mechanisms. On the one hand, it promotes cell cycle arrest and apoptosis in tumor or metastatic cells and on the other hand, it activates an antibody-dependent cellular cytotoxicity (ADCC) response with the aid of natural killer (NK) cells. The NK cells induce cell death by attaching to the Fc domain of antibody and the activity of trastuzumab highly depends on the ability to contact with HER$_2$ antigen as well as NK cells receptors.

ELISA is an appropriate method for simultaneous evaluation of both F$_c$ and F$_{ab}$ fragments of antibody; since, in this analysis method, the structural changes in the antibody are exaggerated. Any change in the F$_{ab}$ or F$_c$ can affect the affinity of antibody to the antigen or secondary antibody. Direct ELISA was applied to evaluate the stability of trastuzumab during the spray drying

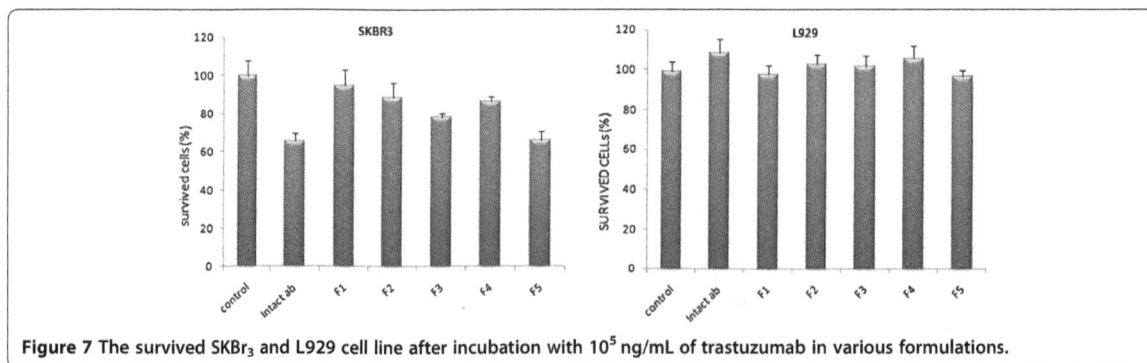

Figure 7 The survived SKBr$_3$ and L929 cell line after incubation with 10^5 ng/mL of trastuzumab in various formulations.

in comparison with unprocessed antibody as positive controls. As presented in Figure 6, just $43.2 \pm 0.2\%$ of the pure antibody was quantified after processing; whereas, presence of excipients in F_2 and F_5 enhanced the affinity of antibody to the antigen up to $79.9 \pm 0.1\%$ and $86.5 \pm 2.3\%$, respectively.

Furthermore, bioactivity of monoclonal antibody was evaluated by means of HER_2-over-expressing breast cancer cell line ($SKBr_3$). The cells were incubated in the presence of 10^5 ng/mL of spray dried samples and unprocessed standard trastuzumab as positive control. The cells viability was evaluated by MTT assay after 48 hours. Statistical comparison of survived cells after incubation showed that the ability of F_1 containing processed pure trastuzumab to kill the cells was the minimum (Figure 7). The 2-side dunnett test indicated no difference between F_1 and negative control. However, the unprocessed trastuzumab presented a great activity to kill the $SKBr_3$ cells (with the minimum cell viability of $65.88 \pm 3.95\%$ after incubation). The ANOVA with the aid of post doc (LSD) test among spray dried formulations indicated the equal ability of F_2, F_3, F_4 with F_5, which showed the greatest ability to preserve the antibody activity ($65.99 \pm 4.6\%$). Also, LSD test indicated no difference between F_5 and positive control. As a result, it could be deduced that combination of various excipients with different properties led to inhibition of aggregation and preservation of antibody structure as well as protection of amino acids in the protein backbone.

Some previous studies indicated the citotoxicity of cyclodextrine and other derivatives on the body cells or on red blood cells [19,20]. The L929 is a fibroblast cell line L929 without any HER_2 antigen on the surface that is suitable for evaluation of toxicity and biocompatibility of formulations. The same concentration of trastuzumab was incubated with this cell line and analysis of cell viability in the presence of different formulations showed no toxic effect at concentrations of 10^5 ng/mL and the 100% of cells were alive after incubation with various formulations after 48 hr (Figure 7). Consequently, we concluded that the death in $SKBr_3$ cells were due to the active trastuzumab rather than formulation excipients. Also the biocompatibility of formulations was confirmed in this experiment.

Conclusion

This report focused on physicochemical stability and biological activity of antibodies after spray-drying. Combination of HPβCD, βCD and trehalose provided the maximum efficacy in protection of the IgG_1 as a general antibody and trastuzumab as a monoclonal antibody. Coexistence of these excipients in the formulations preserved monomers up to 99.1% and 99.9% for IgG and trastuzumab, respectively.

The conformational changes of processed antibodies in dry structure were reversible and it could reform to the native stricter after reconstitution in water. The activity of trastuzumab in best formulation was detected up to 86.46% in ELISA test and it was confirmed by cell culture studies.

Competing interests
The authors declare that they have no competing interests.

Authors' contributions
VR performed the experiment and prepared the manuscript; AV and ARN supervised the project and helped in study design; MASH gave consultation on cell culture and analyzing the antibody bioactivity; AKH gave consultation on ELISA assay; MS helped in statistical analysis and preparation of the manuscript. All authors read and approved the final manuscript.

Acknowledgement
This study (was/has been) funded and supported by Tehran university of medical sciences (TUMS).

Author details
[1]Department of Pharmaceutics, Faculty of Pharmacy, Tehran University of Medical Sciences, Tehran, Iran. [2]Department of Pharmaceutics, Faculty of Pharmacy, Shahid Sadoughi University of Medical Sciences, Yazd, Iran. [3]National Cell Bank of Iran, Pasteur Institute of Iran, Tehran, Iran. [4]Department of Mycology, Pasteur Institute of Iran, Tehran, Iran. [5]Department of Molecular Imaging, The Persian Gulf Biomedical Sciences Research Institute, Bushehr University of Medical Sciences, Bushehr, Iran.

References
1. An Z: Monoclonal antibodies-a proven and rapidly expanding therapeutic modality for human diseases. *Protein Cell* 2010, **1**:319–330.
2. Hacha J, Tomlinson K, Maertens L, Paulissen G, Rocks N, Foidart JM, Noel A, Palframan R, Gueders M, Cataldo DD: Nebulized anti-IL-13 monoclonal antibody Fab' fragment reduces allergen-induced asthma. *Am J Respir Cell Mol Biol* 2012, **47**:709–717.
3. Li G, Badkar A, Nema S, Kolli CS, Banga AK: In vitro transdermal delivery of therapeutic antibodies using maltose microneedles. *Int J Pharm* 2009, **368**:109–115.
4. Castle PE, Karp DA, Zeitlin L, Garcia-Moreno EB, Moench TR, Whaley KJ, Cone RA: Human monoclonal antibody stability and activity at vaginal pH. *J Reprod Immunol* 2002, **56**:61–76.
5. Reilly R, Domingo R, Sandhu J: Oral delivery of antibodies. *Clin-Pharmacokinet* 1997, **32**:313–323.
6. Kaye RS, Purewal TS, Alpar OH: Development and testing of particulate formulations for the nasal delivery of antibodies. *J Control Release* 2009, **135**:127–135.
7. Wang W, Singh S, Zeng DL, King K, Nema S: Antibody structure, instability, and formulation. *J Pharm Sci* 2007, **96**:1–26.
8. Daugherty AL, Mrsny RJ: Formulation and delivery issues for monoclonal antibody therapeutics. *Adv Drug Deliv Rev* 2006, **58**:686–706.
9. Schule S, Schulz-Fademrecht T, Garidel P, Bechtold-Peters K, Frieb W: Stabilization of IgG1 in spray-dried powders for inhalation. *Eur J Pharm Biopharm* 2008, **69**:793–807.
10. Chang LL, Pikal MJ: Mechanisms of protein stabilization in the solid state. *J Pharm Sci* 2009, **98**:2886–2908.
11. Maury M, Murphy K, Kumar S, Mauerer A, Lee G: Spray-drying of proteins: effects of sorbitol and trehalose on aggregation and FT-IR amide I spectrum of an immunoglobulin G. *Eur J Pharm Biopharm* 2005, **59**:251–261.
12. Ramezani V, Vatanara A, Rouholamini Najafabadi A, Gilani K, Nabi-Meybodi M: Screening and evaluation of variables in the formation of antibody particles by spray drying. *Powder Technol* 2013, **233**:341–346.
13. Costantino HR, Andya JD, Nguyen PA, Dasovich N, Sweeney TD, Shire SJ, Hsu CC, Maa YF: Effect of mannitol crystallization on the stability and aerosol performance of a spray-dried pharmaceutical protein,

recombinant humanized anti-IgE monoclonal antibody. *J Pharm Sci* 1998, **87**:1406–1411.

14. Hortobagyi GN: **Trastuzumab in the treatment of breast cancer.** *N Engl J Med* 2005, **353**:1734–1736.

15. Montemurro F, Valabrega G, Aglietta M: **Trastuzumab-based combination therapy for breast cancer.** *Expert Opin Pharmacother* 2004, **5**:81–96.

16. Amphlett G, Cacia J, Callahan W, Cannova-Davis E, Chang B, Cleland JL, Darrington T, DeYoung L, Dhingra B, Everett R, Foster L, Frenz J, Garcia A, Giltinan D, Gitlin G, Gombotz W, Hageman M, Harris R, Heller D, Herman A, Hershenson S, Hora M, Ingram R, Janes S, Watanabe C: **A compendium and hydropathy/flexibility analysis of common reactive sites in proteins: reactivity at Asn, Asp, Gln, and Met motifs in neutral pH solution.** *Pharm Biotechnol* 1996, **9**:1–140.

17. Prestrelski SJ, Tedeschi N, Arakawa T, Carpenter JF: **Dehydration-induced conformational transitions in proteins and their inhibition by stabilizers.** *Biophys J* 1993, **65**:661–671.

18. Prestrelski SJ, Arakawa T, Carpenter JF: **Separation of freezing-and drying-induced denaturation of lyophilized proteins using stress-specific stabilization. II. Structural studies using infrared spectroscopy.** *Arch Biochem Biophys* 1993, **303**:465–473.

19. Kiss T, Fenyvesi F, Kovacsne BI, Feher P, Leposane KR, Varadi J, Szente L, Fenyvesi E, Ivanyi R, Vecsernyes M: **Cytotoxic examinations of various cyclodextrin derivatives on Caco-2 cells.** *Acta Pharm Hung* 2007, **77**:150–154.

20. Kiss T, Fenyvesi F, Bacskay I, Varadi J, Fenyvesi E, Ivanyi R, Szente L, Tosaki A, Vecsernyes M: **Evaluation of the cytotoxicity of beta-cyclodextrin derivatives: evidence for the role of cholesterol extraction.** *Eur J Pharm Sci* 2010, **40**:376–380.

Identifying and prioritizing industry-level competitiveness factors: evidence from pharmaceutical market

Hosein Shabaninejad[1], Gholamhossein Mehralian[2], Arash Rashidian[3], Ahmad Baratimarnani[1*] and Hamid Reza Rasekh[2]

Abstract

Background: Pharmaceutical industry is knowledge-intensive and highly globalized, in both developed and developing countries. On the other hand, if companies want to survive, they should be able to compete well in both domestic and international markets. The main purpose of this paper is therefore to develop and prioritize key factors affecting companies' competitiveness in pharmaceutical industry. Based on an extensive literature review, a valid and reliable questionnaire was designed, which was later filled up by participants from the industry. To prioritize the key factors, we used the Technique for Order Preference by Similarity to Ideal Solution (TOPSIS).

Results: The results revealed that human capital and macro-level policies were two key factors placed at the highest rank in respect of their effects on the competitiveness considering the industry-level in pharmaceutical area.

Conclusion: This study provides fundamental evidence for policymakers and managers in pharma context to enable them formulating better polices to be proactively competitive and responsive to the markets' needs.

Keywords: Competitiveness, Pharmaceutical industry, Key factors, Human capital, Iran

Background

Pharmaceutical industry has changed tremendously in recent years [1]. The importance of big changes in pharmaceutical industry should be considered due to intensity in Research and Development (R&D) activities [2,3], uncertainty in drug development process, lack of new products [4], rapid integration [5], rapid development of generic markets [6] and finally increased global competition and technological advances [7]. Moreover, some unique characteristics such as high-regulated setting, the long development process, risky and high level of cost in research phase [8] distinguish the pharmaceutical industry from other industries.

While competition is increasing tremendously, there is an immediate need for the pharmaceutical companies to behave in a good, sharp and speedy manner. With respect to new competitive environment, it is more important to consider the factors affecting competitiveness of pharmaceutical industries in the internationalized and globalized market [9]. This study tries to identify and prioritize key factors that affecting pharmaceutical competitiveness at the industry level, based on pharmaceutical managers' perspective. The rest of the paper proceeds as follows. The first section presents an overview of pharmaceutical industry in the world and Iran. The next section describes the research methodology, followed by the result of the study. The final section presents discussion and concludes by considering the practical implications and limitations of the study.

Global pharmaceutical industry

Throughout the last decades, the global pharmaceutical industry has been one of the most successful and profitable industries [10], but, as mentioned, due to dynamic forces in the competitive as well as regulatory environment, the conditions of the industry have changed.

* Correspondence: abaratim@gmail.com
[1]Department of Health Services Management, School of Health Management and Information Sciences, Iran University of Medical Sciences, Rashidiasemi st, Valiasr st, Vanak sq., P.O.Box: 1995614111, Tehran, Iran
Full list of author information is available at the end of the article

Given to the strong dependency on innovation, some issues such as the high risks in R&D as well as supply chain [11], cause to decrease the attractiveness of pharmaceutical industry [12] compare to other industries.

While expenditure on R&D has increased steadily over the last decade, the number of New Molecular Entities (NMEs) being brought to the market has decreased. It is important since further development depends on the number of new medicines launched from which the profit serves to fund [12], however drug development new medicine and marketing is a costly, time consuming and risky process. Based on studies, an average cost of approximately $800 million is the cost of bringing a new drug to the market [13,14]. Moreover, it is estimated that an average of 12 years would have been passed from the synthesis of the new active pharmaceutical materials to launch a new drug to the market [15]. Thereby, on average, out of every 10,000 ingredients synthesized in the laboratories, only one or two will successfully pass all the steps to become marketable medicines [16]. Meanwhile, international competitiveness is becoming important for the pharmaceutical sector more. Increased competitiveness and the changing structure of competitors impact the strategic direction of the world pharmaceutical companies in world [9]. On the other hand, companies try to increase the profitability of all phases of the value chain from primary discovery research to production phase and logistics as well as sales and marketing phases [17].

Though, managing pharmaceutical industry effectively and efficiently is vital in developing countries for their health system and economy [18], according to the lack of economic motivations and low capacity of the government for covering the costs of innovative drugs in emerging markets, usually the pharmaceutical sector doesn't invest on novel medicines, thereby innovations are limited in such countries.

Iranian pharmaceutical market

Iran pharmaceutical industry experienced the average growth rate of 28.38% over the last 10 years. The value of medicine which locally manufactured is $1.639 billion, while imported products comprise $0.828 billion during the same period [19]. Moreover Iran's pharmaceutical industry has witnessed profound changes in recent years; the producers were working in an atmosphere of ever-increasing demand, and due to lack of competition, no motives remained for marketing, sales and quality improvement of drugs [20]. Recently, the market has become more competitive as a result of foreign medicines importation; as such in 2000, there were only 53 pharmaceutical manufacturing and 12 companies importing to Iran, these figures were increased to 89 and 93, respectively [19].

Methods
Reliability and validity of the questionnaire
To assess the managers' perspective about the status of key factors on competitiveness of pharmaceutical industry, a questionnaire was designed based on an extensive literature review as well as interviews with pharmaceutical experts. Reliability and validity tests were conducted on the questionnaire with multivariate measures. The validity of a tool refers to the extent which it measures what is intended to be measured [21]. To assess the acceptance of the questionnaire, 10 people involved for at least 10 years in the field of pharmaceutical practice were invited to participate in a pilot test. The participants proposed revising parts of the questionnaire. At the end, all participants expressed high agreement with the appropriateness of the questionnaire. The questionnaire finalized after modifying some questions accordingly. Cronbach's alpha reliability was applied to measure the internal consistency of these multivariate scales [21]. The results showed that the Cronbach's alpha for all dimensions was as 0.89, which indicates strong reliability for our survey instrument.

Data collection
Data for this study have been collected using questionnaires distributed to 25 pharmaceutical firms, which were affiliated to three large pharmaceutical holding companies. To gather the viewpoints of the pharmaceutical industry's executives, the questionnaires were sent to managers in marketing, sales, information technology (IT), finance, R&D, quality assurance and quality control departments. As Table 1 shows, most of participants have more than 10 years of job experience in the pharmaceutical industry (80 percent), and a quarter of the participants were top managers. Although, probability sampling

Table 1 Sample characteristics

Construct	Classification	Number	Percentage
Position	Managerial	41	24.3
	Financing	8	4.7
	Production	32	18.9
	R&D	28	16.6
	Marketing	29	17.2
	Human resource	2	1.2
	Regulatory	9	5.3
	QC	20	11.8
Job experience	Under 3 years	11	6.6
	4-9 years	22	13
	10-15 years	68	40.2
	Up 10 years	68	40.2

R&D: Research and Development **QC:** Quality control.

is preferred over non-probability sampling [22], in some cases it is not feasible, practical or theoretically sensible to consider the probability of sampling. Accordingly, we chose the respondents from managers with comprehensive knowledge about pharmaceutical industry, strategy, international pharmaceutical markets, and general pharmaceutical management issues. The number of questionnaires sent out was 240; the number of returned ones was 169 resulting in a response rate of 70 percent. Three percent of the returned questionnaires were incomplete. Non response bias was checked by comparing for all constructs by ANOVA and produced no significant differences. This study was approved by Iran University of Medical Sciences ethics committee. Participants in this study were informed that; participating in this study is voluntary, they are free not to answer some questions they don't like to answer and their biography will be treated as confidential and will not be published. Moreover participants in this study provided informed consent for publication of this work.

The pharmaceutical industry competitiveness factors prioritization questionnaire is included as Additional file 1.

Factor analysis

Factor analysis is a procedure that relies on the use of correlations between data variables [23]. In this study, each factor was individually tested for construct validity. The confirmatory factor analysis (i.e. Pearson's principal component analysis) was tested with and without rotation (i.e. Varimax rotation with Kaiser Normalization). The conservative factor loadings of greater than 0.5 were considered at 95% level of confidence [24].

Data analysis with Fuzzy TOPSIS

We used Fuzzy TOPSIS for analyzing the data. TOPSIS technique of solving the multi-criteria decision chooses tasks that imply full and complete information on criteria, expressed in numerical type [25]. The method is helpful for solving real problems of managerial decisions. It provides us the optimal solution or the alternative's ranking. The TOPSIS technique would explore among the assumed choices and come upon the one closest to the ideal solution but furthest from the anti-ideal point simultaneously [26]. Justification of the method intends to adjust a different mode of finding out the ideal and anti-ideal solution through standardization of lingual features' quantifying and introducing of fuzzy numbers in description of the features for the criteria expressed by linguistic variables [27].

Results

Considering extensive literature review, we found 150 factors affecting the competitiveness. Based upon the

experts' opinions, 44 variables were finalized as factors with impact on competitiveness of pharmaceutical industry and citations for each factor are shown in Table 2. As noted, some items (variables 37 and 38) were developed from experts' opinions.

Based on factor analysis, 10 items were identified as key factors affecting pharmaceutical industry's competitiveness, and we renamed them: human capital, macro-level policies, strategy and operational effectiveness, supporting and related industries and clusters, administrative infrastructure, capacity for innovation, organizational practices, capital market infrastructure, internationalization of firms and context for strategy and rivalry. The variance explained by these factors was as 81.94 percent, and the Cronbach alpha for each construct was larger than 0.7, which indicates an acceptable degree of consistency for constructs determined in this study as the key factors affecting pharmaceutical industry's competitiveness. The results of factor analysis and reliability of factors are shown in Table 3.

Prioritization of key factors affecting competitiveness of pharmaceutical industry with Fuzzy TOPSIS technique is shown in Table 4.

Fuzzy TOPSIS's results show the human capital ranking as the first key factor affecting the competitiveness of pharmaceutical industry followed by macro-level policies and state remaining factors, respectively. Context for strategy and rivalry was ranked as the last key factor.

Discussion

Given to complexity of the pharmaceutical industry in relation with the research, regulatory and healthcare systems, here, a set of key factors including macro-level policies, strategy and operational effectiveness, supporting and related industries and clusters, administrative infrastructure, capacity for innovation, organizational practices, capital market infrastructure, internationalization of firms, context for strategy and rivalry and above all human capital were identified. These factors provide a fairly consistent and coherent explanation about the structure of competitiveness and its determinants in pharmaceutical industry.

The results of this study show human capital with the highest rank affecting the pharmaceutical competitiveness. However, the context of study is in Iran, as a typical of middle-income country, the importance of human capital on productivity and its direct impact on competitiveness were shown by studies [29,35]. On the other hand, pharmaceutical industry as a science-driven and high-tech industry [12], depend highly on skilled human resources [3]. Regarding to the importance of R&D on success of pharmaceutical companies [3,57], as a long-term and risky procedure [4,13,14], they highly rely on good quality of science graduates. Thus, it is important

Table 2 Pharmaceutical competitiveness variables and related citations

Variables	Citations
1- Graduates with degrees in sciences relevant to pharmaceutical industry	
2- Pharmaceutical expertise employment	[28-30]
3- Pharmaceutical managers' experience in internal and international related area	
4- Scientific research publication relevant to pharmaceutical area	
5- Clinical studies	
6- Investment in pharmaceutical high-tech	
7- GMP structure improving investment in pharmaceutical industry	[31-36]
8- Investment in pharmaceutical research & development	
9- Production process sophistication in pharmaceutical area	
10- Using information technology in pharmaceutical industry	
11- Attract capital from market in pharmaceutical industry	
12- Venture capital in pharmaceutical area	[30,31,37]
13- Foreign direct investment in pharmaceutical industry	
14- Pharmaceutical's market approval procedures	
15- Pharmaceutical regulation	
16- Pharmaceutical standards implementation like GMP	
17- Generic system development	[31,38-44]
18- Price regulation in pharmaceutical market	
19- Pharmaceutical intellectual property right	
20- Pharmaceutical corporation tax	
21- Intensity of domestic competition in pharmaceutical market	
22- Mergers and acquisition in pharmaceutical area	[31,37,45-47]
23- Pharmaceutical import tariff	
24- Existence of major pharmaceutical MNCs branches in domestic market	
25- Privatization in pharmaceutical industry	
26- Availability of latest technologies in pharmaceutical industry	
27- Availability of specialized research and training services in pharmaceutical area	[37,48-50]
28- Quantity and quality of local supplier in pharmaceutical market	
29- Extent of cluster policy and collaboration inside clusters in pharmaceutical industry	
30- Extent of marketing in pharmaceutical market	
31- Quality of drugs	
32- NMEs production in pharmaceutical industry	[7,51-54]
33- Diversification of production in pharmaceutical market	
34- Value chain breadth in pharmaceutical industry	
35- Degree of customer orientation of pharmaceutical market	
36- Extent of staff training in pharmaceutical industry	
37- Relationship-based recruitment in pharmaceutical area	[37], (Items 37 and 38 extract from expert opinions)
38- Frequent changes in pharmaceutical industry at the management level	
39- Pharmaceutical companies' joint venture with MNCs	
40- Pharmaceutical companies' alliance with MNCs	[30,37]
41- Breadth of pharmaceutical international market	
42- Macro policy (export incentives, simplifying customs regulations)	
43- Country's political situation	[55,56]
44- Relations with the countries of the region and the world	

GMP: Good Manufacturing Practice MNCs: Multi- national companies NMEs: New molecular entities.

Table 3 Factor analysis and reliability of factors

Key factors	KMO value	Factor loading	Percentage variance Explained	Cronbach's alpha
Human capital	0.57	0.78 - 0.94	0.74	0.92
Capacity for innovation	0.61	0.46 - 0.73	0.54	0.86
Capital market infrastructure	0.48	0.40 - 0.86	0.73	0.79
Administrative infrastructure	0.70	0.12 - 0.78	0.67	0.84
Context for strategy and rivalry	0.48	0.11 - 0.87	0.53	0.78
Supporting and related industries and clusters	0.61	0.46 - 0.81	0.68	0.81
Strategy and operational effectiveness	0.57	0.35 - 0.82	0.59	0.84
Organizational practices	0.54	0.46 - 0.77	0.73	0.85
Internationalization of firms	0.57	0.56 - 0.90	0.76	0.88
Macro-level policies	0.53	0.48 - 0.92	0.63	0.89

to pay more attention on R&D activities in pharmaceutical sector.

The formation of pharmaceutical industry in Iran was along with the government entry in this industry and the selected structure for the industry was based on government support [19]. Thus, pharmaceutical companies' strategies, administrative infrastructure, technologies, market size, human capital and productivity of pharmaceutical companies were affected by this structure. If Iran pharmaceutical industry wants to enter to international market, this structure should be redesigned and the factors determined in this study could be used as a baseline for defining new strategies and policies for making a competitive pharmaceutical industry.

Factors identified in this study were in turn with porter's competitiveness framework [55]. However, in this study, the demand side of the competitiveness was not identified as a key factor affecting pharmaceutical industry's competitiveness. In pharmaceutical industry, the demand side consists of three groups including patients, physicians and hospital boards. The ultimate consumer – the patient – usually does not have much effect on a physician's decision about a certain prescriptive drug, since their knowledge about the respective drug is limited [12]. Moreover, due to payment of drugs cost by health insurance companies, patient normally does not carry the costs of the product. This implies that patients don't have a key role in the demand side of pharmaceutical market.

Like other studies, innovation was identified as a key factor affecting competitiveness [14,32,34]. Considering the nature of pharmaceutical industry, producing new drugs needs high investment and using state of the art technologies, as such, if developing countries want to be competitive in pharmaceutical industry, other factors have more importance than innovation. Moreover, according to the definition of innovation in the literature [58], the results indicate that pharma companies in middle-income countries should rely on incremental innovation more than on the radical one.

Managerial relevance

This study has some managerial applications. First, competitiveness factors constructed in this study will be the starting points for future studies at the industry level in

Table 4 Rank of fuzzy TOPSIS for competitiveness key factors

Pharmaceutical industry's competitiveness key factors	Important level	Distance from positive ideal	Distance from negative ideal	Key factors' rank
Human capital	0.67	0.56	1.15	1
Macro-level policies	0.65	0.61	1.13	2
Strategy and operational effectiveness	0.56	0.73	0.91	3
Supporting and related industries and clusters	0.54	0.76	0.91	4
Administrative infrastructure	0.54	0.74	0.87	5
Capacity for innovation	0.54	0.74	0.87	6
Organizational practices	0.49	0.86	0.82	7
Capital market infrastructure	0.48	0.89	0.82	8
Internationalization of firms	0.42	0.95	0.70	9
Context for strategy and rivalry	0.27	1.17	0.43	10

competitiveness area. Moreover, the valid and reliable tool designed in this study can be used by other researchers to assess industry-level competitiveness in middle-income countries. Since, this study was done in Iran, the generalizability of the results of this study should be considered cautiously to other contexts.

Second, based on key factors identified, the results of this study will help the managers adopting decisions to enhance the competitiveness of the firms. Finally, competitiveness factors identified in this study will be helpful to managers considering them in their decisions and strategic planning at business level.

Limitation of the study

As a first limitation, although we try to identify all related key factors affecting pharmaceutical industry's competitiveness, but the result of the study should be delivered in other contexts with some modifications. On the other hand, while operationalizing of most competitiveness measures are difficult [59], the key factors proposed in this study should be a basis to determine a set of constructs, which are reasonably approximate to other context. Moreover, although our sample is representative for Iranian managers who involved in pharmaceutical companies, a larger sample could help to improve the generalizability of results.

Conclusions

Understanding competitiveness in pharmaceutical industry is a major concern of policymakers and a major challenge to provide evidences for decision making. This study provides fundamental evidence for policymakers in pharma context to enable them formulating better polices to be proactively competitive and responsive to the markets' needs. Moreover, this work provides a tool for governments and national agencies to assess competitiveness in pharmaceutical industry and to develop measures which can be appropriate for their context. Furthermore, it enables us to compare competitiveness status of similar countries according to their strengths and weaknesses.

Additional file

Additional file 1: Pharmaceutical industry competitiveness factors prioritization questionnaire.

Competing interests
The authors declare that they have no competing interests.

Authors' contributions
HRR carried out designing and conceptual modeling of the study. AR helped in designing methodology of the study. GM performed the statistical analysis. HS developed the idea of the study and participated in designing the methodology, data gathering, data analysis and drafting the manuscript. AB helped to draft and edits the manuscript. All authors read and approved the final manuscript.

Acknowledgments
This study was part of a PhD thesis supported by School of Health Management, Iran University of Medical Sciences. Grant no: IUMS/shmis-91/ 38.

Author details
[1]Department of Health Services Management, School of Health Management and Information Sciences, Iran University of Medical Sciences, Rashidiasemi st, Valiasr st, Vanak sq., P.O.Box: 1995614111, Tehran, Iran. [2]Department of Pharmacoeconomics and Pharma Management, School of Pharmacy, Shahid Beheshti University of Medical Sciences, Tehran, Iran. [3]Department of Health Management and Economics, School of Public Health & Knowledge Utilization Research Center, Tehran University of Medical Sciences, Tehran, Iran.

References
1. Munos B: Lessons from 60 years of pharmaceutical innovation. Nat Rev Drug Discov 2009, 8:959–968.
2. Hsieh PH, Mishra CS, Gobeli DH: The return on R&D versus capital expenditures in pharmaceutical and chemical industries. IEEE Trans Eng Manag 2003, 50:141–150.
3. Rasekh HR, Mehralian GH, Vatankhah-Mohammadabadi AA: Situation analysis of R&D activities: an empirical study in iranian pharmaceutical companies. Iran J Pharm Res 2012, 11:1013–1025.
4. Engelhardt HT, Garrett JR: Innovation And The Pharmaceutical Industry: Critical Reflections On The Virtues Of Profit. United States: M & M Scrivener Press; 2008.
5. Schweizer L: Organizational integration of acquired biotechnology companies into pharmaceutical companies: the need for a hybrid approach. Acad Manage J 2005, 48:1051–1074.
6. Karhu A, Yla-Kojola AM: Internationalisation of pharmaceutical retail sector: growth opportunities in emerging markets. Int J Bus Excel 2010, 3:363–382.
7. McAdam R, Barron N: The role of quality management in pharmaceutical development: clinical trials analysis. Int J Health Care Qual Assur 2002, 15:106–123.
8. Cardinal LB: Technological innovation in the pharmaceutical industry: the use of organizational control in managing research and development. Organ Sci 2001, 12:19–36.
9. Kesič D: Strategic analysis of the world pharmaceutical industry. Management 2009, 14:59–76.
10. Kola I, Landis J: Can the pharmaceutical industry reduce attrition rates? Nat Rev Drug Discov 2004, 3:711–726.
11. Jaberidoost M, Nikfar S, Abdollahiasl A, Dinarvand R: Pharmaceutical supply chain risks: a systematic review. Daru 2013, 21:69.
12. Gassmann O, Reepmeyer G, Von Zedtwitz M: Leading Pharmaceutical Innovation: Trends And Drivers For Growth In The Pharmaceutical Industry. Germany: Springer; 2008.
13. DiMasi JA: The value of improving the productivity of the drug development process. Pharmacoeconomics 2002, 20:1–10.
14. DiMasi JA, Hansen RW, Grabowski HG: The price of innovation: new estimates of drug development costs. J Health Econ 2003, 22:151–185.
15. Matías-Reche F, García-Morales VJ, Martín-Tapia I: Staffing services quality and innovativeness in pharmaceutical companies. Int J Sel Assess 2010, 18:342–350.
16. Festel G, Schicker A, Boutellier R: Practitioner's section: performance improvement in pharmaceutical R&D through new outsourcing models. J Bus Chem 2010, 7:89–96.
17. Zarenzhad F, Mehralian GH, Rajabzadeh A: Developing a model for an agile supply in pharmaceutical industry. Int J Pharm Healthc Mark 2014. In press.
18. Narayana SA, Pati RK, Vrat P: Research on management issues in the pharmaceutical industry: a literature review. Int J Pharm Healthc Mktg 2012, 6:351–375.
19. Kebriaeezadeh A, Koopaei NN, Abdollahiasl A, Nikfar S, Mohamadi N: Trend analysis of the pharmaceutical market in Iran; 1997-2010; policy implications for developing countries. Daru 2013, 21:52.

20. Davari M, Walley T, Haycox A: **Pharmaceutical policy and market in iran: past experiences and future challenges.** *J Pharm Health Serv Res* 2011, **2:**47–52.
21. Kaplan RM: *Basic Statistics For The Behavioral Sciences.* Massachusetts: Allyn and Bacon Newton; 1987.
22. Saunders M, Lewis P, Thornhill A: *Research Methods for Business Students.* India: Pearson Education; 2009.
23. Hurley AE, Scandura TA, Schriesheim CA, Brannick MT, Seers A, Vandenberg RJ, Williams LJ: **Exploratory and confirmatory factor analysis: guidelines, issues, and alternatives.** *J Organ Behav* 1997, **18:**667–683.
24. Hair J: *Multivariate Data Analysis with Reading.* Prentice Hall; 1995.
25. Lai YJ, Liu TY, Hwang CL: **Topsis for MODM.** *Eur J Oper Res* 1994, **76:**486–500.
26. Braglia M, Frosolini M, Montanari R: **Fuzzy TOPSIS approach for failure mode, effects and criticality analysis.** *Qual Reliab Eng Int* 2003, **19:**425–443.
27. Wang YM, Elhag T: **Fuzzy TOPSIS method based on alpha level sets with an application to bridge risk assessment.** *Expert Syst Appl* 2006, **31:**309–319.
28. Department of Health and Association of the British Pharmaceutical Industry, Pharmaceutical Industry Competitiveness Task Force: *Competitiveness And Performance Indicators 2005.* London: Department of Health and Association of the British Pharmaceutical Industry; 2005.
29. Kleynhans E: **The role of human capital in the competitive platform of South African industries.** *J Hum Resource Manag* 2006, **4:**55–62.
30. Mehralian GH, Rasekh HR, Akhavan P, Ghatari AR: **Prioritization of intellectual capital indicators in knowledge-based industries: evidence from pharmaceutical industry.** *Int J Inform Manag* 2013, **33:**209–216.
31. Pammolli F, Gambardella A, Orsenigo L: **Global Competitiveness In Pharmaceuticals: A European Perspective.** In *Office for Official Publications of the European Communities.* Belgium; 2001.
32. Agrawal M, Calantone R, Nason RW: **Competitiveness in the global pharmaceutical industry: the role of innovation.** *J Res Pharm Econ* 1998, **9:**5–32.
33. Da Silva JF, Pinho AFDA: **Study On The Competitiveness Of The Brazilian Pharmaceutical Industry Based On Porter's Typology.** In *Management of Engineering and Technology, 2001. PICMET'01. Portland International Conference on.* IEEE; 2001:693–703.
34. Guan JC, Yam RCM, Mok CK, Ma N: **A study of the relationship between competitiveness and technological innovation capability based on DEA models.** *Eur J Oper Res* 2006, **170:**971–986.
35. Kagochi J, Jolly C: **R&D investments, human capital, and the competitiveness of selected US agricultural export commodities.** *Eur J Oper Re* 2010, **7:**58–77.
36. Department of Health and Association of the British Pharmaceutical Industry: *Competitiveness and Performance Indicators 2009.* London: Industry Strategy Group Pharmaceutical Industry; 2009.
37. Sala-i-Martin X, Schwab K, López-Claros A: *The Global Competitiveness Report 2011-2012.* Geneva: World Economic Forum; 2011.
38. ECORYS Research and Consulting for the European Commission: *Competitiveness Of The Eu Market And Industry For Pharmaceuticals; Welfare Implications Of Regulation.* Rotterdam: ECORYS Macro & Sector Policies; 2011.
39. Garattini L, Tediosi F: **A comparative analysis of generics markets in five European countries.** *Health Policy* 2000, **51:**149–162.
40. Hollis A: **The importance of being first: evidence from canadian generic pharmaceuticals.** *Health Econ* 2002, **11:**723–734.
41. Rai RK: **Battling with TRIPS: emerging firm strategies of indian pharmaceutical industry post-TRIPS.** *J Intellect Property Rights* 2008, **13:**301–317.
42. Ravinder J: **Prices of new pharmaceuticals in india: a cross section study.** *Econ Polit Wkly* 2010, **45:**71–78.
43. Roerner-Mahler A: **Business conflict and global politics: the pharmaceutical industry and the global protection of intellectual property rights.** *Rev Int Polit Econ* 2013, **20:**121–152.
44. Wang YR: **Price competition in the chinese pharmaceutical market.** *Int J Health Care Finance Econ* 2006, **6:**119–129.
45. Demirbag M, Ng CK, Tatoglu E: **Performance of mergers and acquisitions in the pharmaceutical industry: a comparative perspective.** *Multinatl Bus Rev* 2007, **15:**41–62.
46. Godfrey N: **Why is competition important for growth and poverty reduction?** *OECD Global Forum on International Investment, Conference Document* 2008.
47. Siggel E: **International competitiveness and comparative advantage: a survey and a proposal for measurement.** *J Ind Compet Trade* 2006, **6:**137–159.
48. Boasson V, Boasson E, MacPherson A, Shin HH: **Firm value and geographic competitive advantage: evidence from the US pharmaceutical industry.** *J Bus* 2005, **78:**2465–2495.
49. Cooke P: **How benchmarking can lever cluster competitiveness.** *Int J Technol Manag* 2007, **38:**292–320.
50. Ketels CH: **Michael Porter's competitiveness framework—recent learnings and new research priorities.** *J Ind Compet Trade* 2006, **6:**115–136.
51. Glass HE, Poli LG: **"Pressure points" on pharmaceutical industry executives: what lies ahead?** *Int J Pharm Healthc Mktg* 2009, **3:**74–783.
52. Artaud L, Long D: **Quality indicators as a management tool in pharmaceutical R and D.** *Drug Inf J* 1994, **28:**1047–1053.
53. Rod M, Ashill NJ, Carruthers J: **Pharmaceutical marketing return-on-investment: a European perspective.** *Int J Pharm Healthc Mktg* 2007, **1:**174–189.
54. Tiggemann RF, Sabel H: **An innovative concept in pharmaceutical drug development.** *Drug Inf J* 1997, **31:**119–124.
55. Porter M: *The Competitive Advantage of Nations.* London: Free Press; 1990.
56. Zhou Y, Mi J, Yu N, Wang C: **Analysis of government policies in the pharmaceutical industry.** *Inf Technol J* 2012, **11:**1272–1278.
57. Demirel P, Mazzucato M: **Innovation and firm growth: is R&D worth it?** *Industry and Innovation* 2012, **19:**45–62.
58. Youndt MA, Snell SA: **Human resource configurations, intellectual capital, and organizational performance.** *J Manag Issues* 2004, **16:**337–360.
59. Depperu D, Cerrato D: **Analyzing International Competitiveness At The Firm Level: Concepts And Measures.** In *Quaderni del Dipartimento di Scienze Economiche e Sociali, Università Cattolica del Sacro Cuore, Piacenza;* 2005.

Selenium nanoparticle-enriched *Lactobacillus brevis* causes more efficient immune responses in vivo and reduces the liver metastasis in metastatic form of mouse breast cancer

Mohammad Hossein Yazdi[1], Mehdi Mahdavi[2], Neda Setayesh[1], Mohammad Esfandyar[1] and Ahmad Reza Shahverdi[1*]

Abstract

Background and the purpose of the study: Selenium enriched *Lactobacillus* has been reported as an immunostimulatory agent which can be used to increase the life span of cancer bearing animals. Lactic acid bacteria can reduce selenium ions to elemental selenium nanoparticles (SeNPs) and deposit them in intracellular spaces. In this strategy two known immunostimulators, lactic acid bacteria (LAB) and SeNPs, are concomitantly administered for enhancing of immune responses in cancer bearing mice.

Methods: Forty five female inbred BALB/c mice were divided into three groups of tests and control, each containing 15 mice. Test mice were orally administered with SeNP-enriched *Lactobacillus brevis* or *Lactobacillus brevis* alone for 3 weeks before tumor induction. After that the administration was followed in three cycles of seven days on/three days off. Control group received phosphate buffer saline (PBS) at same condition. During the study the tumor growth was monitored using caliper method. At the end of study the spleen cell culture was carried out for both NK cytotoxicity assay and cytokines measurement. Delayed type hypersensitivity (DTH) responses were also assayed after 72h of tumor antigen recall. Serum lactate dehydrogenase (LDH) and alkaline phosphatase (ALP) levels were measured, the livers of mice were removed and prepared for histopathological analysis.

Results: High level of IFN-γ and IL-17 besides the significant raised in NK cytotoxicity and DTH responses were observed in SeNP-enriched *L. brevis* administered mice and the extended life span and decrease in the tumor metastasis to liver were also recorded in this group compared to the control mice or *L.brevis* alone administered mice.

Conclusion: Our results suggested that the better prognosis could be achieved by oral administration of SeNP-enriched *L. brevis* in highly metastatic breast cancer mice model.

Keywords: Selenium enriched *L. brevis*, Immune responses, 4T1 breast cancer, Liver metastasis

* Correspondence: Shahverd@sina.tums.ac.ir
[1]Department of Pharmaceutical Biotechnology, Faculty of Pharmacy and Biotechnology Research Center, Tehran University of Medical Sciences, Tehran, Iran
Full list of author information is available at the end of the article

Introduction

Using the immunomodulatory agents in the field of cancer treatment has a growing trend during last decades [1,2]. This strategy is also known as adjuvant therapy and some studies have demonstrated the advantages of this strategy for cancer treatment [3]. Immunomodulatory agents are divided in two groups of immunosupressors and immunostimulators. Chemical immunomodulators like levamizole have been used in order to stimulate immune response against cancer and AIDS [4]. Natural immunomodulators like glucan or other oligosaccharide components which are mostly derived from microbial source are being applied to stimulate the immune response against cancers [5].

Lactic acid bacteria (LAB) are Gram positive normal flora which shows variety of beneficial effects on their host's health including the prevention of tumor growth [6]. Many studies which include the effects of orally administered lactobacilli and bifidobacteria on the immune system have been performed in animal models (e.g., tumor, infection, and allergy models) [7,8]. An increase in natural killer (NK) cell activity was observed in mice which were administered orally with some strains of LAB [9]. The activation of the systemic and secretary immune response by LAB requires many complex interactions among the different constituents of the intestinal ecosystem (microflora, epithelial cells and immune cells). It also seems that some of these immunological effects may be related to the cell components of LAB bacteria [10]. As many studies have demonstrated it is notably interesting that immune system can be optimized through oral supplementation of specific Lactobacillus strains [11,12]. Depending on their intuitive properties, orally applied lactobacilli have been reported to affect T-helper 1 and T-helper 2 pathways by local cytokine production in the gut and systemic specific antibody formation [13,14].

On the other hand selenium (Se), as an essential micronutrient element which exhibit anticarcinogenic effects, can prevent the transformation of normal cells to malignant cells and the activation of oncogenes in transformed cells [15,16]. Consumption of Se affects the development and expression of nonspecific, humoral, and cell-mediated immune responses and deficiency in Se appears to result in immunosuppression, whereas supplementation with low doses of Se appears to result in augmentation or restoration of immunologic functions [17]. SeNP-enriched Lactobacillus can be considered as a new form of Se organic products. Recently we reported the effect of SeNP-enriched Lactobacillus plantarum on the immune response and lifespan of 4T1 breast cancer bearing mice and show this can increase host immune response (i.e. NK cell cytotoxicity) and enhanced the survival rate of animals for 130 days [18].

To obtain a better survival rate, in the current study we isolated and characterized another immunostimulant lactic acid bacterium (Lactobacillus brevis) and used for intracellular reduction of Se ions. These SeNP-enriched probiotic has been administered in mice bearing 4T1 breast cancer tumor and the effect of this administration on the survival of cancerous animals, immune responses and liver metastasis was compared to L. brevis alone.

Materials and methods

Animals

Forty five female inbred BALB/c mice with six to eight weeks old and each weighing from 25 to 30 g, were purchased from the Pasture Institute of Iran (Tehran, Iran). They were divided into three groups of test and control, each containing 15 mice. The mice were kept in plastic cages, allowed free access to water, and maintained on a 12:12 h light and dark cycle during the study period. The temperature and humidity were controlled at 23 ± 1°C and 55 ± 10%, respectively, and all mice were fed via a standard mouse pellet diet. The control mice in this study were kept separated from the test group, but at the same temperature and humidity, and they were fed the same food.

Lactobacillus isolation and characterization

The Lactobacillus bacterium was isolated from human feces and characterized by 16s rDNA sequence analysis [19]. Genomic DNA was extracted from bacterial cells using PrimePrep Genomic DNA isolation kit according to the manufacturer's instructions. It was then subjected to PCR amplification using universal primers 27F (5′ GA GTTTGATCCTGGCTCAG-3′) and 1492R (5′-GGTTA CCTTGTTACGACTT-3′) targeting the conserved regions of bacterial 16S ribosomal RNA gene. The amplification program consisted of one cycle of 94°C for 3 min; 30 cycles of 94°C for 20 s, 55 for 30 s, and 72°C for 2 min; and finally one cycle of 72°C for 5 min. The amplified DNA fragment was purified from 1% agarose gel using the QIAquick Gel Extraction Kit (Qiagen, USA) according to the supplier's instructions and was sent for automated sequencing using the above primers (GenFanAvaran Co., Iran). Sequence similarity searches were done with the BLAST database (National Center for Biotechnology Information), and the sequence was submitted to GenBank.

Preparation of SeNP-enriched and non-enriched probiotics

The isolated LAB bacterium which was identified as Lactobacillus brevis was inoculated into 10 ml of DeMan–Rogosa–Sharpe (MRS) broth (Merck, Germany) and cultivated overnight at 37°C under anaerobic conditions. One mL of a stock solution of SeO_2 (254 mM) was then added to 100 ml of Lactobacillus broth culture to reach a final concentration of 200 mg/L Se ions (corresponding to a 2.54 mM solution of SeO_2), and incubation at 37°C was continued for 72h. During this time, the Se ions were reduced to form intracellular red elemental selenium. The bacteria were then collected by centrifugation at $4000 \times g$ for 30 min at 4°C, washed three times with sterile phosphate buffer saline (PBS), and used for the animal study.

Animal study

The SeNP-enriched *L. brevis* alone was separately re-suspended in PBS solutions to obtain the desired bacterial cell concentration of 2.7×10^8 CFU/ml. 0.5 ml of this suspension (containing about 100 μg/ml of Se ions) was orally administered to the mice by using a standard gastric feeding gavage as follows:

The test group of mice was daily administered with 0.5 ml of SeNP-enriched *L. brevis* suspension for three consecutive weeks prior to tumor challenge. This daily feeding was continued for three repeated cycles of seven days on/three days off. Same above protocol was also concomitantly repeated for *L .brevis* alone. Also the control mice (PBS-received mice) were given an equal volume of PBS solution in a similar procedure.

Tumor challenge

The $4T_1$ cell line ATCC CRL-2539 (originated from mice breast tumor and is routinely applied to simulate the end stage of human breast cancer in animal model) was used for the induction of tumors in inbred Balb/c mice. For this purpose, 200 μl of RPMI, containing $4T_1$ cells at a concentration of 1×10^6 cell/ml, was injected subcutaneously near the mammary glands of female mice. All mice were followed until a tumor nodule was observed (10 days after injection).

The tumor growth measurement

Tumor growth was measured twice during this study firstly when tumors became palpable and at last before mice scarification by caliper measurement of the tumor length in two different dimensions. The tumor volumes of 15 mice in each test and control groups were determined using the formula: $V = 0.5 \times d^2 \times D$ [20] where V is the tumor volume (mm^3), d is the shorter diameter, and D is the longer diameter. Finally average tumor volumes of last time measurement were subtracted from the first time and reported as related tumor volume.

Providing the tumor antigen

The tumor antigen was prepared from the tumor of one of the mice. The tumor was removed from the body, dissected into small sections (1 mm^3), and homogenized in sterile PBS. This homogenized sample was washed with sterile PBS, 100 μl/ml of PMSF was added to inhibit

the endogenous proteases, and the sample was sonicated (Hielscher Ultrasonics GmbH, Germany) for 10 minute. The sample was then dialyzed against 1000 ml of PBS buffer for 24 h at 4°C using a cellulose membrane with a 14 kD cutoff (Sigma, Germany) and the PBS was changed every eight hours. After dialysis, the concentrated sample was collected and the protein concentration was determined using the conventional Bradford method. The sample was used to stimulate splenocytes in the cytokine production tests and delayed type hypersensitivity response (DTH) assay.

Evaluation of DTH response

The DTH response was measured according to a method described by Jin et al. [21]. Briefly, 30 days after tumor challenge, 7 mice from each group were challenged with the tumor antigen (20 μg) in the left footpad and with the PBS in the right footpad. Footpad induration was measured at 72 h later using caliper measurements.

Cytokine determination in spleen cell culture

One month after tumor challenge, spleens of eight mice from each group were removed aseptically and dissected. Spleen cells were then prepared using an appropriate nylon mesh screen and the remaining RBCs in the spleen cell collection were disrupted with conventional RBC lysis buffer. The spleen cell counts were adjusted to 2.5×10^6 cell/ml in RPMI1640 (Gibco Life Technologies, Germany) supplemented with 10% fetal bovine serum (Invitrogen, Paisley Germany), 100 μg/ml streptomycin, and 100 IU/ml penicillin (Sigma, Germany). These cells were then stimulated with 20 μg/ml of the tumor antigen (the amount was determined in a previous study) for 72 h [4] at 37°C in a humidified atmosphere of 5% CO_2. The levels of IL-17 and IFN-γ in the spleen cell culture supernatants were determined using ELISA kits (R&D Systems, Minneapolis, MN), according to the manufacturer's instructions. The limit of detection for IFN-γ was 2 pg and for IL-17 was 5 pg.

Natural killer cell activity by LDH assay

The NK cell activity was evaluated in eight mice from each group (these mice were also used for the cytokine determination test). An aliquot containing 2.5×10^6 splenocytes was removed and mixed with target K562 cells at a ratio of 1:100 (Target:Effector) in 96-well culture plates with U-shaped bottoms (Corning, Corning, NY) in 0.2 ml of RPMI1640 containing 2% BSA. The release of LDH was measured using an LDH assay kit (Takara, Japan) by first gently centrifuging the plates for 5 min at $250 \times g$ and then incubating them for four h at 37°C in 5% CO_2. After incubation, the plates were centrifuged for 10 min at $250 \times g$, and the supernatant was transferred from each well of the culture plate to the corresponding well of a new 96 well plate. One hundred microliters of reaction solution (prepared according to the kit instructions) was then added to each well, and the plate was incubated with gentle shaking on an orbital shaker for 30 min. The absorbance of each well was then read at 490 nm. The specific release of LDH was calculated as a percentage using the following formula [22]:

$$Experimental\,value-low\;control\,/\,high\,control-low\,control \times 100$$

LDH and ALP determination in blood circulation

Blood was collected from pre-orbital cavity of eight mice from each group (these mice were also used for spleen cell culture). Each mouse was placed under the anesthesia induced by ether and the blood samples (one ml) were collected from the pre-orbital cavity into

appropriate microtubes. Serum samples were prepared by storing the blood at 4°C for one hour, and the resulting coagulated blood cells were then separated from the serum by centrifugation for 20 min at $4000 \times g$. The serum was transferred to a new microtube, and the lactate dehydrogenase (LDH) and alkaline phosphatase (ALP) levels in each sample was determined using the IFCC method [23,24].

Histopathological studies

After cervical dislocation of experimental mice (these mice were also used for spleen cell culture) the liver was taken for histopathological analysis. Tissues were fixed in 10% formalin in PBS solution, in embedded paraffin, and cut into 3-5-μm thick sections. The sections were stained with hematoxylin eosin for general analysis using light microscope with 400× magnification. Pathological assay was done after preparation of H&E stained slides from tumor and liver tissues. In next step, the 10 microscopic fields in each slide were carefully observed and proportions (%) of metastasis and necrosis cells were

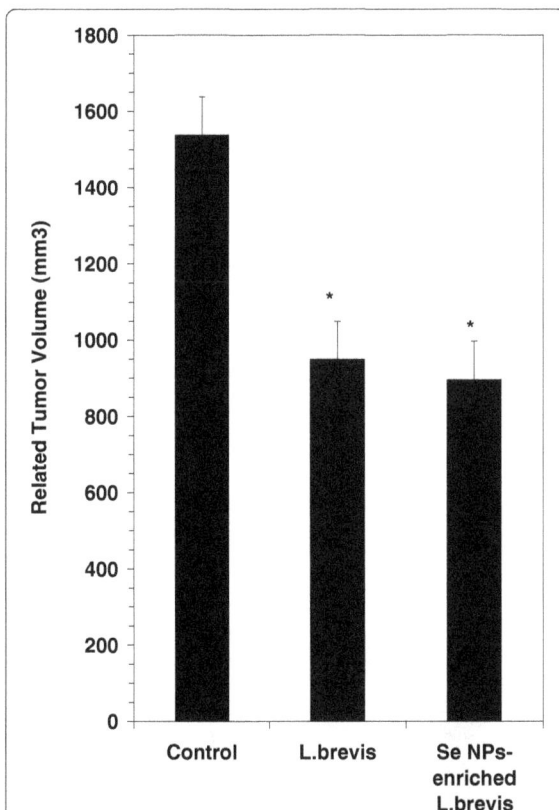

Figure 1 Related tumor volume in tumor-bearing mice which received SeNP-enriched *L. brevis*, *L. brevis* alone and PBS buffer (control group). Tumor growth was measured twice a week and evaluated by caliper measurement of the tumor length. The tumor related volume which refers to the measurement of 15 tumors in each group was achieved by subtraction of first measurement from the latest. Asterisks indicate statistical significance (P ≤ 0.05 significance).

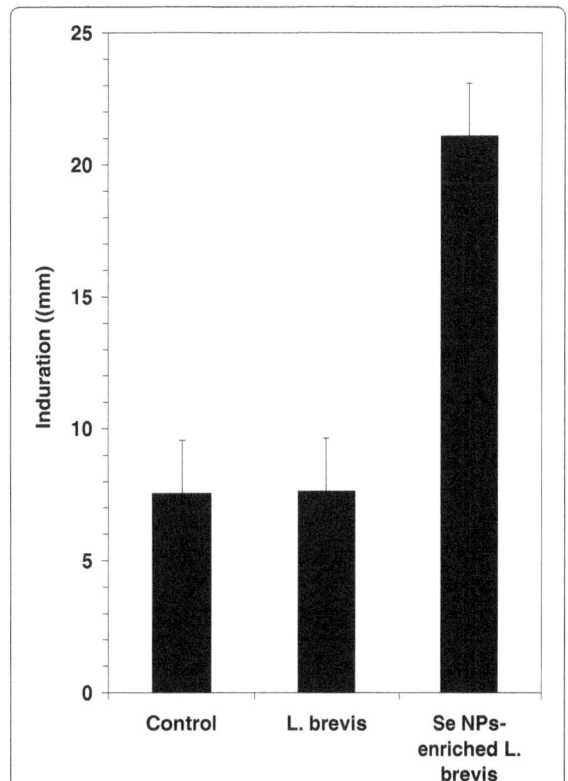

Figure 2 Foot pad induration in tumor-bearing mice which received SeNP-enriched *L. brevis*, *L. brevis* alone and PBS buffer (control group). Footpad induration was measured at 72 h after tumor antigen re-challenge using caliper measurements.

estimated from microscopic evaluation of the mentioned selected fields.

Survival rate

At the end of the study period (one month after tumor challenge), seven mice from each group (these mice were also used for the DTH assay) were kept in standard conditions and fed with standard diet, with free access to water, and maintained under a 12:12 h light dark cycle until they died. Daily deaths were recorded; after the last death in both groups, the data were analyzed with a Kaplan-Meier test.

Statistical analysis

All of the statistical analyses, except for survival rate, were conducted using SPSS software (Version 15.0) and ANOVA tests. The survival rate data were analyzed by the Kaplan-Meier test using also SPSS software (Version 15.0). The values are presented as mean ± SD.

Ethical approval

The experimental procedures carried out in this study were in compliance with the guidelines of the Tehran University of Medical Science (Tehran, Iran) for the care and use of laboratory animals.

Results

Identification of the microorganism

BLAST search of the 16S rDNA sequence against the NCBI Nucleotide database was conducted for identification of isolate. Alignment results containing 180 characters revealed 100% identity with *L. brevis*. The 16S rRNA gene sequence of the *L. brevis* isolate has been submitted to GenBank under accession number JX966418.

The tumor volumes growth measurement and DTH response

Tumor growth was evaluated by twice-weekly caliper measurements of the tumors from 15 mice from each group. The tumor volume was calculated as described in the Materials and Methods section. Data analysis showed a significant ($P \le 0.05$) decrease in the growth rate of tumors in the test mice when compared to the control mice (Figure 1). The tumor mass has been enlarged to 1550 mm^3 in control mice while in test groups, which received SeNP-enriched *L. brevis* or *L. brevis* alone, the tumor volumes were decreased to 890 and 950 mm^3, respectively. Also the antigen-specific Th1 recalling response was assessed by evaluating the DTH reaction in the tumor antigen rechallenged mice. Also as mentioned before, these mice were challenged with tumor antigen in the left footpad and with PBS solution

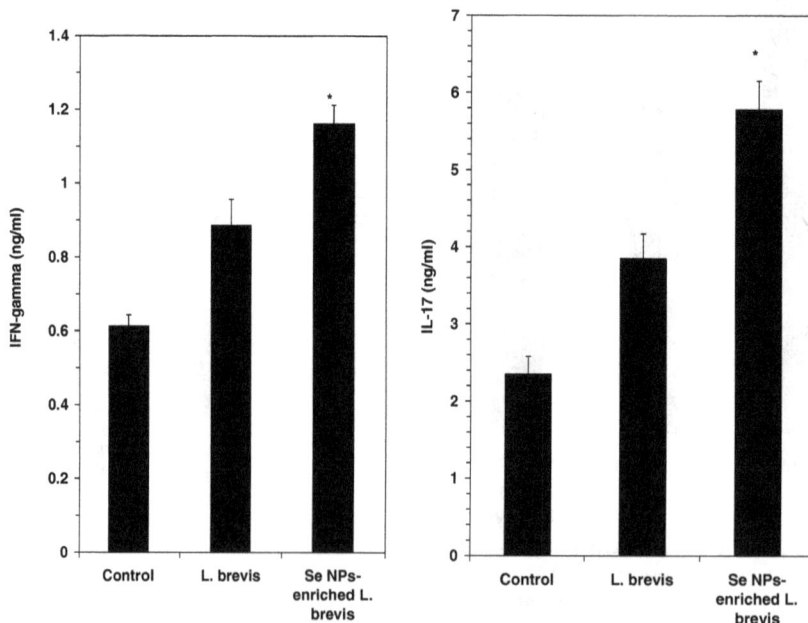

Figure 3 Inductions of IFN-γ (left illustration) and IL17 (right illustration) by administration of SeNP-enriched *L. brevis* in a spleen cell culture. The spleen cells were stimulated with tumor antigen for 72 h and then the levels of IFN-γ and IL-17 in the culture supernatants were determined by ELISA. Data represent the means ± standard deviations for triplicate cultures of eight animals per group * ($P \le 0.05$).

in the right footpad 30 days after tumor injection. The results showed a greater swelling and thickness in the left footpad 72h after the tumor antigen challenge in the test group which received SeNP-enriched *L. brevis* compared with the other groups (Figure 2). In contrast, no significant increase in DTH response was observed in those test mice which received *L. brevis* alone compared to control mice. It may show that the prescription of *L. brevis* alone could not significantly enhance the Th1 recalling response.

Cytokine determination in spleen cell culture

The levels of IFN-γ and IL-17 in the spleen cell culture supernatants were measured using a sandwich ELISA assay (R&D Systems, Minneapolis, MN). As shown in right illustration of Figure 3, the level of IFN-γ was significantly higher in the test groups than in the control group ($P \leq 0.05$). The IL-17 level in the test groups was also significantly elevated when compared to the control level (Left illustration of Figure 3).

Natural killer cell activity by LDH assay

We investigated and compared the effects of administration of SeNP-enriched *L. brevis* and *L. brevis* alone on NK cells by using K562 cells as target cells and evaluating the release of LDH from these cells after 4 h of exposure to the NK cells that were present among the harvested splenocytes. The mice treated with SeNP-enriched *L. brevis* showed a significantly increased level of NK cell activity ($P \leq 0.001$) compared to other groups (Figure 4) which received probiotic alone or PBS solution (control mice).

Serum levels of LDH and ALP

Analysis of serum showed a decrease in the levels of LDH and ALP in the mice which received SeNP-enriched *L. brevis* when compared to the other groups received *L. brevis* alone or PBS solution (control mice). The decrease in serum LDH may have directly contributed to the decrease in the rate of tumor development and tumor cell division in the groups treated by SeNP-enriched *L. brevis* or *L. brevis* alone (left illustration of Figure 5). Also the decrease in the ALP level in test mice shows better liver prognosis in both treated groups compared to control group (right illustration of Figure 5).

Histopathological studies

As it observes in left illustration of Figure 6 the rate of tumor necrosis in test mice which received SeNP-enriched *L. brevis* was considerably increased in comparison to other test or control groups. On the other hand the highest decreasing rate in the level of liver metastasis was diagnosed in histopathological slides (Figures not shown) prepared from liver tissue of mice

which received SeNP-enriched *L. brevis* (right illustration of Figure 6).

Survival rate

The results of survival analysis in Figure 7 show the decrease in the rate of mortality among the SeNP-enriched *L. brevis* administered mice group in comparison to other groups. In the test group which received SeNP-enriched *L. brevis*, it was observed a remarkable decrease in mortality rate and indicated that administration of this formulation could enhance the survival rate of tumor bearing mice over 230 days period. The effect of *L. brevis* without SeNPs was also investigated on the survival rates of tumor bearing mice. Oral administration of *L. brevis* alone also enhanced the survival rate of 4T1 tumor bearing mice over 75 days period, but this enhancement was not as same as the

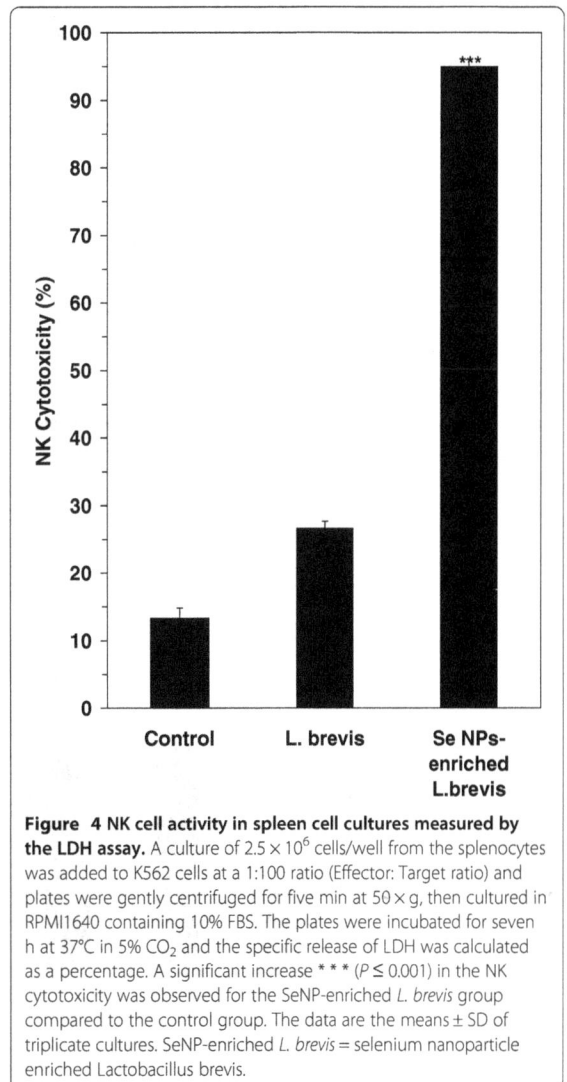

Figure 4 NK cell activity in spleen cell cultures measured by the LDH assay. A culture of 2.5×10^6 cells/well from the splenocytes was added to K562 cells at a 1:100 ratio (Effector: Target ratio) and plates were gently centrifuged for five min at $50 \times g$, then cultured in RPMI1640 containing 10% FBS. The plates were incubated for seven h at 37°C in 5% CO_2 and the specific release of LDH was calculated as a percentage. A significant increase * * * ($P \leq 0.001$) in the NK cytotoxicity was observed for the SeNP-enriched *L. brevis* group compared to the control group. The data are the means ± SD of triplicate cultures. SeNP-enriched *L. brevis* = selenium nanoparticle enriched Lactobacillus brevis.

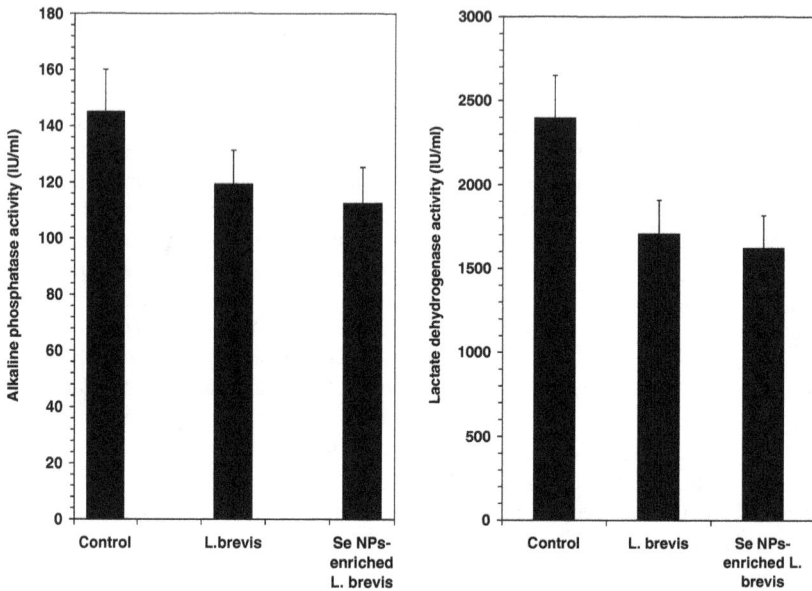

Figure 5 Differences between the levels of ALP and LDH in the serum of mice, measured using the conventional IFCC method. Data are shown in the range of U/L.

survival rate observed in the mice treated with SeNP-enriched *L. brevis* (230 days). This result even is more considerable than the survival time of cancerous mice which received purified biogenic SeNPs (90 days) [25] or SeNP-enriched *L. plantarum* (130 days) [18].

Discussion

Tumor development in cancer patients has been reported to attenuate immunological response in cancer bearing patients [26]. Also routine chemotherapy and irradiation treatment can considerably decrease the host immunity and are main reasons to weak immune system in cancer bearing patients [27] attenuate immunological response in cancer bearing patients. It also weakens the natural defense against foreign threats such as pathogenic or opportunistic microorganisms. Therefore using some immunomodulatory agents in immunosuppressed patients seems to be helpful to decrease the cancer development

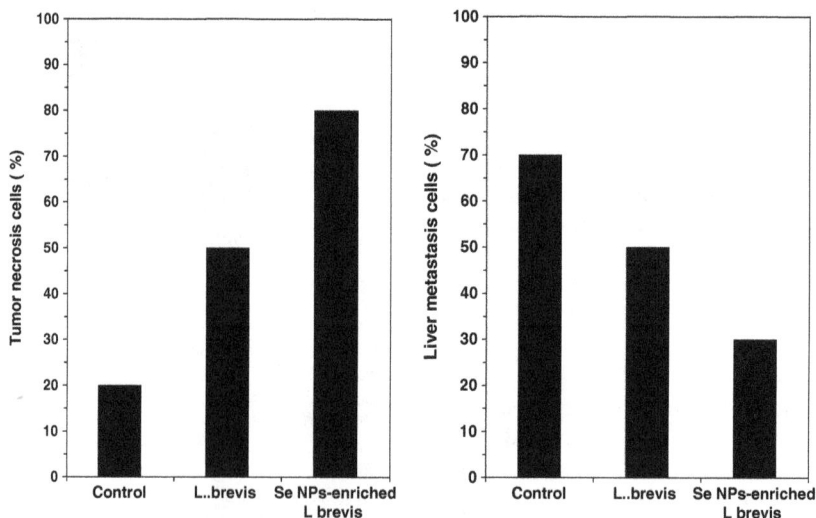

Figure 6 The levels of tumor necrosis (left illustration) and liver metastasis (right illustration) cells were diagnosed in histopathological slides prepared from tissue samples removed mice which received SeNP-enriched *L. brevis*.

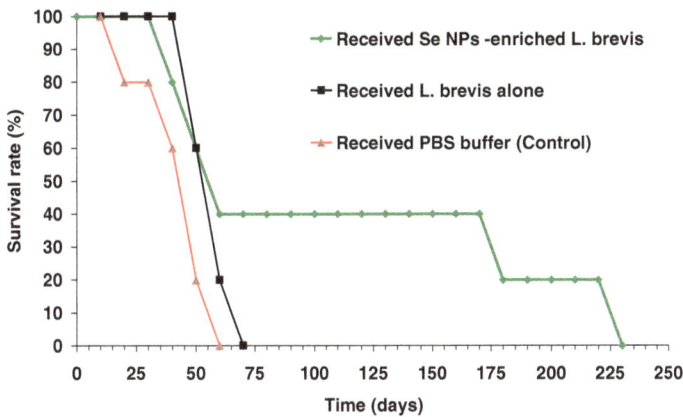

Figure 7 Survival rates of mice administered SeNP-enriched *L. brevis* and *L. brevis* alone when compared with control mice at the end of the study. A total of seven mice from each experimental group were kept under standard conditions until they died. The rate of death was registered every day and the obtained data were analyzed with a Kaplan-Meier test after the last death in both test and control groups. The lifespans of animals that received SeNP-enriched *L. brevis* or *L. brevis* alone were considerably increased compared to the lifespans of control mice.

and prevent additional complications such as infectious diseases. On the other hand, metastasis is major cause of death among cancer bearing patient and can worsen the prognosis of cancer especially for those who are suffering from advanced level of cancer.

Recently we reported the immunostimulatory effect of purified biogenic SeNPs [25] and SeNP-enriched *L. plantarum* on the life span of 4T1 breast cancer animal model [18]. Both formulations have increased the survival rate of cancerous animals but the effect of SeNP-enriched *L. plantarum* on the survival rate of 4T1 cancer bearing mice was more remarkable than purified biogenic SeNPs or *L. plantarum* alone [18]. Oral administration of SeNP-enriched *L. plantarum* delayed the mortality of some cancerous animals for 130 days which was 40 days longer than the survival time of animals received purified biogenic SeNPs. Although the immunomodulatory effect of LAB is currently established [28,29] but still it should not be ignored that this effect is variable in different species of these bacteria [30]. So the oral supplementation with other SeNPs LAB strain may lead to obtain a better survival rate in cancerous animals. Regarding to above fact, in this study another strain of LAB was isolated from human feces and identified as *L. brevis*. In next step this bacterium was enriched by elemental Se and used for oral supplementation of breast cancer bearing animals. Then the effect of this type of supplementation and supplementation of *L. brevis* alone on the immune responses and the liver metastasis have been investigated and compared in breast cancer bearing animals.

SeNP-enriched *Lactobacillus* is an organoselenium agent and a new form of Se which is synthesis and accumulated in intracellular space of bacteria, this form of Se

also considered as biogenic SeNPs [31]. Although results of some studies implied to the protective effect of Se enriched *lactobacillus* on the CCL$_4$ liver injury but as a best of the authors' knowledge it still no more understood about immunostimulatory effect of this new form of LAB [32]. Cytokine assay in the current study showed an increase in the level of IFN-γ through the oral administration of SeNP- enriched *L. brevis*. On the other hand IL-17 as another Th1 known cytokine also raised due to this administration. Moreover, NK cell activity was enhanced in the test mice which received SeNP-enriched *L. brevis* and could be related to the increase in the level of IFN-γ in some way.

NK cells play a major role in the rejection of tumors and cells infected by viruses [32,33]. Also any decrease in tumor volume occurred in SeNP-enriched *L. brevis* administered mice can address to engaging of antitumor immune responses such as NK cytotoxicity (Figure 4). Enhancement of tumor necrosis as well as higher DTH response in test mice which received SeNP- enriched *L. brevis* can further confirm this hypothesis (Figure 2).

In the other hand, although the serum levels of aspartate aminotransferase (AST) and alanine aminotransferase (ALT) as two types of liver function enzymes were similar in test and control groups (data are not shown) but regarding to the result of histopathological study the tumor metastasis into liver of SeNP-enriched *L. brevis* treated mice was considerably lower than control group which received PBS buffer. Moreover, it observed that by administration of SeNP- enriched *L. brevis* the serum level of ALP and LDH, which are considered for cancer monitoring, have been reduced. Conclusively, the enhancement of life span in SeNP- enriched *L. brevis* administered mice which observed during this investigation as a promising result can introduce this oral formulation as a good candidate for future prevention and immunotherapy of cancer. But still more studies are needed to develop this formula.

Competing interests
The authors declare that they have no competing interests.

Authors' contribution
YMH: Conducting experiments and manuscript preparation, MM: Supervising Immunoassay experiments, NS: Conducting molecular experiment, ME: Participating in animal experiments, ShAR: Project design, supervising experiments and manuscript preparation. All authors read and approve the final manuscript.

Acknowledgment
This work was supported by the Biotechnology Research Center, Tehran University of Medical Sciences (Tehran, Iran).There is no conflict of interest for authors in this work.

Author details
[1]Department of Pharmaceutical Biotechnology, Faculty of Pharmacy and Biotechnology Research Center, Tehran University of Medical Sciences, Tehran, Iran. [2]Department of virology, Pasteur Institute of Iran, Tehran, Iran.

References
1. Yazdi MH, Soltan Dallal MM, Hassan ZM, Holakuyee M, Agha Amiri S, Abolhassani M, Mahdavi M: Oral administration of Lactobacillus acidophilus induces IL-12 production in spleen cell culture of BALB/c mice bearing transplanted breast tumor. Br J Nutr 2010, 104(2):227–232.
2. Motta G, Cea M, Carbone F, Augusti V, Moran E, Nencioni PFA: Current standards and future strategies in immunochemotherapy of non-Hodgkin's lymphoma. J BUON 2011, 16(1):9–15.
3. Mark N, Levine MD: Timothy Whelan BM, B Ch: Adjuvant Chemotherapy for Breast Cancer 30 Years Later. N Engl J Med 2006, 355:1920–1922.
4. Turowski RC, Triozzi PL: Application of chemical immunomodulators to the treatment of cancer and AIDS. Cancer Invest 1994, 12(6):620–643.
5. Vetvicka V, Saraswat-Ohri S, Vashishta A, Descroix K, Jamois F, Yvin JC, Ferrières V: New 4-deoxy-(1 → 3)-β-d-glucan-based oligosaccharides and their immunostimulating potential. Carbohydr Res 2011, 346(14):2213–2221.
6. De Roos NM, Katan MB: Effects of probiotic bacteria on diarrhea, lipid metabolism, and carcinogenesis: a review of papers published between 1988 and 1998. Am J Clin Nutr 2000, 71:405–411.
7. Shida K, Makino K, Morishita A, Takamizawa K, Hachimura S, Ametani A, Sato A, Kumagai Y, Habu S, Kaminogawa S: Lactobacillus casei inhibits antigen-induced IgE secretion through regulation of cytokine production in murine splenocyte cultures. Int Arch Allergy Immunol 1998, 115:278–287.
8. Shu Q, Lin H, Rutherfurd KJ, Fenwick SG, Prasad J, Gopal PK: Dietary Bifidobacterium lactis (HN019) enhances resistance to oral Salmonella typhimurium infection in mice. Microbiol Immunol 2000, 44:213–222.
9. Takagi A, Matsuzaki T, Sato M, Nomoto K, Morotomi M, Yokokura T: Inhibitory effect of oral administration of Lactobacillus casei on 3-methylcholanthrene-induced carcinogenesis in mice. Med Microbiol Immunol 1999, 188:111–116.
10. Grangette C, Nutten S, Palumbo E, Morath S, Hermann C, Dewulf J, Pot B, Hartung T, Hols P, Mercenier A: Enhanced antiinflammatory capacity of a Lactobacillus plantarum mutant synthesizing modified teichoic acids. Proc Natl Acad Sci USA 2005, 102(29):10321–10326.
11. Bengmark S: Immunonutrition: role of biosurfactants, fiber, and probiotic bacteria. Nutrition 1998, 14:585–594.
12. Dugas B, Mercenier A, Lenoir-Wijnkoop I, Arnaud C, Dugas N, Postaire E: Immunity and probiotics. Immunol Today 1999, 20:387–390.
13. Maassen CB, van Holten JC, Balk F, den Bak-Glashouwer MJ H, Leer R, Laman JD, Boersma WJ, Claassen E: Orally administered Lactobacillus strains differentially affect the direction and efficacy of the immune response. Vet Q 1998, 3:81–83.
14. Maassen CB, van Holten-Neelen C, Balk F, den Bak-Glashouwer MJ, Leer RJ, Laman JD, Boersma WJ, Claassen E: Strain-dependent induction of cytokine profiles in the gut by orally administered Lactobacillus strains. Vaccine 2000, 18:2613–2623.
15. Schrauzer GN: Anticarcinogenic effects of selenium. Cell Mol Life Sci 2000, 57:1864–1873.
16. Schrauzer GN: Nutritional selenium supplements: product types, quality, and safety. J Am Coll Nutr 2001, 20:1–4.
17. Kiremidjian-Schumacher L, Stotzky G: Selenium and immune responses. Environ Res 1987, 42(2):277–303.
18. Yazdi MH, Mahdavi M, Kheradmand E, Shahverdi AR: The preventive oral supplementation of a selenium nanoparticle-enriched probiotic increases the immune response and lifespan of 4T1 breast cancer bearing mice. Arzneimittel-forsch 2012, 62(11):525–531.
19. Bergey DH, Holt JG: Bergey's Manual of Determinative Bacteriology. 9th edition. Philadelphia: Lippincott Williams and Wilkins Press; 1994.
20. Attia M, Weiss DW: Immunology of spontaneous mammary carcinomas in mice. Acquired tumour resistance and enhancement in strain mice infected with mammary tumour virus. Cancer Res 1996, 26:1787–1792.
21. Jin H, Li Y, Ma Z, Zhang F, Xie Q, Gu D, Wang B: Effect of chemical adjuvants on DNA vaccination. Vaccine 2004, 22:2925–2935.
22. Subleski JJ, Wiltrout RH, Weiss JM: Application of tissue-specific NK and NKT cell activity for tumor immunotherapy. J Autoimmun 2009, 33:275–281.
23. Bakker AJ, Mirchi B, Dijkstra JT, Reitsma F, Syperda H, Zijlstra A: IFCC Method for lactate dehydrogenase measurement in heparin plasma Is unreliable. Clin Chem 2003, 49:662–666.
24. Strömme JH, Björnstad P, Eldjarn L: Improvement in the quality of enzyme determinations by scandinavian laboratories upon introduction of scandinavian recommended methods. Scand J Clin Lab Invest 1976, 36(6):505–511.
25. Yazdi MH, Mahdavi M, Varastehmoradi B, Faramarzi MA, Shahverdi AR: The Immunostimulatory effect of biogenic selenium nanoparticles on the 4T1 breast cancer model: an In Vivo study. Biol Trace Elem Res 2012, 149(1):22–28.
26. O'Hara RJ, Greenman J, MacDonald AW, Gaskell KM, Topping KP, Duthie GS, Kerin MJ, Lee PW, Monson JR: Advanced colorectal cancer is associated with impaired interleukin 12 and enhanced interleukin 10 productions. Clin Cancer Res 1943, 1998(4):1948.
27. Rasmussen L, Arvin A: Chemotherapy-induced immunosuppression. Environ Health Perspect 1982, 43:21–25.
28. Kim SY, Lee KW, Kim JY, Lee HJ: Cytoplasmic fraction of Lactococcus lactis ssp. lactis induces apoptosis in SNU-1 stomach adenocarcinoma cells. Biofactors 2004, 22:119–122.
29. Vintiñi EO, Medina MS: Host immunity in the protective response to nasal immunization with a pneumococcal antigen associated to live and heat-killed Lactobacillus casei. BMC Immunol 2011, 11:12–46.
30. Fujiwara D, Inoue S, Wakabayashi H, Fujii T: The Anti-Allergic Effects of Lactic Acid Bacteria Are Strain Dependent and Mediated by Effects on both Th1/Th2 Cytokine Expression and Balance. Int Arch Allergy Immunol 2004, 135:205–215.
31. Shakibaie M, Khorramizadeh MR, Faramarzi MA, Sabzevari O, Shahverdi AR: Biosynthesis and recovery of selenium nanoparticles and the effects on matrix metalloproteinase-2 expression. Biotechnol Appl Biochem 2010, 56:7–15.
32. Chen L, Pan D-D, Zhou J, Jiang Y-Z: Protective effect of selenium-enriched lactobacillus on CCl4-induced liver injury in mice and its possible mechanisms. World J Gastroenterol 2005, 11(37):5795–5800.
33. Wang G, Zhao J, Liu J, Huang Y, Zhong JJ, Tang W: Enhancement of IL-2 and IFN-gamma expression and NK cells activity involved in the anti-tumor effect of ganoderic acid Me in vivo. Int Immunopharmacol 2007, 7(6):864–870.

Tribulus terrestris for treatment of sexual dysfunction in women: randomized double-blind placebo - controlled study

Elham Akhtari[1], Firoozeh Raisi[2*], Mansoor Keshavarz[1], Hamed Hosseini[3,4], Farnaz Sohrabvand[5], Soodabeh Bioos[1], Mohammad Kamalinejad[6] and Ali Ghobadi[7]

Abstract

Background: Tribulus terrestris as a herbal remedy has shown beneficial aphrodisiac effects in a number of animal and human experiments. This study was designed as a randomized double-blind placebo-controlled trial to assess the safety and efficacy of Tribulus terrestris in women with hypoactive sexual desire disorder during their fertile years. Sixty seven women with hypoactive sexual desire disorder were randomly assigned to Tribulus terrestris extract (7.5 mg/day) or placebo for 4 weeks. Desire, arousal, lubrication, orgasm, satisfaction, and pain were measured at baseline and after 4 weeks after the end of the treatment by using the Female Sexual Function Index (FSFI). Two groups were compared by repeated measurement ANOVA test.

Results: Thirty women in placebo group and thirty women in drug group completed the study. At the end of the fourth week, patients in the Tribulus terrestris group had experienced significant improvement in their total FSFI ($p < 0.001$), desire ($p < 0.001$), arousal ($p = 0.037$), lubrication ($p < 0.001$), satisfaction ($p < 0.001$) and pain ($p = 0.041$) domains of FSFI. Frequency of side effects was similar between the two groups.

Conclusions: Tribulus terrestris may safely and effectively improve desire in women with hypoactive sexual desire disorder. Further investigation of Tribulus terrestris in women is warranted.

Keywords: Tribulus terrestris, Sexual dysfunction, Women, Traditional medicine

Background

Hypoactive sexual desire disorder (HSDD) is a multi factorial and multifaceted disorder which has been entangled with biologic and psychological considerations and interpersonal relations. HSDD is a common sexual complaint affecting approximately 1 in 10 adult women in the USA [1,2], and its prevalence appears to be similar in Europe (7%-16%) [3] and Australia (16%) [4]. According to some scientific reports the prevalence in Iran is 30% [5].

Currently there are two therapeutic modalities for women who suffer from the lack of libido: psychotherapy and pharmacotherapy. Several drugs have been suggested for treating women's loss of libido including estrogen, methyl testosterone [4], phenethylamin [5], bupropion [6] and saffron [7]. However, there is no Food and Drug Administration (FDA) approved drug for treating women's HSDD [8,9].

Avicenna's *The Canon of Medicine* (1025 AD) provides a full chapter to the description of libido, its disorders and treatments. Twentieth chapter of the book discusses the libido under rubric of "*Bah*", its disorders and causes that may boost and reduce the sex drive as well as treatments for each cause [10]. According to *the Canon of Medicine* and Aghili Khorasani's *Makhzan al-Advia* (The treasury of Spices) (18th AD), Bindii or *Tribulus terrestris* influences libido [11] and is able to boost sex drive in human beings. According to the Iranian Traditional Medicine (ITM) deregulation and disorders of libido in both sexes is considerably common. It is worthy to mention that, ITM is based on principles of Humorist school and

* Correspondence: Fraisi@gmail.com
[2]Psychiatry, Fellow of the European Committee of Sexual Medicine (FECSM), Roozbeh Psychiatric Hospital, Psychiatric and Clinical Psychology, Research Center, Tehran University of Medical Sciences, South Kargar Street, Tehran 13337, Iran
Full list of author information is available at the end of the article

four humors (black bile, yellow bile, phlegm and blood), but the mentioned herbal medicine, Tribulus terrestris, has been classified as an experimental remedy because it affects all four humors and boosts the libido.

Recent scientific studies on medicinal herbs have referred to Tribulus terrestris as an effective drug of women's sex drive [12]. A study on mice hypothesized that the drug may affect follicle-stimulating hormone (FSH) and luteinizing hormone (LH); injecting 10 mg of Tribulus extract into female mice resulted in significant increase in both growth rate and size of follicles in comparison to the control mice [13].

The aim of our clinical trial was to analyze the effect of Tribulus on women with HSDD in childbearing age.

Methods
Trial design
This was a randomized, double-blind, placebo-controlled clinical trial study, performed in two medical centers in Tehran Province, Rostamabad Neighborhood Health Center, part of the 1st district of the greater Tehran Municipality, and Sajjad Hospital in city of Shahryar. This study was approved by the ethics committee of School of Medicine, Tehran University of Medical Sciences (TUMS), and it was registered in the clinical trial center under reg. no. of IRCT20121111111425N1

Participants
Participants of the study were selected after responding to this specific question *"Do you suffer from loss of libido?"* in a direct and face to face encounter, and the study was conducted from June 2012 to July 2013. Then a phone interview was scheduled for all 96 women who were selected; and subsequently they were invited for a screening visit after verification of their disorder. The inclusion criteria of the study were: being married and actively living with a partner at least 15 days per month, being in childbearing age, lack and or loss of libido which causes distress, having normal pelvic exam, negative pap smear test conducted at least within past six months, and having normal breast exam. The exclusion criteria were: lack of steady sexual partner, suffering from a serious medical condition (any disease which may force the participant to use drugs during the study), any history of genital tract or breast cancers, suffering from major depression disorder or other psychiatric disorders, menopause, pregnancy, husband's sexual problems and active plans for divorce. Participants with the mentioned inclusion criteria were allowed to start the next stage which was a face to face interview based on Diagnostic and Statistical Manual of Mental Disorders (DSM-IV-TR) codes for HSDD [14]. Finally patients were asked to sign the informed consent forms.

Preparations of tribulus terrestris
Tribulus is widely scattered across the planet a herbal plant [15]. Tribulus belongs to Zygophyllaceae family. Alpha amyrin constitutes over 60% of active ingredient (AI) of the herb [16]. Dried leaves of Tribulus were obtained from a licensed distributer of herbs and natural remedies in Tehran. They were approved and registered by the SHUM herbarium (voucher number: SHUM 8051).

Preparations of syrup and placebo
Traditional Medicine Department, School of Medicine, TUMS used the whole vaporized ethanolic extract of Tribulus terrestris for preparing the syrup. There was 3.5 grams of ethanolic extract in every 5 ml of the syrup. The placebo was prepared via the same method without Tribulus terrestris extract as a sucrose syrup.

Treatment and assessment
Each participant was initially asked to fill the Female Sexual Function Index (FSFI) (21) a self-reported questionnaire under supervision of an Iranian traditional medicine intern who was already trained by a gynecologist and a psychiatrist for conducting the trial, and then she was provided with a drug bottle with specific coding. Drug Product Information Form (DPIF) was inscribed on a label attached to the bottle. The specific code was recorded on both questionnaire and participant's data sheet. The DPIF instructions included this information: 7.5 ml of the drug should be used two times a day for four full weeks since the day after the completion of menstruation period. Two days after submitting the drug, the patient was checked by a physician through a phone call in order to make sure that the drug was used correctly. Again, after a week a second phone call was made to make sure of continuity of the mentioned order. Patients, who forgot to use more than three doses of their drugs, were excluded. Another interview according to the DSM-IV-TR criteria for HSDD was made four weeks after completion of the drug therapy, side effects (if any) were checked and FSFI questionnaire was refilled. The participants were allowed to call their therapist during the treatment period.

Outcomes
The participants filled the FSFI questionnaire [1,17] two times: 1) at the beginning of the study, 2) four weeks after finishing their drug. The questionnaire have 19 questions with six domains included desire, arousal, lubrication, orgasm, satisfaction and pain, and a general score in which higher scores reflected better sexual activity. Questions 1 and 2 were related to the sexual desire and its score varied between 1.2 and 6. Questions 3, 4, 5 and 6 analyzed arousal of the patient. Another domain of the questionnaire was lubrication which covered questions 7, 8, 9, and 10. The orgasm domain included questions 11, 12 and 13. Questions

14, 15 and 16 all were related to the sexual satisfaction and finally questions 17, 18 and 19 analyzed pain.

The initial outcome was the assessment of desire and total score of our samples with FSFI before and after intervention. Likewise, different subscales including arousal, lubrication, orgasm, satisfaction and pain were compared as the secondary targets using the questionnaire before and after treatment. The FSFI question contained 19 questions which analyzed five domains of women's sexual function. Side effects were recorded systematically within the trial period through visits made within 1, 2 and 4 weeks and after the end of pharmacotherapy.

Sample size
The statistical power was set at 80% in order to achieve a minimum score of 3, to improve the "sexual desire" score in the intervention (experimental) group in comparison with the control group. The standard deviation (SD) was 3.5 (resulted from our pilot study). In regards to possibility of loss measuring 20% during the study period, we achieved significance level of 95% and a bilateral t-test.

Randomization, allocation concealment, and blinding
The randomized sequence was produced by a methodology using randomization permuted block technique with blocks size of 4 which was submitted to therapists with ratio 1:1 divided in two groups. The randomized sequence for allocating the main or placebo treatment was concealed through producing unknown codes; hence, pre-provided drugs and placebo were submitted through similar packs but different codes, as neither therapists nor patients were aware of the active ingredient of the drug packs.

Statistical analysis
Descriptive baseline characteristics for two groups comparisons were tabulated as means and SD or as percentages. All analyses comparing the efficacy of our primary and secondary outcomes were by intention-to-treat principles. Using General Linear Model (GLM) score of desire, arousal, lubrication, orgasm, satisfaction, and pain between two groups were compared by repeated measurement ANOVA test. Compound symmetry assumption was tested using Mauchley's Sphericity test. The time groups cross-product (interaction term) was considered as group differences in their response over time with the baseline values as a covariate in this model. Significance level of 5% (alpha = 0.05) was used for all statistical tests.

Results
A total of 96 women were enrolled for the study (Figure 1), and 67 women were identified as qualified (out which two women decided not to participate after acquiring DSM IV codes and upon issuing the informed consent, three other women stopped participating at the second phone call time point despite receiving drug and answering the first phone call. According to the code recorded on the questionnaire, (before taking drug) it was turned out that two women were from the placebo group and another one was from the drug group. Their reasons for stopping participating at the studying included very sweet taste of the drug (one woman) and anxiety due to using an investigational drug (two women). Another two women were not available after getting off the study; they signed the consent form, but there was no drug available at that time when they were in the center, and they never came back to receive their ration. Between June 2012 and July 2013, participants took part in an interview and then they filled the FSFI questionnaire; then they were assigned randomly in drug and placebo groups. There was a second visit a week after starting pharmacotherapy and third visit was made four weeks after termination of the treatment which was accompanied with the filling of the questionnaire for the second time. Hence patients in average were followed up for two consecutive months (Figure 1).

60 women out of 67 participants completed their treatment process and the results were analyzed according to what was recorded in their questionnaires. The mean ages of drug and control groups were 36 ± 6.24 years and 36.13 ± 5.88 years, respectively. 70% and 66.6% of participants in drug and control groups had bachelor or higher educational degrees (Table 1). 30 members of Tribulus and 30 members of the placebo group completed their treatment process.

Patients' desire was the main measured outcome of the study in both groups (Table 2) which was measured after four weeks of pharmacotherapy process by using the Female Sexual Function Index (FSFI) questionnaire and the following scores were gained: score of placebo group, before and after intervention, respectively: 2.66 ± 0.75 and 2.86 ± 0.79; scores of Tribulus group, before and after intervention, respectively: 3.06 ± 0.69 and 3.90 ± 0.71. After matching the effect of the possible effective variables (age, pregnancy rate, method of delivery, method of contraception), the difference became significant statistically ($p < 0.001$).

Another variable analyzed in this study was arousal which was measured four weeks after completion of the treatment process through the FSFI questionnaire. Scores of placebo group before and after pharmacotherapy were 3.16 ± 0.95 and 3.17 ± 0.75; Scores of intervention group before and after using Tribulus terrestris were 3.61 ± 0.92 and 4.21 ± 0.67. After matching the effect of the possible effective variables (age, pregnancy rate, method of delivery, method of contraception), the difference became significant statistically ($p = 0.037$).

According to the FSFI another secondary variable was lubrication. Similar to two previous variables lubrication

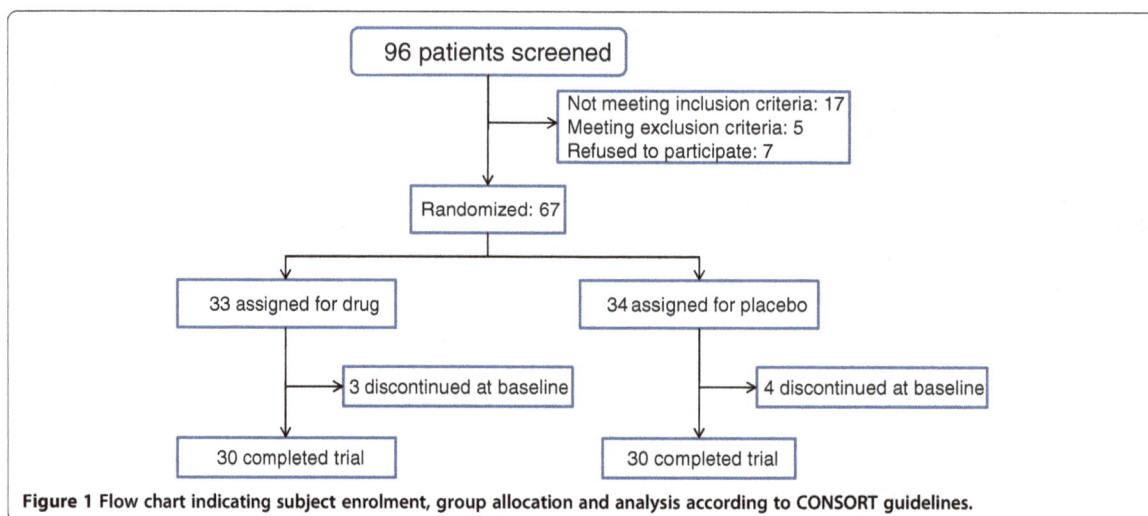

Figure 1 Flow chart indicating subject enrolment, group allocation and analysis according to CONSORT guidelines.

was analyzed four weeks after completion of the treatment. Scores of this domain gained by placebo group before and after usage were 4.15 ± 1.15 and 4.18 ± 0.79 while scores won by intervention group were 4.15 ± 1.13 and 4.66 ± 0.87. After matching the effect of the possible effective variables (age, pregnancy rate, method of delivery, method of contraception), the difference became significant statistically ($p < 0.001$).

Orgasm was analyzed using the FSFI questionnaire after four weeks of completion of treatment with Tribulus terrestris. Scores of this domain gained by placebo group

before and after usage were 3.31 ± 0.97 and 3.59 ± 0.85 while scores won by intervention group were 3.21 ± 0.98 and 4.20 ± 0.72. After matching the effect of the possible effective variables (age, pregnancy rate, method of delivery, method of contraception), the difference became significant statistically ($p < 0.001$).

Satisfaction was measured four weeks after completion of treatment process through the FSFI questionnaire. Scores of this domain gained by placebo group before and after pharmacotherapy were 3.43 ± 1.13 and 3.75 ± 1.12; scores won by intervention group before and after

Table 1 Demographic and baseline characteristics of patients

		Tribulus (n = 30)	Placebo (n = 30)
Age (years), mean ± SD		36 ± 6.24	36.13 ± 5.88
Partner age, mean ± SD		39.87 ± 7.13	40.43 ± 7.74
BMI kg/m^2		26.25 ± 3.75	24.67 ± 2.92
Education	Diploma	9	10
	Bachelor	21	17
	MA	0	3
Delivery (mean ± SD)			
Type of delivery	No	10%	6.7%
	NVD	60%	40%
	C/S	30%	53.3%
Contraception	Natural	33.3%	43.3%
	OCP	10%	6.7%
	Candom	23.3%	13.3%
	IUD	16.7%	13.3%
	None	10%	3.3%
	Tubectomy	6.7%	20%
Marriage years mean ± SD		14 ± 5.97	12.73 ± 6.22

Table 2 Summary results for each study group

	Control Mean ± SD	Baseline Mean ± SD	Mean differences (CI 95%) Control mean ± SD	Placebo N = 30 Baseline mean ± SD	Tribulus terrestris N = 30
Desire	3.66 ± 0.69	3.90 ± 0.71	2.66 ± 0.75	2.86 ± 0.79	0.71 (0.41 – 1.01) p < 0.001
Arousal	3.61 ± 0.92	4.21 ± 0.67	3.16 ± 0.95	3.17 ± 0.75	0.75 (0.47 – 1.46) p = 0.037
Lubrication	4.15 ± 1.13	4.66 ± 0.87	4.15 ± 1.15	4.18 ± 0.79	0.50 (0.32 – 0.68) p < 0.001
Orgasm	3.21 ± 0.98	4.20 ± 0.72	3.31 ± 0.97	3.59 ± 0.85	0.85 (0.56 – 1.14) p < 0.001
Satisfaction	3.44 ± 1.15	4.61 ± 0.93	3.43 ± 1.13	3.75 ± 1.12	1.10 (0.73– 1.48) p < 0.001
Pain	4.19 ± 1.56	5.07 ± 1.01	4.19 ± 1.51	4.87 ± 1.42	0.37 (0.16 – 0.73) p < 0.001
General score	22.41 ± 2.87	26.80 ± 3.03	20.39 ± 4.64	21.25 ± 4.72	4.32 (3.33 – 5.31) p = 0.040

using Tribulus terrestris were 3.44 ± 1.15 and 4.61 ± 0.93. After matching the effect of the possible effective variables (age, pregnancy rate, method of delivery, method of contraception), the difference became significant statistically ($p < 0.001$).

Pain was measured four weeks after completion of treatment process through the FSFI questionnaire. Scores of this domain gained by placebo group before and after pharmacotherapy were 4.19 ± 1.51 and 4.87 ± 1.42; scores won by intervention group before and after using Tribulus terrestris were 4.19 ± 1.56 and 5.07 ± 1.01. After matching the effect of the possible effective variables (age, pregnancy rate, method of delivery, method of contraception), the difference became significant statistically ($p = 0.041$).

Finally general scores of both drug and placebo groups were analyzed and compared based on FSFI questionnaire four weeks after completion of intervention. The general scores in placebo and intervention groups before using Tribulus terrestris were 20.89 ± 6.46 and 21.25 ± 4.72, respectively; and four weeks after its completion were 22.41 ± 2.87 and 26.80 ± 3.03, respectively ($p = 0.040$). These results confirmed by the interviews using DSM-IV-TR (Table 2).

Safety assessment
Possible side effects including abdominal pain, cramping, nausea, vomiting, diarrhea or constipation were recorded using Common Terminology Criteria for Adverse Events (CTCAE) Version 4.02 during the scheduled visits. Only one patient reported grade 1 abdominal cramp.

Discussion
Our findings showed that Tribulus terrestris was effective in improving women's sex drive based on the questions of FSFI questionnaire. Since the basic findings of two groups were similar, the improved score of the Tribulus group can be attributed to libido boosting effects of the plant. Our findings confirmed what has already been described in the Iranian Traditional Medical textbooks

about libido boosting effects of Tribulus. There is also more recent evidence that Tribulus can be used as a libido booster plant in women [12]. There may be a possible synergy between Tribulus and FSH-LH mechanism. For instance, one animal experiment showed that mice, injected with 10 mg Tribulus extract, developed thicker theca internal layer and more follicles in comparison with control mice in the same period of time [13].

Prescribing Tribulus extract for women can increase desire score in women who suffer from loss of sex desire. However, according to our knowledge there has not been any similar research on the impact of Tribulus extract in improving women's sex desire in childbearing age. The effect of testosterone in improving desire in menopausal women has been confirmed by studies that have looked at women's sex drive and how to boost it [18,19]. The role of conjugated testosterone in treating lack of sex drive has been emphasized [20]. Currently testosterone is the only approved drug for treatment of HSDD in menopausal women, particularly for those have surgically-induced menopause [21]. In one study on women with SSRI induced desire disorder, it was shown that Saffron was an effective herbal remedy which could improve desire [7]. Another study showed that Bupropion was effective in improving women's desire [6]. However, Tribulus is the only drug which not only improves the sexual desire in women but also it does not have any unexpected side effects in patients.

Our study showed very clearly through acquired scores of the FSFI questionnaire that patients had significant increase in their scores related to questions about desire, arousal and satisfaction. Our results indicated a considerable improvement in scores of desire. Thus, Tribulus had apparent boosting effects on desire, and it was able to improve sexual satisfaction and sexual behavior.

Although our study showed the effect of Tribulus on improving the desire, it must be noticed that Iranian women are generally modest and shy because of their cultural beliefs about sexual concepts, and our sample size was small. In order to produce consistent results and more reliable evidence, more studies with a large sample size must be carried out.

Conclusion

Tribulus terrestris may safely and effectively improve desire in women with HSDD. Further investigation of Tribulus terrestris in women is warranted.

Competing interests

The authors do not have any financial/commercial competing interest in the study presented here. This study was supported with Tehran University of Medical Sciences, School of Traditional Medicine.

Authors' contribution

EA was responsible for recruiting, visiting and evaluating patients; she was also involved in designing the study, analyzing the data and writing the manuscript. FR (the corresponding author) supervised the trial and was involved in all aspects of the study including designing and coordinating the study as well as analyzing the data and drafting the manuscript. MK gave his valuable comments throughout the study and was involved in the original design of the proposal, and also the final revision of the manuscript. HH performed all statistical analysis of the data and interpreted the results of the study. FS was the consultant gynecologist who recommended and supervised the gynecological evaluations of the patients. SB was consulted for a list of medications or herbal products that could interfere with the results of this study. MK participated in the identification of the plants, plant extraction and supervised preparing the placebo and Tribulus terrestris extract. AG prepared the placebo and Tribulus terrestris extract under supervision of MK. All authors read and approved the final manuscript.

Acknowledgements

This study was part of Dr. Elham Akhtari's postgraduate dissertation. The authors like to thank Dr. Roshanak Mokaberinejad at Shahid Behehshti University of Medical Sciences and Dr. Padideh Ghaeli at Tehran University of Medical Sciences for their valuable help throughout the study.

Author details

[1]Department of Traditional Medicine, School of Medicine, Tehran University of Medical Sciences, Tehran, Iran. [2]Psychiatry, Fellow of the European Committee of Sexual Medicine (FECSM), Roozbeh Psychiatric Hospital, Psychiatric and Clinical Psychology, Research Center, Tehran University of Medical Sciences, South Kargar Street, Tehran 13337, Iran. [3]School of Public Health, Tehran University of Medical Sciences, Tehran, Iran. [4]Clinical Trial Center, Tehran University of Medical Sciences, Tehran, Iran. [5]Department of Gynecology and Infertility, Imam Khomeini Hospital, Tehran University of Medical Sciences, Tehran, Iran. [6]Department of Pharmacognosy, School of Pharmacy, Shaheed Beheshti University of Medical Sciences, Tehran, Iran. [7]Department of Traditional Medicine, School of Traditional Pharmacology, Tehran University of Medical Sciences, Tehran, Iran.

References

1. Shifren JL, Monz BU, Russo PA, Segreti A, Johannes CB: Sexual problems and distress in United States women: prevalence and correlates. Obstet Gynecol 2008, 112(5):970–978.
2. Leiblum SR, KKoochaki PE, Rodenberg CA, Barton IP, Rosen RC: Hypoactive Sexual desire disorder in postmenopausal women: US results from the Women's International Study of Health and Sexuality (WISHeS). Menopause 2006, 13(1):46–56.
3. Dennerstein L, Koochaki P, Barton I, Graziottin A: Hypoactive sexual desire disorder in menopausal women: a survey of western European women. J Sex Med 2006, 3(2):212–22.
4. Hayes RD, Dennerstein L, Bennett CM, Fairley CK: What is the "true" prevalence of female sexual dysfunctions and does the way we assess these conditions have an impact? J Sex Med 2008, 5(4):777–778.
5. Safarinejad MR: Female sexual dysfunction in population based study in Iran: prevalence and associated risk factors. Int J Impot Res 2006, 18(4):382–395.
6. Davis SR, van der Mooren MJ, van Lunsen RH, Lopes P, Ribot J, Rees, Moufarege A, Rodenberg C, Buch A, Purdie DW: Efficacy and safety of a testosterone patch for the treatment of hypoactive sexual desire disorder in surgically menopausal women: a randomized, placebo-controlled trial. Menopause 2006, 13(3):387–396.
7. Berman JR, Berman LA, Werbin TJ, Goldstein I: Female sexual dysfunction: anatomy, physiology, evaluation and treatment options. Curr Opin Urol 1999, 9(6):563–568.
8. Segraves RT, Clayton A, Croft H, Wolf A, Warnock J: Bupropion sustained release for the treatment of hypoactive sexual desire disorder in premenopausal women. J Clin Psychopharmacol 2004, 24(3):339–342.
9. Kashani L, Raisi F, Saroukhani S, Sohrabi H, Modabbernia A, Nasehi AA, Jamshidi A, Ashrafi M, Mansouri P, Ghaeli P, Akhondzadeh S: Saffron for treatment of fluoxetine-induced sexual dysfunction in women: randomized double-blind placebo-controlled study. Hum Psychopharmacol 2013, 28(1):54–60.
10. Simon JA: Opportunities for intervention in HSDD. J Fam Pract 2009, 58(7 Suppl Hypoactive):S26–30.
11. Basson R, Leiblum S, Brotto L, Derogatis L, Fourcroy J, Fugl-Meyer K, Graziottin A, Heiman JR, Laan E, Meston C, Schover L, van Lankveld J, Schultz WW: Definitions of women's sexual dysfunction reconsidered: advocating expansion and revision. J Psychosom Obstet Gynaecol 2003, 24(4):221–229.
12. Clayton AH: The pathophysiology of hypoactive sexual desire disorder in women. International J of Gynecol Obstet 2010, 110(1):7–11.
13. Ibn-e-sina (Avicenna Husain): Al-Qanun fit-tib [The Canon of Medicine], (Research of Ebrahim Shamsedine). Beirut, Lebanon: Alaalami Beirut library Press; 2005.
14. Aghili Khorasani MH: Makhzan al Advieh. Tehran, Iran: Bavardaran Press. Research Institute for Islamic and Complementary Medicine, Iran University of Medical Sciences; 2001.
15. Mazaro-Costa R, Andersen ML, Hachul H, Tufik S: Medicinal plants as alternative treatments for female sexual dysfunction: Utopian vision or possible treatment in climacteric women? J Sex Med 2010, 7(11):3695–3714.
16. Esfandiari A, Dehghan A, Sharifi S, Vesali E: Effect of Tribulus Terresteris extract on ovarian activity in immature wistar rat: a histological evaluation. J Anim Vet Adv 2011, 7(10):883–886.
17. Brotto LA: The DSM4 diagnostic criteria for hypoactiove sexual desire disorder in women. Arch Sex Behav 2010, 39(2):221–239.
18. Zargari A: Medicinal plants, Vol 1; Tehran. Iran: Tehran University of Medical Sciences Press; 1989.
19. Abirami P, Rajendran A: GC-MS analysis of Tribulus terrestris. 1. Asian J Plant Sci Res 2011, 1(4):13–16.
20. Wiegel M, Meston C, Rosen R: The female sexual function index (FSFI): cross validation and development of clinical cutoff scores. J Sex Marital Ther 2005, 31(1):1–20.
21. Rosen R, Brown C, Heiman J, Meston C, Shabsigh R, Ferguson D, Agostino R Jr: The female sexualfunction index (FSFI): a multidimensional self-report instrument of female sexual function. J Sex Marital Thera 2000, 26(2):191–208.

Quantification of verbascoside in medicinal species of *Phlomis* and their genetic relationships

Parisa Sarkhail[1], Marjan Nikan[2], Pantea Sarkheil[1], Ahmad R Gohari[2,3], Yousef Ajani[4], Rohollah Hosseini[5], Abbass Hadjiakhoondi[2,6] and Soodabeh Saeidnia[2,3*]

Abstract

Background: The genus *Phlomis* (Lamiaceae) is introduced by its valuable medicinal species, of which 17 species are growing wildly and ten of them are exclusively endemic of Iran. The main phytochemical characteristic of this genus is presence of iridoid glycosides including ipolamide, auroside, lamiide and also phenylethanoids such as verbascoside (acetoside) found in Lamiales order.

Due to the broad range of biological and pharmacological activities of verbascoside and lack of any report on quantification of this compound within Iranian species of *Phlomis*, we conducted a research to achieve two main goals, finding a genetic biodiversity by RAPD (Randomly Amplified Polymorphic DNA), as well as detecting and quantifying verbascoside in nine species of *Phlomis* growing wildly in Iran.

Results: The results showed that various samples of *P.olivieri* possess different genetic distances from each other. Also, various species of *P.olivieri* display close relationships to *P.anisodonta* and *P. persica*. Phytoanalysis of *Phlomis* species by means of TLC scanner using verbascoside as a phytochemical marker showed that the highest concentration of verbascoside was found in *P. anisodonta*, however, *P. bruguieri* and *P. olivieri* (from Mazandaran) were in the second and third places. Interestingly, the lowest concentration of verbascoside was detected in *P. olivieri* (from Azerbayjan), exhibiting the effect of various growing areas and conditions on the measured levels of this compound.

Conclusions: verbascoside can be found in various species of Iranian *Phlomis*, of which *P. anisodonta*, *P. bruguieri* and *P. olivieri* might be the best choices. In addition, although the concentration of verbascoside in these plants may be affected by the growing areas and conditions, there are a good agreement between genetic relations and verbascoside levels.

Keywords: *Phlomis*, RAPD, Verbascoside, Quantification, TLC scanner

Background

The genus *Phlomis* (Lamiaceae) is introduced by its valuable medicinal properties. Seventeen species of *Phlomis* are growing wildly and ten of them are exclusively endemic of Iran [1,2]. The medicinal importance of *Phlomis* species (called: Gush-e Barreh in Persian language) had described by Dioscorides (first century B.C.) in "*De MateriaMedica*", and these plants have been employed in herbal medicine for respiratory tract disorders or wound healing till date [3].

However, a number of *Phlomis* species have been consumed in folk medicine as antitussive remedies, and also for gastrointestinal complains, tonic, sedative, carminative and astringent agents a well [4].

A survey on phytochemical characteristics of this genus revealed that *Phlomis* species are rich in iridoids, flavonoids, terpenoids, phenolic compounds and their glycosides, which are attributed to various biological and pharmacological effects of them including antinociceptive, antioxidant, antimicrobial and anti-diabetic effects [3-6]. The main phytochemical characteristics of this genus are presence of the iridoid glycosides including ipolamide, auroside, lamiide and also phenylethanoids such as verbascoside (acetoside), which is a caffeic acid

* Correspondence: saeidnia_s@tums.ac.ir
[2]Medicinal Plants Research Center, Faculty of Pharmacy, Tehran University of Medical Sciences, Tehran, Iran
[3]Division of Pharmacy, College of Pharmacy and Nutrition, University of Saskatchewan, Saskatoon, Canada
Full list of author information is available at the end of the article

sugar ester and can be found in plant species of Lamiales order [7-9].

Regarding to remarkable role of verbascoside in generation of a broad range of biological and pharmacological activities [10-12] and lack of any report on quantification of this compound within Iranian species of *Phlomis*, we tried to conduct a research to achieve two main goals, detection and quantification of verbascoside in nine species of *Phlomis* growing wildly in Iran, as well as finding a genetic biodiversity among them by RAPD analysis (Randomly Amplified Polymorphic DNA) appraising to the presence of a chemotaxonomic marker, verbascoside, whether or not it will be in agreement with phylogenetic cladogram.

Methods

Sample collection

Locations, altitudes and collection periods of the plant materials used in this study are given in Table 1. The plants were identified by Mr. Yousef Ajani from Institute of Medicinal Plants, Karaj, Iran. The voucher specimens have been deposited at two Herbariums located at Faculty of Pharmacy, Tehran University of Medical Sciences, and Institute of Medicinal Plants (IMP), Iranian Academic Centre for Education, Culture and Research (ACECR) in Iran. Plant materials were dried in shadow and the leaves of the plants were separated from the stem, and were ground to powder in porcelain mortars with liquid nitrogen. Then, the powdered plant material was used for DNA extraction.

DNA extraction

Genomic DNA(s) were extracted from the plant materials using a modified method, which was already described

[13]. Approximately 150 mg of each plant sample was frozen in liquid nitrogen (in 2-ml Eppendorf tubes). 500 ml of DNA extraction buffer (contains, 2% CTAB {cetyl trimethylammonium bromide}, 100 mM TrisHCl (pH = 8), 20 mM EDTA {ethylene diamine tetra acetic acid}, 1.4 M NaCl, 0.2% 2-mercaptoethanol and 4% PVP {polyvinylpyrrolidone}) was added to each Eppendorf tube and mixed well. The mixture was incubated at 65°C in a water bath for 60 min with intermittent shaking at 5 to 10 min intervals. The mixture was mixed with equal volume of phenol: cloroform: isoamylalchol (25:24:1), and centrifuged at $13000 \times g$ for 10 min at 24°C. The supernatant was transferred into a new 1.5-ml tube and 800 µl cold isopropanol (from freezer) was added and inverting until thoroughly mixed and placed in the freezer (-20°C) for 20 min. The mixture centrifuged at $13000 \times g$ for 5 min at 4°C. The supernatant was removed and the precipitate was kept at room temperature for 15 min and then, mixed gently with 300 µl ammonium acetate (7.5 M) for 20 min at room temperature. After centrifugation at $13000 \times g$ for 10 min at 4°C, the supernatant was removed and 600 µl of ethanol (70%) was added then centrifuged at $6000 \times g$ for 10 min at 4°C. The DNA was pelleted by centrifugation and the ethanol was poured off, the DNA was allowed to air-dry before being dissolved in 200 µl of TE buffer.

Primers

Thirty RAPD primers (ten-mers) were purchased from two companies: Operon Technologies, Alameda, California, USA and Cinnagen, Tehran, Iran. The primers were tested for amplification in a preliminary study, because in RAPD analysis, some primers will work and some may not. In preliminary study, quickly screening of three sets of primers,

Table 1 Locations, altitudes and collection periods of the plant materials used in RAPD analysis

Number	Herbarium No.	Species	Location	Altitude (m)	Date
1	1612	*P. olivieri*	Marivan to paveh, 51 km a paveh 35°14′27.7″N, 46°11′45.6″E	2448	07, 2011
2	1611	*P. persica*	Sanandaj to marivan, 108 km a marivan 35°24′53.9″N, 46°53′12.5″E	1766	07, 2011
3	1557	*P .rigida*	Sanandaj to marivan,between sheikh attar and baghan 35°30′54.0″N, 46°27′32.5″E	1598	07, 2011
4	1582	*P.kurdica*	Sanandaj to marivan, 41 km a sanandaj 35°22′51.7″N, 46°42′46.7″E	1595	07, 2011
5	1610	*P.persica*	Olalan region, 5 km a kargabad to salavatbad 35°17′13.6″N, 47°09′42.3″E	2218	07, 2011
6	1581	*P. bruguieri*	Sanandaj to marivan,in the beginning of the road 35°22′35.4″N, 47°00′11.5″E	1519	07, 2011
7	1580	*P. anisodonta*	Marivan to paveh between dezli and hanigarmohalleh 35°16′39.4″N, 46°11′11.2″E	2246	07, 2011
8	1648	*P. caucasica*	Ahar; Khoy to qotur, 45 km a qotur, 35° 22′51.7″N, 46°42′ 46.7″E	-	07, 2011
9		*P. olivieri*	Shabestar (details are not available)	-	07, 2010
10	1631	*P. olivieri*	Azerbayjan; Khoy to qotur, 45 km a qotur, 35°22′51.7″N, 46°42′46.7″E	1297	06, 2011
11	—	*P. olivieri*	Tabriz (details are not available)	-	07, 2010
12	1634	*P. anisodonta*	Mazandaran, 5 km after pol-e zanguleh toward yush, 36°12′0.3.3″N, 51°20′50.7″E	2558	06, 2011
13	6532	*P. persica*	North of Iran (details are not available)	-	07, 2002
14	6534	*P. olivieri*	Mazandaran (details are not available)	-	07, 2001
15	6531	*P. anisodonta*	North of Iran, pol-e- zangule	-	07, 2002

which previously used successfully for RAPD analysis of other Labiatae species [14,15], was performed using some samples of *Phlomis*, and then those which were giving good profiles for analysis of a large number of samples were selected. Some of the primers were chosen for further analysis (Table 2) based on their ability to produce distinct and polymorphic amplified products within the samples [14]. As a matter of fact, RAPD does not need any particular knowledge of the DNA sequence of the target organism and the amplification is randomly performed. Because the identical 10-mer primers can (or cannot) amplify a segment of DNA, relating to the positions, which are complementary to the primers' sequence. For instance, when a mutation has occurred in one of the samples (DNAs) just at the site that was already

complementary to the primer, a PCR product would not be produced, therefore a different pattern of amplified DNAs might be observed.

RAPD assay

Polymerase chain reactions (PCR) with single primer were carried out in a final volume of 20 µl containing 20 ng template DNA, 20 ng of primer (0.5 to 1 µl), 6 µl of RNase-free water and 10 µl of Taq PCR Master Mix kit (includes 1.5 mM $MgCl_2$, 125 units of TaqDNA Polymerase, and 200 µM each dNTP), purchased from Qiagen, USA. Amplification was performed in a Primus 25 (Peqlab, Germany) thermal cycler, programmed for a preliminary 3 min denaturation step at 94°C, followed by 44 cycles of denaturation at 94°C for 30 s, annealing at 36 +

Table 2 Sequencing primers used for RAPD analysis together with total number of amplified fragments and the polymorphism percentage

Primer	Sequences 5' to 3'	Total bands	Polymorphism percentage
Zo1	GGT-CGG-AGA- \<A\>	11	100
Zo2	TCG-GAC-GTG- \<A\>	8	100
Zo3	AGA-CGT-CCA- \<C\>	7	87
Zo4	GGA-AGT-CGC- \<C\>	13	88
Zo5	AGT-CGT-CCC- \<C\>	10	100
Zo6	CTG-CAT-CGT– \<G\>	11	100
Zo7	GAA-ACA-CCC- \<C\>	9	90
Zo8	TGT-AGC-TGG- \<G\>	7	98
Zo9	ACG-CGC-ATG- \<T\>	13	78
Zo10	GAC-GCC-ACA- \<C\>	10	96
Zo11	ACC-AGG-TTG- \<G\>	13	100
Zo12	AAT-GGC-GCA- \<G\>	16	100
Zo13	CAC-TCT-CCT- \<C\>	12	100
Zo14	GAA-TCG-GCC- \<A\>	13	89
Zo15	CTG-ACC-AGC- \<C\>	7	99
Zo16	GGG-AGA-CTA- \<C\>	8	98
Zo17	ACA-ACG-CGA- \<G\>	10	89
Zo18	CCG-CCT-AGT- \<C\>	13	100
Zo19	GGA-GGA-GAG- \<G\>	7	100
Zo20	TCA-TCC-GAG- \<G\>	5	100
Zo21	CAG-AAG-CCC- \<A\>	9	90
Zo22	AAG-GCG-GCA- \<G\>	10	96
Zo23	CAG-CGA-CAA- \<G\>	6	100
Zo24	TGG-AGA-GCA- \<G\>	7	100
Z025	ACA-TGC-CGT- \<G\>	4	100
Zo26	CTG-GGG-CTG- \<A\>	10	100
Zo27	TGA-CGG-AGG- \<T\>	9	98
Zo28	TCT-CCG-CCC- \<T\>	9	78
Zo29	TGC-CCA-GCC- \<T\>	13	90
Zo30	AAA-GTG-CGG- \<G\>	7	96

4°C/ 30 s and extension at 72°C for 1 min, finally at 72°C for 2 min for amplification. PCR products (alongside the negative control and GelPilot DNA Mulecular Weight Marker: 100 bp) were separated by 1% (w/v) agarose gel electrophoresis for RAPD respectively. Green viewer (4 µl) was used to visualize under UV light (Benchtop 3 UV™ Transilluminator) and photographs were recorded by a Canon digital camera. Data were summarized based on the presence or absence of unique and shared polymorphic bands from the photographs. Each amplification fragment was detected by approximate size in base pairs. The DNA profiles were scored visually from photographs of the gels. Reproducible bans (observed at least for two times) were considered for analysis. A pair-wise difference matrix between samples was determined for the RAPD data using simple matching coefficient (Ssm) followed by calculation of genetic distances (d) [15]. UPGMA (unweighted pair-group method arithmetic average) was used to construct the dendrogram. UPGMA employed a sequential clustering algorithm, in which genetic distances were used in order to show similarity, and the phylogenetic tree was built in a stepwise manner [16]. Also, the number of unique bands in various samples by each primer is shown in a table as Additional file 1. In this method, the first cluster is built on the pair of plant DNAs with the smallest distance, then following the first cluster is considered as a single composite and the new distance matrix can be calculated as follows:

$$Distance(A, B), C = (distance\,AC + distance\,BC)$$

Again, a new distance matrix is recalculated using the newly calculated distances and the whole cycle is being repeated. The final step consists of clustering the last Plant DNA sample with the composite of all others.

The cladogram constructed base on genetic distances, derived from RAPD analysis, shown in Figure 1. The indicated cladogram was designed by the software Dendroscope which is freely available from http://dendroscope.org [17,18]. Also, Figure 2 exhibits a gel electrophoresis of RAPD pattern of the plant DNA samples with primer Zo21.

HPTLC (High Performance Thin Layer Chromatography) analysis
Reagents and Instruments
Silica gel 60 F_{254} pre-coated plates (Merck) were used for preliminary TLCs. The spots were detected by spraying anisaldehyde-H_2SO_4 reagent followed by heating.

All the chemicals and reagents used for TLC were purchased from Merck by analytical grades. The instrument for HPTLC was from CAMAG. The TLC scanner was CS-9000, Dual Wavelength, Flying-spot Scanner (Shimadzu).

Sample preparation for TLC scanner
Dried and powdered leaves of *Phlomis* species (100 g) were extracted twice with MeOH (80%, 1500 ml) in percolator for one week. The combined methanol extracts were evaporated by Rotary Evaporator. Dried crude extract was dissolved in water and the water soluble portion was successively fractionated using dichloromethane, diethyl ether and n-butanol, respectively. The n-butanol layers were combined and concentrated to dryness in vacuo at <45°C. The n-butanol extracts (80 mg/mL) and the standard solutions of verbascoside were prepared in MeOH.

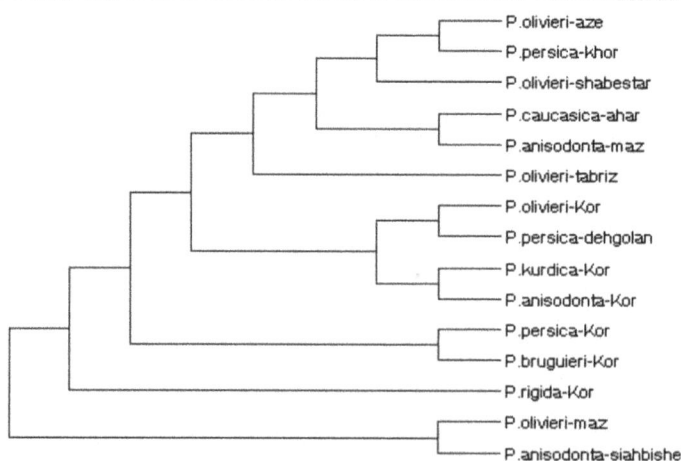

Figure 1 Cladogram of *Phlomis* samples based on the UPGMA analysis. (1) *P. olivieri-kor* (Kordestan), (2) *P. persica-kor* (Kordestan), (3) *P. rigida-kor* (kordestan) , (4) *P. kurdica-kor* (Kordestan) , (5) *P. persica-dehgolan* (kordestan) (6) *P. bruguieri-kor* (Kordestan), (7) *P. anisodonta-kor* (Kordestan), (8) *P. caucasica* (Ahar), (9) *P. olivieri-shabestar* (Shabestar), (10) *P. olivieri-azer* (Azerbayjan), (11) *P. olivieri-tabriz* (Tabriz), (12) *P. anisodonta-maz* (Mazandaran), (13) *P. persica-khor* (Khorasan), (14) *P. olivieri-maz* (Mazandaran), (15) *P. anisodonta-siahbishe* (Pole zangole).

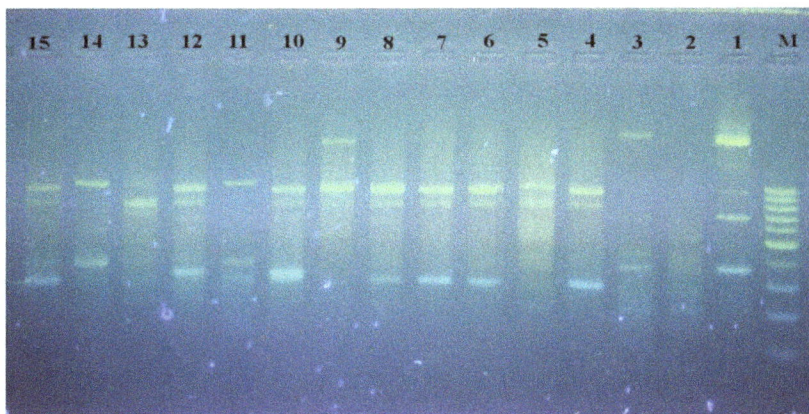

Figure 2 RAPD profile produced from the primer, Zo 21; M: DNA size marker. (1) *P. olivieri* (Kordestan), (2) *P. persica* (Kordestan), (3) *P. rigida* (kordestan), (4) *P. kurdica* (Kordestan) , (5) *P. persica* (dehgolan) (6) *P. bruguieri* (Kordestan), (7) *P. anisodonta* (Kordestan), (8) *P. caucasica* (Ahar), (9) *P. olivieri* (Shabestar), (10) *P. olivieri* (Azerbayjan), (11) *P. olivieri* (Tabriz), (12) *P. anisodonta* (Mazandaran), (13) *P. persica* (Khorasan), (14) *P. olivieri* (Mazandaran), (15) *P. anisodonta* (Pole zangole).

Thin - layer chromatography

The plates were pre washed with methanol and dried for 24 h at room temperature. Before use they were activated at 120°C for 30 min. The activated plates were manually spotted with 1 μL aliquots of the solutions. The mobile phase (ethylacetate: water: formic acid, 10:3:2) was used per development. Plates were developed to a distance of 15 mm in chromatographic chamber. Then the plates were dried in a current of air by means of an air dryer. Densitometer scanning was then performed at λmax = 234 nm. The radiation source was a deuterium lamp emitting a continuous UV spectrum between 200-370 nm. Each analysis was repeated five times, whilst each track scanned three times, and baseline correction (lowest slope) was used. The start wavelength was 200 nm and the end wavelength was 370 nm. The verbascoside was quantified by densitometric scanning of the developed plate at 270 nm.

Validation of the method
Linearity of detector response

The linearity of the TLC method was evaluated by analysis of 4 standard solutions of verbascoside at concentrations 1.2, 0.9, 0.6 and 0.3 mg/mL. The solutions were applied on the same plate. The plate was developed using the above-mentioned mobile phase.

Specificity

The specificity of the method was ascertained by comparing the Rf values and the spectrum of verbascoside standard with the spectrum obtained from a sample of the extract, at three different positions on the bands, i.e. peak start (S), peak apex (M), and peak end (E) [19]. The Rf value for verbascoside and the relative spots in the

plant samples was equal to 0.65 in the mobile phase as ethylacetate: water: formic acid, (10:3:2) (Figure 3).

Results and discussion

RAPD markers have been widely used in the analysis of genetic relationships and genetic diversity in a number of plant taxa because of its simplicity, speed and relatively low cost compared to other DNA-based markers. Pairwise comparison of all RAPD profiles revealed a similarity matrix. Simple matching coefficients (Ssm) and genetic distances (d), derived from RAPD banding patterns, are shown in Figure 4. The range of genetic distances between different species of *phlomis* from Iran was calculated between 316-988.Actually, the most far away genetic distance (d = 0.990) has been observed between *P. bruguieri* (Kordestan) and *P. olivieri* from Mazandaran followed by the distance between *P. anisodonta* (Kordestan) and *P. persica* from Khorasan (d = 0.988), as well as *P. persica* (Kordestan) and *P. anisodonta* (Mazandaran) (d = 0.988), while the closest distance (d = 316) has been observed for *P. persica* from Dehgolan and *P. olivieri* from Kordestan. The farthest and closest distances are indicated in the Figure 4 by bold and underlined numbers, respectively. The genetic distance between the two samples, *P. olivieri* (Azerbayejan) and *P. persica* (Khorasan), was observed to be short (0.622) and their RAPD banding patterns were quite similar to each other; also there is a close relationship between these two samples of *Phlomis* with *P. olivieri* from Shabestar.

As shown in the dendrogram, various species of *P. olivieri* display close relationships to *P. anisodonta* and *P. persica*. On the other hand, *P. anisodonta* species represents the closest relationship with *P. Caucasica* and *P. kurdica*. It is interesting to note that different samples of *P. olivieri*,

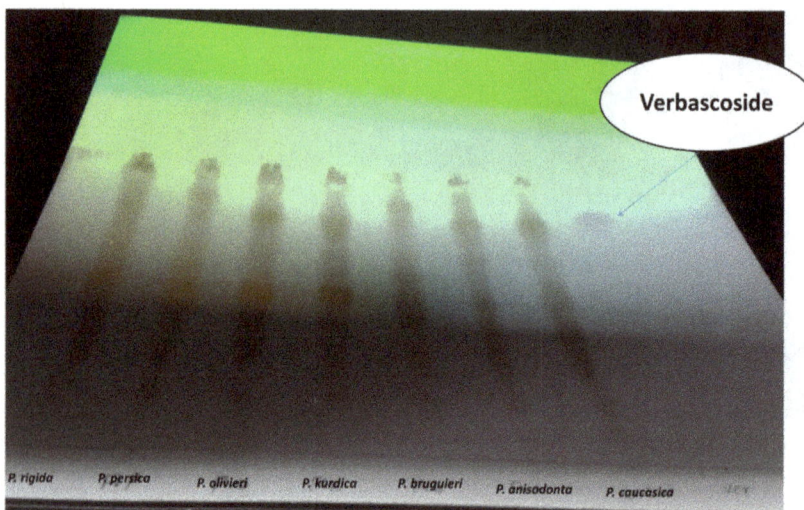

Figure 3 Verbascoside and the relative spots in the plant samples on a TLC plate under UV chamber (254 nm) in the mobile phase, ethylacetate: water: formic acid (10:3:2).

Samples	1	2	3	4	5	6	7	8	9	10	11	12	13	14	15
1		0.12	0.072	0.213	0.1	0.109	0.231	0.166	0.089	0.343	0.172	0.095	0.357	0.03	0.082
2	0.938		0.064	0.12	0.084	0.141	0.128	0.094	0.151	0.085	0.112	0.139	0.058	0.058	0.088
3	0.963	0.967		0.059	0.064	0.092	0.055	0.051	0.079	0.061	0.059	0.094	0.022	0.024	0.039
4	0.887	0.938	0.97		0.075	0.089	0.171	0.14	0.098	0.316	0.154	0.098	0.326	0.121	0.088
5	0.316*	0.957	0.967	0.961		0.092	0.073	0.064	0.088	0.05	0.084	0.09	0.077	0.056	0.097
6	0.943	0.926	0.952	0.954	0.952		0.08	0.105	0.137	0.118	0.125	0.189	0.03	0.032	0.052
7	0.876	0.933	0.972	0.91	0.962	0.959		0.144	0.083	0.295	0.115	0.112	0.302	0.018	0.057
8	0.913	0.951	0.974	0.927	0.967	0.946	0.925		0.052	0.226	0.227	0.308	0.052	0.022	0.056
9	0.954	0.921	0.959	0.949	0.954	0.928	0.957	0.973		0.151	0.17	0.252	0.043	0.046	0.075
10	0.810	0.915	0.969	0.827	0.974	0.939	0.839	0.879	0.921		0.259	0.092	0.46	0.041	0.06
11	0.909	0.942	0.97	0.919	0.957	0.935	0.94	0.879	0.911	0.86		0.064	0.068	0.039	0.078
12	0.951	0.927	0.951	0.949	0.953	0.900	0.942	0.831	0.864	0.952	0.967		0.053	0.063	0.093
13	0.801	0.970	**0.988**	0.820	0.96	0.984	0.835	0.973	0.978	0.734	0.965	0.973		0.142	0.119
14	0.984	0.970	0.987	0.937	0.971	0.983	**0.990**	**0.988**	0.976	0.979	0.980	0.967	0.926		0.236
15	0.958	0.954	0.98	0.954	0.950	0.973	0.971	0.971	0.961	0.969	0.960	0.952	0.938	0.874	

Figure 4 Simple matching coefficient (S_{sm}, above the diagonal) and genetic distances (d, below the diagonal) between pairs of *Phlomis* samples resulted from RAPD. (1) *P. olivieri* (Kordestan), (2) *P. persica* (Kordestan), (3) *P. rigida* (kordestan), (4) *P. kurdica* (Kordestan), (5) *P. persica* (dehgolan), (6) *P. bruguieri* (Kordestan), (7) *P. anisodonta* (Kordestan), (8) *P. caucasica* (Ahar), (9) *P. olivieri* (Shabestar), (10) *P. olivieri* (Azerbayjan), (11) *P. olivieri* (Tabriz), (12) *P. anisodonta* (Mazandaran), (13) *P. persica* (Khorasan), (14) *P. olivieri* (Mazandaran), (15) *P. anisodonta* (Pole zangole); * The underlined number shows the closest genetic distance; ** The bold numbers exhibit the farthest genetic distances.

gathered from different habitats, did not exhibit so much close relationship to each other. Figure 2 shows a photo sample from a gel electrophoresis of all DNA samples alongside a DNA size marker in the presence of primer Zo21. RAPD molecular markers exhibited significant differences between various samples of the same species growing in different areas.

The results of quantification of verbascoside in different *Phlomis* species by using TLC scanner revealed that the highest concentration of verbascoside was found in *P. anisodonta*, however, *P. bruguieri* and *P. olivieri* (from Mazandaran) were in the second and third places (Table 3). Interestingly, the lowest concentration of verbascoside was detected in *P. olivieri* (from Azerbayjan), exhibiting the effect of various growing areas and conditions on the measured levels of this compound. Although the concentration of verbascoside in these plants may be affected by the growing areas and conditions, there are a good agreement between genetic relations and verbascoside levels. For instance, the concentration of verbascoside in three samples of *P.olivieri* (Azerbayjan, Shabestar, Tabriz) is significantly different (Table 3), alongside the far distances of these samples from the same species (Figure 1). Another example is almost equal level of verbascoside in *P. caucasica* and *P. olivieri* (Azerbayjan) (4.1 and 3.9 mg/mL, respectively) that support the close relationship between these two species (d = 0.879), in compared to those of Mazandaran and Kurdistan or Shabestar (Figure 4).

Verbascoside was previously isolated and identified from various species of *Phlomis*, of which *P. sieheana*, *P. samia*, *P. monocephala* and *P. carica* are recently reported from Turkey [20,21]. Furthermore, verbascoside is a phenylpropanoid glycoside well-known for its antioxidant, anti-inflammatory and photoprotective activity, and recently applied in dermocosmetic preparations. Moreover, verbascoside is used in formulation of suppositories for probable applications in treatment of inflammation in the intestinal mucosa [10,22]. A recent report reveals that verbascoside possesses stronger affinity for negatively charged membranes composed of phosphatidylglycerol than for phosphatidylcholine membranes. However, this compound can promot phase separation of lipid domains in phosphatidylcholine membranes and formed a stable lipid complex [23]. Regarding the importance of verbascoside as an active ingredient in *Phlomis* species, quantification of this compound is a successful method for standardization of the *Phlomis* extracts. Actually, the quantitative determination of phenylethanoid glycosides in methanolic extracts of five species of the genus *Phlomis* has been already investigated by using HPLC method combined with photodiode-array detection and electrospray/MS analysis. In that study, forsythoside B, verbascoside, samioside, alyssonoside, isoverbascoside, leucosceptosides A and B and martynoside were employed for detection. Although the results of that report is not comparable with the present study due to using different method of quantification as well as different species Phlomis, the investigators demonstrated that the content of phenylethanoid glycosides contributes to the chemotaxonomy of this genus [24]. Moreover, phenylethanoid glycosides like verbascoside, forsythoside B, and leucosceptoside A have been reported from *P. longifolia* [25]. However, acteoside and forsythoside B were also isolated from *P. tuberosa* [26].

Actually, plant secondary metabolite pathways have extensively been studied at the level of intermediates and enzymes that mainly lead to pharmaceutically important products. However, only a relatively small number of genes have been identified so far [27]. In fact, the idea about the probable link between plant genotype and its

Table 3 The concentration of verbascoside determined by using TLC-scanner in different species of *Phlomis*

Plant Samples/or Standards	Calculated Area	Concentration (mg/mL) Mean ± SD
P. olivieri (Azerbayjan)	257559.8	3.9 ± 0.2
P. olivieri (Tabriz)	461645.8	8.6 ± 0.2
P. olivieri (Mazandaran)	479058.9	9.1 ± 0.4
P. bruguieri	506145.9	9.6 ± 0.5
P. kurdica	393148.1	7.0 ± 0.1
P. rigida	515808.8	9.8 ± 0.1
P. anisodonta	578081.9	11.3 ± 0.2
P. persica	463498.0	8.6 ± 0.4
P. caucasica	264396.1	4.1 ± 0.2
Verbascoside (1.2 mg/mL)	614373.5	12.0 ± 0.6
Verbascoside (0.9 mg/mL)	462891.9	9.0 ± 0.3
Verbascoside (0.6 mg/mL)	363006.8	6.0 ± 0.4
Verbascoside (0.3 mg/mL)	212619.3	3.0 ± 0.2

phytochemistry has been demonstrated by different studies so far. For instance, when genetic distance between genotypes of cottonwoods increased, the phytochemistry and arthropod community composition changed accordingly [28]. RAPD method, which can be used as one of the molecular biological techniques to determine genetic distances, has many advantages as follows: There is no need to knowledge of the DNA sequence for the targeted gene; It can be used for most genetic marker applications; The procedure is streamlined compared to other molecular analysis; It needs only thermocycler and agarose gel so is cost effective with less labor [29].

The present study demonstrates that RAPD analysis can be used beside phytochemical analysis of secondary metabolites in plants, due to the relationship between phytochemistry and genetic distances, and may create the useful fingerprints and molecular profiles to support phytochemical diversity data from plants.

Conclusions

In conclusion, the present study reveals that verbascoside can be found in various species of Iranian *Phlomis*, of which *P. anisodonta*, *P. bruguieri* and *P. olivieri* might be the best choices. In addition, although the concentration of verbascoside in these plants may be affected by the growing areas and conditions, there are a good agreement between genetic relations and verbascoside levels.

Additional file

Additional file 1: The number of unique bands in different samples of *Phlomis* produced by each primer.

Competing interests
The authors declared that there is no conflict of interests.

Authors' contributions
PP: Interpreting of the HPTLC data; MN: DNA extraction and analysis; PP: Participating in TLC scanner analysis; ARG: Plant gathering and HPTLC advising; YA: Plant identification; SRH: Standardization of the HPTLC method; AH: Advising the plant extraction and verbascoside analysis; SS: Participating in manuscript drafting and interpreting of RAPD data. All authors read and approved the final manuscript.

Acknowledgements
This research has been supported by Tehran University of Medical Sciences and Health Services Grant (No. 14177).

Author details
[1]Pharmaceutical Sciences Research Center, Tehran University of Medical Sciences, Tehran, Iran. [2]Medicinal Plants Research Center, Faculty of Pharmacy, Tehran University of Medical Sciences, Tehran, Iran. [3]Division of Pharmacy, College of Pharmacy and Nutrition, University of Saskatchewan, Saskatoon, Canada. [4]Institute of Medicinal Plants (IMP), Iranian Academic Centre for Education, Culture and Research (ACECR), Karaj, Iran. [5]Department of Toxicology and Pharmacology, Faculty of Pharmacy, Tehran University of Medical Sciences, Tehran 1417614411, Iran. [6]Department of Pharmacognosy, Faculty of Pharmacy, Tehran University of Medical Sciences, Tehran 1417614411, Iran.

References
1. Albaladejo RG, Aparicio A, Silvestre S: Variation patterns in the *Phlomis* × composite (Lamiaceae) hybride complex in Iberian Peninsula. *Bot J Linn Soc* 2004, 145:97–108.
2. Rechinger KH: *Flora Iranica*. Graz-Austria: Akademic Druck-u Verlagsanstalt; 1982.
3. Couldis M, Tanimanidis A, Tzakou O, Chinou IB, Harvala C: Essential oil of *Phlomis lanata* growing in Greece: chemical composition and antimicrobial activity. *Planta Med* 2000, 66:670–672.
4. Sarkhail P, Abdollahi M, Fadayevatan S, Shafiee A, Mohammadirad A, Dehghan G, Esmaily H, Amin G: Effect of *Phlomis persica* on glucose levels and hepatic enzymatic antioxidants in streptozotocin-induced diabetic rats. *Pharmacogn Mag* 2010, 6(Suppl 23):219–224.
5. Sarkhail P, Abdollahi M, Shafiee A: Antinociceptive effect of *Phlomis olivieri* Benth., *Phlomis anisodonta* Boiss. and *Phlomis persica* Boiss. total extracts. *Pharmacol Res* 2003, 48(Suppl 3):263–266.
6. Dellai A, Mansour HB, Limem I, Bouhlel I, Sghaier MB, Boubaker J, Ghedira K, Chekir-Ghedira L: Screening of antimutagenicity via antioxidant activity in different extracts from the flowers of *Phlomis crinita* Cav. Ssp *mauritanica* munby from the center of Tunisia. *Drug ChemToxicol* 2009, 32:283–292.
7. Kamel MS, Mohamed KM, Hassanean HA, Ohtani K, Kasai R, Yamasaki K: Iridoid and megastigmane glycosides from *Phlomis aurea*. *Phytochemistry* 2000, 55:353–357.
8. Ersoz T, Saracoglu I, Harput US, Calis I: Iridoid and Phenylpropanoid Glycosides from *Phlomis randiflora* var. *mbrilligera* and *Phlomis fruticosa*. *Turk J Chem* 2002, 26:171–178.
9. Sarkhail P, Monsef-Esfehani HR, Amin G, Salehi Surmaghi MH, Shafiee A: Phytochemical study of *Phlomis olivieri* Benth. and *Phlomis persica* Boiss. *Daru* 2006, 14(Suppl 3):115–121.
10. Vertuani S, Beghelli E, Scalambra E, Malisardi G, Copetti S, Dal Toso R, Baldisserotto A, Manfredini S: Activity and stability studies of verbascoside, a novel antioxidant, in dermo-cosmetic and pharmaceutical topical formulations. *Molecules* 2011, 16(Suppl 8):7068–7080.
11. Santos-Cruz LF, Ávila-Acevedo JG, Ortega-Capitaine D, Ojeda-Duplancher JC, Perdigón-Moya JL, Hernández-Portilla LB, López-Dionicio H, Durán-Díaz A, Dueñas-García IE, Castañeda-Partida L, García-Bores AM, Heres-Pulido ME: Verbascoside is not genotoxic in the ST and HB crosses of the Drosophila wing spot test, and its constituent, caffeic acid, decreases the spontaneous mutation rate in the ST cross. *Food ChemToxicol* 2012, 50(Suppl 3–4):1082–1090.
12. Isacchi B, Iacopi R, Bergonzi MC, Ghelardini C, Galeotti N, Norcini M, Vivoli E, Vincieri FF, Bilia AR: Antihyperalgesic activity of verbascoside in two models of neuropathic pain. *J Pharm Pharmacol* 2011, 63(Suppl 4):594–601.
13. Doyle JJ, Doyle JL: Isolation of plant DNA from fresh tissue. *Focus* 1990, 12:13–15.
14. Saeidnia S, Gohari AR, Ito M, Honda G, Hadjiakhoondi A: Phylogenetic analysis of Badrashbu species using DNA polymorphism. *J Med Plants* 2005, 4(Suppl 15):66–72.
15. Saeidnia S, Sepehrizadeh Z, Gohari AR, Jaberi E, Amin GR, Hadjiakhoondi A: Determination of genetic relations among four Salvia L. species using RAPD analysis. *World Appl Sci J* 2009, 6(Suppl 2):238–241.
16. Nei M, Li WH: Mathematical modes for studying genetic variation in terms of restriction endonucleases. *Proc Natl Acad Sci U S A* 1979, 76(Suupl 10):5269–5273.
17. Huson DH, Richter DC, Rausch C, Dezulian T, Franz M, Rupp R: Dendroscope: an interactive viewer for large phylogenetictrees. *BMC Bioinform* 2007, 8:460.
18. Saeidnia S, Faraji H, Sarkheil P, Moradi-Afrapoli F, Amin G: Genetic diversity and relationships detected by inter simple sequence repeat (ISSR) and randomly amplified polymorphic DNA (RAPD) analysis among *Polygonum* species growing in North of Iran. *Afr J Biotechnol* 2011, 10(Suppl 82):18981–18985.
19. Gohari AR, Saeidnia S, Hadjiakhoondi A, Abdoullahi M, Nezafati M: Isolation and quantificative analysis of oleanolic acid from *Satureja mutica* Fisch. & C.A. Mey. *J Med Plants* 2009, 8(Suppl 5):65–69.
20. Ersoz T, Harput US, Calis I: Iridoid, phenylethanoid and monoterpene glycosides from *Phlomis sieheana*. *Turk J Chem* 2002, 26:1–8.

21. Yalcin FN, Ersoz T, Akbay P, Calis I: **Iridoid and phenylpropanoid glycosides from *Phlomissamia, P. monocephala* and *P. carica*.** *Turk J Chem* 2003, **27**:295–305.

22. Algieri F, Zorrilla P, Rodriguez-Nogales A, Garrido-Mesa N, Bañuelos O, González-Tejero MR, Casares-Porcel M, Molero-Mesa J, Zarzuelo A, Utrilla MP, Rodriguez-Cabezas ME, Galvez J: **Intestinal anti-inflammatory activity of hydroalcoholic extracts of Phlomis purpurea L. and *Phlomis lychnitis* L. in the trinitrobenzenesulphonic acid model of rat colitis.** *J Ethnopharmacol* 2013, **146**:750–709.

23. Funes L, Laporta O, Cerdán-Calero M, Micol V: **Effects of verbascoside, a phenylpropanoid glycoside from lemon verbena, on phospholipid model membranes.** *Chem Phys Lipids* 2010, **163**(Suppl 2):190–199.

24. Kirmizibekmez H, Montoro P, Piacente S, Pizza C, Dönmez A, Caliş I: **Identification by HPLC-PAD-MS and quantification by HPLC-PAD of phenylethanoid glycosides of five *Phlomis* species.** *Phytochem Anal* 2005, **16**:1–6.

25. Ersöz T, Schühly W, Popov S, Handjieva N, Sticher O, Caliş I: **Iridoid and phenylethanoid glycosides from *Phlomis longifolia* var. *longifolia*.** *Nat Prod Lett* 2001, **15**:345–351.

26. Ersöz T, Ivancheva S, Akbay P, Sticher O, Caliş I: **Iridoid and phenylethanoid glycosides from *Phlomis tuberosa* L.** *Z Naturforsch C* 2001, **56**:695–698.

27. Verpoorte R, van der Heijden R, Memelink J: **Engineering the plant cell factory for secondary metabolite production.** *Transgenic Res* 2000, **9**:323–343.

28. Iason GR, Dicke M, Hartley SE: *The Ecology of Plant Secondary Metabolites: From Genes to Global Processes.* New York: Cambridge University Press; 2012:311.

29. Saeidnia S, Gohari AR: *Pharmacognosy and Molecular Pharmacognosy in Practice.* Germany: LAP Lambert Academic Publishing; 2012.

Current approaches of the management of mercury poisoning: need of the hour

Mehrdad Rafati-Rahimzadeh[1], Mehravar Rafati-Rahimzadeh[2], Sohrab Kazemi[3] and Ali Akbar Moghadamnia[3,4*]

Abstract

Mercury poisoning cases have been reported in many parts of the world, resulting in many deaths every year. Mercury compounds are classified in different chemical types such as elemental, inorganic and organic forms. Long term exposure to mercury compounds from different sources e.g. water, food, soil and air lead to toxic effects on cardiovascular, pulmonary, urinary, gastrointestinal, neurological systems and skin. Mercury level can be measured in plasma, urine, feces and hair samples. Urinary concentration is a good indicator of poisoning of elemental and inorganic mercury, but organic mercury (e.g. methyl mercury) can be detected easily in feces. Gold nanoparticles (AuNPs) are a rapid, cheap and sensitive method for detection of thymine bound mercuric ions. Silver nanoparticles are used as a sensitive detector of low concentration Hg^{2+} ions in homogeneous aqueous solutions. Besides supportive therapy, British anti lewisite, dimercaprol (BAL), 2,3-dimercaptosuccinic acid (DMSA. succimer) and dimercaptopropanesulfoxid acid (DMPS) are currently used as chelating agents in mercury poisoning. Natural biologic scavengers such as algae, azolla and other aquatic plants possess the ability to uptake mercury traces from the environment.

Keywords: Mercury compounds, Chelating agents, Poisoning, Gold nanoparticles, Natural biologic scavengers

Introduction

Mercury (Hg) atomic number 80, is a liquid metal at room temperature and pressure. Mercury freezes at -38.9°C and boils at 357°C. It is sometimes called quick silver and is easily alloyed with many other metals, such as gold, silver and tin [1]. It exists in the environment in three forms: elemental mercury (poisonous as vapor), organic mercury (methyl mercury and ethyl mercury) and inorganic mercury (mercuric mercury) and all these forms have toxic health effects [2].

In recent years, due to abundant availability of various chemicals, the rate of intoxication has been surprisingly increased [3,4]. People can overuse or misuse drugs, chemicals, and may get poisoned intentionally or accidentally [5,6]. Similarly, heavy metals, either released from natural sources or from industries wastes pose a consistent health threat to human being [7].

Mercury could be found in different commercial forms [8]. Mercury and its related compounds are being circulated and concentrated in soil and distributed into the air via coal fuels, industrial furnaces or active volcanoes. It then returns to the soil, water, or living organisms. Recycling from atmospheric emission, deposition in water reservoirs and exposure and bioaccumulation in animals and humans is a known example of mercury cycle in the environment [9] (see Figure 1).

Epidemiology

Humans exposure to mercury usually take place via eating mercury contaminated food, dental care procedures (using amalgams in endodontics) using mercury based, thermometers, and sphygmomanometer), occupational exposure (e.g. mining) and others (using fluorescent light bulbs and batteries) [10].

Metallic mercury intoxication was known in ancient times by Aristotle, but that large scale occupational poisoning with mercury had occurred when the great statue of Buddha of Nara was constructed in 8th century in Japan [11].

* Correspondence: moghadamnia@yahoo.com
[3]Department of Pharmacology, Faculty of Medicine, Babol University of Medical Sciences, Babol, Iran
[4]Cellular and Molecular Research Center, Babol University of Medical Sciences, Babol, Iran
Full list of author information is available at the end of the article

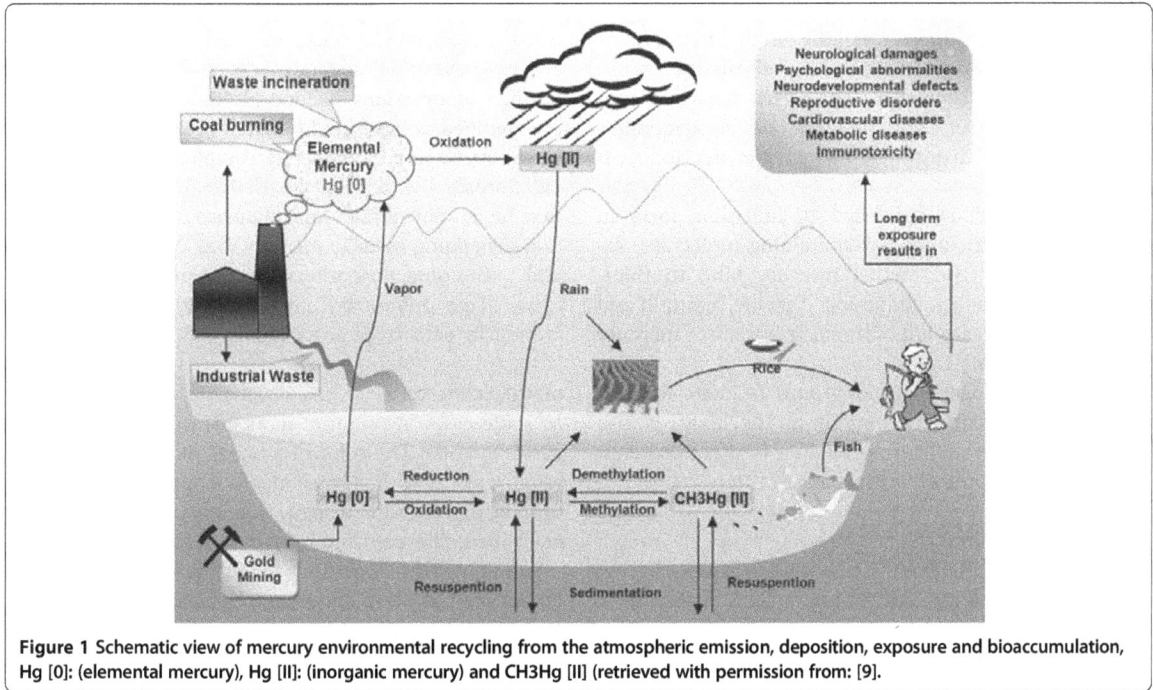

Figure 1 Schematic view of mercury environmental recycling from the atmospheric emission, deposition, exposure and bioaccumulation, Hg [0]: (elemental mercury), Hg [II]: (inorganic mercury) and CH3Hg [II] (retrieved with permission from: [9].

In 20th century, two big disasters of mercury poisoning had been reported. The first, Minamata disease; poisoning of 2200 peoples due to consumption of mercury contaminated fishes and shell fish in Kyushu Japan. Also other cases of mercury intoxication had been reported in Niigata (the main island of Honshu, Japan) with approximately 700 victims, during 1950's and 1960's [9,12-14].

The third, three epidemics of mercury poisoning cases have been reported in Iraq during 1955-1956, 1959-1960, and largest outbreak in 1971-1972 in the rural population following the consumption of mercury contaminated homemade. Based on official reports, 6530 patients were hospitalized and 459 persons died [13,14].

There is a serious concern of environmental pollution following handling of mercury compounds, for example; dumping inorganic mercury along the Amazon River in Brazil, pit-working in gold mines in Tanzania, Indonesia, and the Philippines, Ecuador, Faroe islands, French Guiana, New Zealand, Peru, Seychelles island and Slovenia [15,16].

Some sea foods e.g. tuna fish may concentrate mercury compounds and its chronic use may cause poisoning. Similarly, in coastal provinces of Iran (e.g. Khuzestan) [17-19] mercury compounds have been reported in tap and agricultural water sources in Shiraz and Mashhad, two populous cities in Iran [20,21]. Persian Gulf and Caspian Sea are the main seafood sources in Iran. Although, mercury concentration in marginal countries of

Caspian Sea except the Republic of Azerbaijan and with coast line of the Persian Gulf and Oman Sea are generally quite low by international standard, but large consumption pattern may result in increased health risks [22-24].

According to recent studies it has been shown that mercury vapors from handling of amalgam, can be hazardous for dental staffs [25,26].

Mercury poisoning is a known topic in various regions of the world, but the incidence of new cases of poisoning in Iran has created an opportunity to reconsider to this silent threat.

Governmental and nongovernmental organizations should prepare basic data about mercury poisoning and design informative and educational programs on mercury poisoning in order to substantially reduce the incidence of poisoning with mercury. This review can be helpful in achieving the purpose to manage the various aspects of poisoning by mercury compounds.

Mechanisms of toxicity

Mercury compounds exert toxic health effects by different mechanisms such as; interruption of microtubule formation, changing intracellular calcium balance and membrane potential, altering cell membrane integrity, disturbing or inhibition of enzymes, inducing oxidative stress, inhibition of protein and DNA synthesis and disturbing immune functions [27].

Mercury binds to phosphoryl, carboxyl and amide groups in biological molecules [28]. Methyl mercury induces oxidative stress and the free radicals may cause neurotoxicity. On the other hand, it has been reported that accumulation of serotonin, aspartate, and glutamate has a role in mechanism of methyl mercury induced-neurotoxicity [29].

Methyl mercury is converted to inorganic form in CNS that binds to sulfhydryl-containing molecules. Inorganic mercury and methyl mercury bind to thiol-containing protein e.g. glutamine, cysteine, albumin and etc. These complexes affect the distribution of mercury in the body [30].

Binding to endogenous thiol-groups facilitate the distribution of mercury compounds in the body. It also protects the compounds from binding to other proteins, thus providing a protective mechanism [31].

Clinical manifestations
Different forms of mercury compounds have different clinical manifestations and adverse effects that will be explained in the details below.

Elemental mercury
Inhaling elemental mercury vapors causes acute symptoms such as cough, chills, fever, and shortness of breath, and also GIT complaints such as nausea, vomiting and diarrhea accompanied by a metallic taste, dysphagia, salivation, weakness, headaches and visual disorders [28]. Long-term inhalation of elemental mercury may cause cognitive impairment including decreased performance intellectual functioning, impairments of attention and short term memory, visual judgment of angles and directions, psychomotor retardation and personality changes including depression and willing to be alone, anxiety and lack of sensitivity to physical stimuli [32]. Whenever elemental or metallic mercury is ingested, it rarely confronts to clinical consequences in normal GIT mucosa. However, people having abnormal GIT mucosa absorb enough elemental mercury during exposure, producing severe irritation [2]. Corrosive injuries will start immediately after mercuric salts ingestion. Oral cavity problems such as inflammation of the mouth, ulcerative gingivitis, loose teeth, gingival bleeding and metallic taste may be observed [33]. Also, a grayish discoloration of mucous membranes, nausea, vomiting, local oropharyngeal pain, bloody diarrhea may be seen. Released mercury from dental amalgams may even induce stomatitis [34,35].

Elemental mercury crosses the alveolar membrane during respiration and readily absorbs into blood, and then distributed and transferred into the tissues [36]. The clinical manifestations of intoxication include: chest pain, dyspnea, dry cough, hypoxemia and altered carbon monoxide diffusing capacity and ventilatory patterns [37].

Mercury vapor at higher concentrations have caused necrotizing bronchitis, bronchiolitis and pneumonitis. It can also progress to pulmonary edema, respiratory failure and death. Complications include multiple pneumothoraces, pneumomediastinum, and subcutaneous emphysema [38]. In survivors, severe pulmonary complication like; interstitial fibrosis and residual restrictive pulmonary diseases may be developed [28]. Subcutaneous injection of a solution containing metallic mercury may cause local abscess and granuloma formations. IV (intravenous) injection cause acute pulmonary embolism and systemic microembolism with respiratory failure [38].

Inorganic mercury
In acute cases ingestion of inorganic mercury salts cause gastroenteritis. The color of mucous membranes changes rapidly along with development of metallic taste, local oropharyngeal pain, nausea, vomiting, bloody diarrhea, colic abdominal pain and renal dysfunction [15].

Subsequently, stomatitis, hematemesis, and hematochezia may be seen, chronic inorganic mercury salts intoxication may lead to development of tremor of the lips, tongue, severe salivation, losing teeth, anorexia, and weight loss [28,39].

In addition to salivation, gingivitis, gingival bleeding, oral stomatitis, corrosive damage to the mouth and throat have also been observed. The symptoms of acute inorganic mercury inhalation include dyspnea, chest pain, tightness, and dry cough, which are followed by acute chemical pneumonitis and bronchiolitis. Another clinical manifestation is shock that causes to massive fluid loss, and acute tubular necrosis. The predominant manifestations of sub-acute or chronic mercury intoxication include GI symptoms, neurologic abnormalities and renal dysfunction [15,28,39].

The first visible lesion of atherosclerosis in arterial wall is the fatty streak or the foam cell. These cells penetrate into the sub-endothelial space. This penetration can predispose uptake and storage cholesterol, and may result in atherogenesis [40]. Oxidation of LDL in the arterial intima has an important role in athrogenesis. Oxidized LDL increases pro-inflammatory genes expression that causes to aggregate monocyte in the vessels wall and may induce vessel dysfunction. This behaves to generate free radicals [41]. Mercury compounds catalyze peroxidation, e.g. mercuric chloride increases hydrogen peroxide formation and depletes glutathione. This process is increased at the risk of coronary heart disease [42]. The clinical finding of mercury toxicity include coronary heart disease (CHD), myocardial infarction (MI), increases in carotid intimal medial thickness (IMT), carotid obstruction and hypertension [43].

When inorganic mercury compounds are absorbed into bloodstream, the highest concentration (about 85-90%) is found in the kidneys. Inorganic mercury salts are taken up and accumulated in the proximal tubules of the kidneys [44,45]. Clinical findings are polyuria and proteinuria (especially low molecular proteinuria) which are the main indicators of tubular damage in kidneys. In severe conditions, patients suffer from nephrotic syndrome with hematuria and anuria [44]. Chronic inorganic mercury exposure can cause immune complex nephritis, especially membranous nephropathy [46]. In humans, long term exposure to mercury has been accompanied with immunological glomerular diseases which is responsible for mercury-induced nephropathy [47].

Organic mercury

In mild exposure, organic mercury compounds especially methyl mercury do not produce severe symptoms, but high exposure to organic mercury compounds leads to acute GIT symptoms and delayed neurotoxicity, regional destruction of neurons [28,48]. Ethyl mercury is rapidly metabolized into inorganic mercury that can induce nephrotoxicity [49]. CNS manifestation including autism syndrome which may appear after ethyl mercury intoxication [50,51]. Poisoning with organic mercury often occurs after eating some sea food containing mercury. Organic mercury is divided into three forms; aryl, short chain alkyl, and long chain alkyl compounds. Aryl and long chain alkyl have similar properties to inorganic mercury toxicity, but they are slightly corrosive (organic mercury is less corrosive than inorganic mercury) [33,52]. Also, in contaminated areas, most of the fresh water and salt water fish contain methyl mercury and this agent has acute GI symptoms, in which the above subjects have been pointed out [52].

Toxic effects on CNS

Toxic effects of mercury compounds on the human central nervous system are well known and in experimental animals it has been shown that mercury cross the placenta and reach fetal brain and get accumulated in the CNs and subsequent neurological disturbance occur in fetus [53,54].

Toxic effects on skin

Mercury compounds show toxic effects on the skin in many ways. Most common symptoms of contact dermatitis after exposure to mercury compounds include mild swelling, vesiculation, scaling, irritation, urticaria and erythema. Allergic contact dermatitis accompanied by pain, is the most important form of mercurial reaction in skin that can occur by both topical and systemic exposure [34]. In case of injection these mucocutaneous hyperpigmentation results and also purpura may be seen in advanced stage [34,35].

Diagnostic evaluation

Mercury exists in several physical and chemical statuses and may undergo biotransformation. In clinical laboratories, mercury levels in blood and urine are often determined as the total mercury, without paying attention to the physical and chemical forms [55].

Urine

Urine is a good sample for assaying elemental and inorganic mercury. Quantity more than 100 µg/L, produce neurological signs while concentration greater than 800 µg/L are often associated with death. Organic mercury such as methyl mercury is excreted mainly in feces, so the urine sample test is not a reliable indicator of the level of organic mercury in the body [56].

Blood

In acute intoxication, concentration of methyl mercury in red blood cells is high, but it varies in chronic toxicity. The whole blood mercury concentration is often less than 10 µg/L, but it normally may reach to 20 µg/L. After long term exposure to mercury vapors, the blood mercury concentration may be increased to 35 µg/L [27].

Hair and nail

Hair has high sulfhydryl groups and mercury compounds have high tendency to bind sulfur. After exposure to methyl mercury, total mercury levels in hair and blood will be used as biomarkers to evaluate the extent of poisoning. Hair: blood ratio in human is 250:1 [57]. It may be noted that hair analysis should not be used alone for confirming mercury exposure or its toxicity. In general, mercury concentrations in the hair do not exceed 10 mg/kg. In moderate intoxications, hair mercury concentration is in the range of 200-800 mg/kg but in severe case it may reach to 2400 mg/kg. WHO has advised monitoring of hair levels of methyl mercury in pregnant women and the concentrations equal or greater than 10 ppm increase the risk of neurological deficits in the next generation [33]. Meanwhile, the Methyl mercury easily crosses the blood-placenta barrier and accumulates more in the fetus than the mother. Methyl mercury binds to hemoglobin, its concentration in cord blood is higher than mother's blood. The umbilical cord is formed and developed mainly in the second and third trimesters. Both inorganic and methyl mercury are detected in the regular analysis of total mercury concentration, but the methylated form of mercury is detected in cord blood. Based on this result, the National Research Council (NRC) recommended the cord blood mercury concentration as the best available biomarker for fetal exposure to methyl mercury [58,59]. According to Brockman et al. [60] report the Hg/Selenium molar ratio is suggested to assess methyl mercury exposures in rats' nails. Therefore, in human studies the nails may simultaneously be used to evaluate methyl mercury exposures [60].

Application of nano-medicine in the diagnosis of mercury poisoning

Nanotechnology has revolutionized drug and medical sciences. This technology can cover a wide spread application such as tissue, cell and gene structures, medical instruments and tools, drugs delivery [61] and in biomedical researches, diagnosis evaluations and treatments [62]. Efficient methods have been presented in the literature regarding diagnosis of mercury poisoning. The use of gold nanoparticles (AuNPs) which is a rapid, cheap and sensitive detection method. This method detect DNA and RNA sequences [63,64]. Some studies have reported that Hg^{2+} bind thymine (thymine-mercury-thymine). This interaction may form base pairs in DNA. These bases are absorbed onto AuPNs surfaces. This combination develops Hg2+ sensors, based on the function of DNA and lysozyme gold. After the combinations of DNA with gold nanoparticles, then Hg2+ is detected by colorimetric sensors [63].

Silver nanoparticles (AgNPs) have been used as antibacterial, sunscreens and cosmetic agents. Also, AgNPs have been used as a biosensor or sensitive detector of low concentration Hg2+ ions in homogeneous aqueous solutions [65]. On the other hand, ultrasensitive surface-enhanced Raman scattering (SERS) nanosensor developed for mercury ion (Hg^{2+}) detection based on 4-mercaptopyridine (4-MPY) functionalized silver nanoparticles (AgNPs) (4-MPY-AgNPs) in the presence of spermine [66]. This reagent determine mercury up to 0.34 nM. Other Sensors for Mercury (Hg, HgI, HgII) determine concentration levels up to parts-per-billion [67,68].

Other diagnostic evaluation

Diagnostic tests depend on the clinical situation that includes: complete blood cell count, electrolytes assay, renal and liver function tests initially in acute elemental mercury vapor. Chest X ray (CXR) may show interstitial or alveolar abnormalities. Thereafter, acute respiratory distress syndrome (ARDS) may appear. Other diagnostic procedures are electrocardiography (ECG), pulmonary function test (PFT), cardiovascular monitoring, electroneuromyography and neuropsychologic tests [27].

Treatment of mercury poisoning
Immediate considerations and decontamination

Monitoring of vital organs is needed in primary management of acute exposure to elemental mercury vapors. Supplemental oxygen or endotracheal intubation and mechanical ventilation are recommended [38]. After pulmonary aspiration bronchial lavage must not be done,

because the particles of mercury can disperse further into the lungs and the level of absorption may increase. Chest X-rays determine the extent of dispersion. The small mercury droplets are absorbed faster than the bigger ones [39]. In acute ingestions of inorganic mercury, vascular access for IV fluid replacement is required to prevent shock. Inorganic mercury produces severe corrosive injuries. For corrosive injury, endoscopic examination is needed because it causes oropharyngeal edema and upper airway obstruction. To overcome obstruction of the airway, IV fluid therapy and endotracheal intubation and/or tracheostomy are needed [38,39]. The skin should be washed with soap and water in case of direct contact with mercury.

Gastrointestinal decontamination should be implemented for inorganic mercury salt because of systemic absorption, but the important problem is the corrosive property of these compounds. In spite of the corrosiveness of inorganic mercury and the risk for perforation, the removal of inorganic mercury is still beneficial. Whole-bowel irrigation with polyethylene glycol solution may be useful for removing residual mercury. Serial abdominal radiographies are needed to follow -up of the patients [28]. Activated charcoal (AC) may be used but its efficacy is controversial in case of mercury poisoning. The usual oral dose of AC is 0.5-1 gr/kg, with a maximum dose of 100 gr [69]. Many organic and inorganic contaminants are removed with this method [70]. It is believed that AC has been used to absorb different agents, except hydrocarbons, acids-alkalis, ethanol and heavy metal. Unlike in the cases of heavy metal poisoning, charcoal tightly binds with metallic compounds [38,69].

Chelating agents
Penicillamine

It is a white crystalline, water-soluble derivative of penicillin. D-penicillamine (DPA) is preferred to L isomer, because DPA is less toxic than the L isomer [71]. D-penicillamine is the drug of choice in Wilson's disease, and also useful in the management of other heavy metal toxicity [72].

Penicillamine increase urinary excretion of lead and mercury. The dosage schedule of DPA is: adults 250 mg qid, po, for 1-2 weeks, children 20-30 mg/kg/daily in 4 divided doses (maximum 250 mg/dose). D-penicillamine is only used for elemental and inorganic mercury toxicity and is not useful for organic mercury toxicity [73]. Hypersensitivity and nephrotoxicity are the most common adverse effects of penicillamine [71]. N-acetyl-d, l, penicillamine (NAP) is an analog of DPA, that it is more effective chelator of mercury. Recently succimer has replaced penicillamine, because of its strong metal-mobilizing capacity and lower side-effects [27,71].

Dimercaprol or British anti-Lewisite (BAL)

Since more than 60 years, BAL has been prescribed by physicians for the treatment of heavy metal poisonings, both accidental and iatrogenic. During World War II, BAL decreased the risk of damage or death of the allied soldiers. In 1951, BAL was applied to treat Wilson's disease. Nowadays, BAL is one of the prominent drugs used in the management of heavy metals poisoning [74] (Figure 2).

In poisoning cases with elemental and inorganic mercury salts, dimercaprol (BAL) may be administered 5 mg/kg IM once, 2.5 mg/kg IM every 8 to12 hours for 1 day, and then 2.5 mg/kg IM every 12 to 24 hours for 7 days [38]. Dimercaprol is ineffective and it may even increase mercury levels in the brain and aggravate CNS symptoms in case of organic mercury poisoning [75]. The common side effects of dimercaprol include nausea, vomiting, hypertension, tachycardia, pain at the injection site, headache, diaphoresis and convulsions [38].

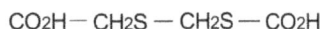

Meso 2,3-dimercaptosuccinic acid (Succimer,DMSA)

It is a water-soluble analog of BAL, with chemical formula $C_4H_6O_4S_2$, approved by FDA in 1991. Meso 2,3-dimercaptosuccinic acid inhibit activity of sulfhydryl-containing enzymes and prevents mercury induced symptoms [71,76]. In humans, *DMSA* is rapidly metabolized and excreted via urine and a small amount via bile and lungs [77]. In the United States, BAL or DMSA is preferred for treatment of inorganic mercury poisoning [28]. WHO recommends that DMSA should be started in children with urine mercury levels equal or greater than 50 µg/mL creatinine, if they are even asymptomatic [78]. DMSA has a half-life of 3.2 h [77].

DMSA is given via oral administration or IV injection. Adult doses are 10 mg/kg tid for the first 5 days, then 10 mg/kg bid for the next 14 days. Children dose is calculated based on the body surface area (BSA), 350 mg/m^{2}tid for the first 5 days, then 350 mg/m^2 bid for the next 14 days. If necessary, it may be repeated,

with a 2- week interval between treatments [38]. The dimercapto chelating agents are least toxic. But in some patients, neutropenia has been reported, therefore CBC, renal and hepatic functions should be checked before starting and during the treatment. The side effects of DMSA include GI disorders, skin rashes and flu-like symptoms [77].

2,3-dimercapto-1-propane sulfonic acid (Unithiol, DMPS)

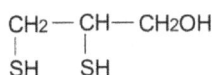

It is a water-soluble analog of the dimercaprol with chemical formula $C_3H_7O_3S_3Na$,. It has been approved for use in Russia and other former Soviet countries since 1958, in Germany since 1976, and in the USA since 1999 [71,76]. It has replaced DMSA in Europe [28]. In the body, DMPS is oxidized to disulfide forms. At least 80% of DMPS is oxidized within the first 30 minute. Approximately, 84% of total DMPS is excreted by the renal system. It reduces the renal mercury burden when it enters the renal tubular cells [79]. DMPS penetrates into the kidney cells, and removes the mercury accumulated in renal tissues and excrete mercury into the urine. Based on clinical and experimental evidences, it has been shown that DMPS remove mercuric mercury deposits in human tissues except brain [76,77]. All of the complexes of inorganic mercury and chelating agents are excreted via renal system [80].

DMPS is given either orally or IV injection. The adult dose is: 250 mg IV every 4 hours for the first 48 hours is administered, then 250 mg IV every 6 hours for the second 48 hours and next 250 mg IV every 8 hours. After IV administration, oral therapy may be started with 300 mg tid for 7 weeks. Duration of treatment depends on the concentration of mercury in blood and urine. Side effects are rare but, rash, nausea, and leucopenia may be observed [38].

New DMSA analogues

Recently, many studies have shown that esters of DMSA may be more effective antidotes for heavy metal poisoning.

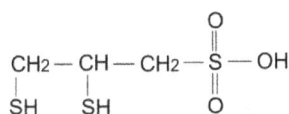

Figure 2 Chemical formula of BAL and their analogs meso-2,3-Dimercaptosuccinic acid (DMSA) and 2,3 Dimercapto-1-propanesulfonic acid (DMPS).

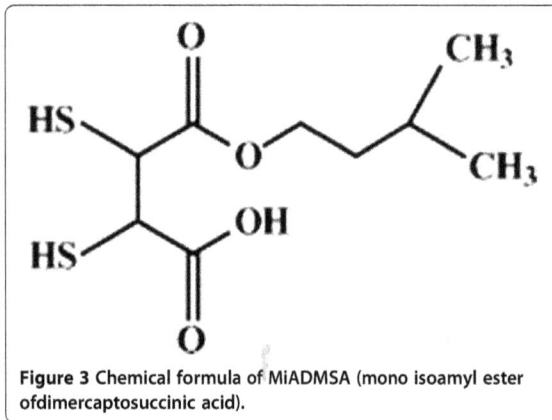

Figure 3 Chemical formula of MiADMSA (mono isoamyl ester ofdimercaptosuccinic acid).

These compounds are mono and di esters of DMSA that can enhance tissue elimination of mercury [81]. DMSA removes mercury both from the kidneys and bile. Its sulfhydryl group binds very tightly to mercury [82]. DMSA has hydrophilic and lipophobic properties. It cannot pass through cell membrane. *Mono isoamyl ester of DMSA (MiADMSA)* is a water-soluble lipophilic chelating agent and it is C_5 branched chain ester (Figure 3). It may be a more effective chelating agent for reducing lead, mercury and cadmium burden [83]. MiADMSA can penetrate to intracellular space and has an extensive cellular distribution. It removes heavy metals from both intra and extra cellular sites [84].

MiADMSA can decrease the oxidative stress in tissue by two ways. First, it removes the heavy metal from the target organ and second, it scavenges ROS (reactive oxygen species) via sulfhydryl groups [84]. Heavy metals

such as mercury, lead and selenium have a high affinity for sulfhydryl groups [85]. MiADMSA has lipophilic property and its molecular size may allow removing heavy metals and producing better therapeutic efficacy [83]. It is administered via oral and intraperitoneal route at doses 25,50 and 100 mg/kg. Although, based on histopathological studies of liver and kidneys in experimental animals, oral administration has been found better than intraperitoneal injection [81].

Other new DMSA analogous are *Monomethyl DMSA (MmDMSA)* and *Monocyclohexyl DMSA (MchDMSA)*. MmDMSA has a straight and branched chain of methyl groups, whereas MchDMSA has a cyclic carbon chain (Figure 4). Both are lipophilic and penetrate into cells. Both of them are chelating agents and are administrated through oral route. However, more studies are required to evaluate their efficacy [86].

Combination therapy with chelating agents

Nowadays, one of the main subjects in the treatment of heavy metal toxicity is the combination therapy. Co-administration of DMSA with MiADMSA has been found more effective than mono-therapy with MiADMSA, not only in controlling lipid peroxidation but also in controlling decreased catalase activity. It helps to reduce the dose of chelator agent, provides better clinical recoveries and minimize the possible side effects [81,87].

Plasma exchange-hemodialysis-plasmapheresis

Plasma exchange is initiated about 24-36 hours after the clinical diagnosis, when the patient's life is in danger and there is no suitable alternative therapy. Plasma exchange may be used in emergency condition, if there is a high

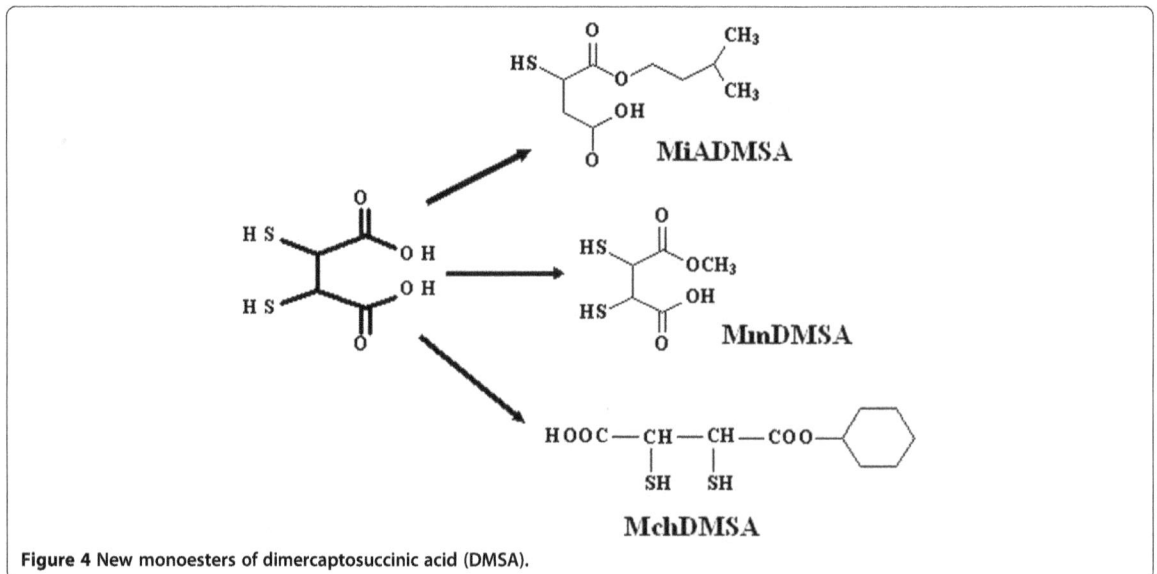

Figure 4 New monoesters of dimercaptosuccinic acid (DMSA).

plasma concentration of pathogenic substances. Therefore, plasma exchange can potentially be useful in heavy metals toxicity e.g. mercury [88]. Hemodialysis is the best way for water-soluble and dialyzable substances, also if renal failure occurs, hemodialysis maybe necessary [38,89]. Some of the toxic substances can strongly bind to plasma proteins and cannot be removed by hemodialysis. Plasmapheresis is eventually able to remove protein- bound heavy metals in plasma, such as mercury. Some toxicologists suggest using these procedures with chelating agents. In mono-therapy the elimination half- life of inorganic mercury may vary from 30 to100 days. When DMPS and hemodialysis are co-administered, the elimination half-life may be decreased between 2 to 8 days [89,90].

Managements of mercury contaminations
Natural and chemical decontamination
Algae, Azolla and other aquatic plants possess the ability to uptake toxic agents from the environment [91,92]. Chlorella increases elimination of mercury from the GIT, muscles, ligaments, connective tissue, and bone [93]. Chlorella and cilantro as food materials can detoxify some neurotoxins such as heavy metals (e.g. mercury) and toxic chemicals (e.g. phthalates, plasticizers and insecticides [94,95]. Photoinduced electron transfer (PET) sensor has been used for the detection of mercury ions [96]. It shows high selectivity for mercury ions in buffer solution (pH = 7). This sensor can selectively bind to very low concentration Hg^{2+} to form stable complexes [96]. The complexes of AgNPs with polyethylene glycol (PEG) and polyvinylpyrrolidone (PVP) are other systems that show high selectivity for Hg^{2+} [65].

Nano filtration
Nanotechnology may help to decrease water pollution problems by removing microorganisms, pesticides, insecticides and heavy metals (lead, mercury, cadmium, zinc). Nano-catalysts and nano-filters can eliminate toxic contaminants from waste waters [97]. Removing mercury by carbon nanotubes (CNTs) is an effective method in this field. Oxidized CNTs can absorb cations, because in this form the surface of absorption of CNTs is increased along with chemical and electrostatic binding [98].

Finally, long term administration of nano-medicines is still waiting to be approved by FDA and other authorized international organizations. In addition, removal of vapor-phase elemental mercury from stack emissions with sulfur-impregnated activated carbon has been under consideration.

Conclusion
Mercury exposure leads to harmful effects on almost every organ and system. It should be considered as a silent threat to environment and human life, through the world. The main concern is with the more subtle effects arising from prenatal to adult's period, and exist delay development and cognitive changes in children and clinical manifestations in adults. New protocols for the treatment of poisoning such as access to new antidotes, chelating agents, combination therapy of different chelating agents and specific nano-sorbents can help in the management of mercury poisoning. There are risks of mercury compounds for health in the worldwide. Therefore governmental and non-governmental organizations need to identify highly prone people to mercury exposure, and make sure safe food and drinking water.

In addition, it is necessary to pay attention to the safe transport and handling of mercury compounds.

Competing interest
The authors declared that they have no competing interests.

Author contributions
MRR: drafted the review article; MRR: searched in literature and arranged the information; SK: arranged references and edited figures and inserted the references using endnote software; AAM; he is corresponding person and carried out the final writing and editing of the manuscript, sending the manuscript, he responded to the reviewers and corrected and supervised all parts of the manuscript writing All authors read and approved the final manuscript.

Acknowledgement
We would like to thank the staffs of Shahid Beheshti Hospital and Zahravy Central library at Babol University of Medical Sciences, Dr. Haji Bahadar from International Campus of Tehran University of Medical sciences, Iran and Miss Yasaman Moghadamnia for editing the text and Dr. Evangeline Foronda for the proof reading.

Author details
[1]Department of Nursing, Babol University of Medical Sciences, Babol, Iran. [2]Department of Medical Physics, Kashan University of Medical Sciences, Kashan, Iran. [3]Department of Pharmacology, Faculty of Medicine, Babol University of Medical Sciences, Babol, Iran. [4]Cellular and Molecular Research Center, Babol University of Medical Sciences, Babol, Iran.

References
1. Stwertka AA: *A Guide to the Elements*. 2nd edition. Oxford: Oxford University Press.
2. Ibrahim D, Froberg B, Wolf A, Rusyniak DE: **Heavy metal poisoning: clinical presentations and pathophysiology.** *Clin Lab Med* 2006, **26**:67–97. viii.
3. Rafati-Rahimzadeh M, Moghaddamnia AA: **Organophosphorus compounds poisoning.** *J Babol Univ Med Sci* 2010, **12**:71–85 [in Persian].
4. Moghadamnia AA: **Survey of acute suicidal poisoning in the west of Mazandaran province during the years 1994-97.** *J Mazandaran Univ Med Sci* 1999, **22–23**:18–25 [in Persian].
5. Moghadamnia AA, Abdollahi M: **An epidemiological study of poisoning in northern Islamic Republic of Iran.** *East Mediterr Health J* 2002, **8**:88–94.
6. Paudyal BP: **Poisoning: pattern and profile of admitted cases in a hospital in central Nepal.** *JNMA J Nepal Med Assoc* 2005, **44**:92–96.
7. Rafati-Rahimzadeh M, Rafati-Rahimzadeh M, Moghaddamnia AA: **Arsenic compounds toxicity.** *J Babol Univ Med Sci* 2013, **15**:51–68 [in Persian].
8. Neustadt J, Pieczenik S: **Heavy-metal toxicity-with emphasis on mercury.** *Integrative Med* 2007, **6**:26–32.
9. Mostafalou S, Abdollahi M: **Environmental pollution by mercury and related health concerns: Renotice of a silent threat.** *Arh Hig Rada Toksikol* 2013, **64**:179–181.

10. Saint-Phard D, Van Dorsten B: **Mercury toxicity: clinical presentations in musculoskeletal medicine.** *Orthopedics* 2004, 27:394–397. quiz 398-399.

11. Satoh H: **Occupational and enviromental toxicology of mercury and its compounds.** *Ind Health* 2000, 38:153–164.

12. Clifton JC II: **Mercury exposure and public health.** *Pediatr Clin North Am* 2007, 54:237–245.

13. Grandjean P, Satoh H, Murata K, Eto K: **Adverse effects of methylmercury: environmental health reserch implication.** *Environ Health Perspect* 2010, 118:1137–1145.

14. Watanabe C, Satoh H: **Evolution of our understanding of methykmercury as a health threat.** *Environ Health Perspect* 1996, 104:367–379.

15. Asano S, Eto K, Kurisaki E, Gunji H, Hiraiwa K, Sato M, Sato H, Sato H, Hasuike M, Hagiwara N, Wakasa H: **Review article: acute inorganic mercury vapor inhalation poisoning.** *Pathol Int* 2000, 50:169–174.

16. Dourson ML, Wullenweber AE, Poirier KA: **Uncertainties in the reference dose for methylmercury.** *Neurotoxicology* 2001, 22:677–689.

17. Tayebi L, Sobhanardakani S, Farmany A, Cheraghi M: **Mercury Content in Edible Part of Otolithes Ruber Marketed in Hamadan, Iran.** *World Acad Sci Eng Technol* 2011, 59:1527–1529.

18. Rahimi E, Hajisalehi M, Kazemeini HR, Chakeri A, Khodabakhsh A, Derakhshesh M, Mirdamadi M, Ebadi AG, Rezvani SA, Kashkahi MF: **Analysis and determination of mercury, cadmium and lead in canned tuna fish marketed in Iran.** *Afr J Biotechnol* 2010, 9:4938–4941.

19. Askary Sary A, Mohammadi M: **Comparison of mercury and cadmium toxicity in fish species from marine water.** *Res J Fish Hydrobiol* 2012, 7:14–18.

20. Yousefzadeh H, Mousavi R, Sadeghi M, Namaei Ghassemi M, Eshaghian K, Moradi VA, Mokhtari MA, Danay G, Fakhary M, Balali-Mood M: *Toxic elements of mercury, lead, chromium, arsenic, aluminium and cadmium in drinking and agricultural water wells of Mashhad, Iran.* Penang, Malaysia: Paper presented at: 10th Scientific Congress of the Asia Pacific Association of Medical Toxicology (APAMT); 2011.

21. Karimi A, Moniri F, Nasihatkon A, Zarepoor MJ, Alborzi A: **Mercury exposure among residents of a building block in Shiraz, Iran.** *Environ Res Section* 2002, 88:41–43.

22. De Mora S, Sheikholeslami MR, Wyse E, Azemard S, Cassi R: **An assessment of metal contamination in coastal sediment of the Caspian Sea.** *Mar Pollut Bull* 2004, 48:61–77.

23. De Mora S, Fowler SW, Wyse E, Azemard S: **Distribution of heavy metals in marine organisms from Mosa Bay, Persian Gulf.** *Int J Environ Res* 2004, 5:757–762.

24. Mortazavi MS, Sharifian S: **Mercury bioaccumulation in some commercially valuable marine organisms from Mosa Bay.** *Persian Gulf Int J Environ Res* 2011, 5:757–762.

25. Neghab M, Choobineh A, Hassanzadeh J, Ghaderi E: **Symptoms of intoxication in dentist associated with exposure to low levels of mercury.** *Ind Health* 2011, 49:249–254.

26. Zolfaghari G, Esmaili-Sari A, Ghasempouri SM: **Evaluation of environmental and occuptional exposure to mercury among Iranian dentists.** *Sci Total Environ* 2007, 381:59–67.

27. Klaassen CD: *Casarett & Daull's toxicology the basic science of poisons.* New York: McGrowHill; 2007.

28. Nelson LS, Lewin NA, Howland MA, Hoffman RS, Goldfrank LR, Flomenbaum NE: *Goldfrank's toxicological emergencies.* New York: McGrawHill; 2011.

29. Yee S, Choi BH: **Oxidative stress in neurotoxic effects of metylmercury poisoning.** *Neurotoxicology* 1996, 17:17–26.

30. Davidson PW, Myers GJ, Weiss B: **Mercury exposure and child development outcomes.** *Pediatrics* 2004, 113:1023–1029.

31. Patrick L: **Mercury toxicity and antioxidants: part I: role of glutathione and alpha-lipoic acid in the treatment of mercury toxicity.** *Altern Med Rev* 2002, 7:456–471.

32. Hua MS, Huang CC, Yang WJ: **Chronic elemental mercury intoxication: neuropsychological follow-up case study.** *Brain Inj* 1995, 10:377–384.

33. Alhibshi EA: **Subclinical neurotoxicity of mercury: a behavioural, molecular mechanisms and therapeutic perspective.** *Res J Pharmaceut Biol Chem Sci* 2012, 3:34–42.

34. Dantzig PI: **A new cutaneous sign of mercury poisoning?** *J Am Acad Dermatol* 2003, 49:1109–1111.

35. Boyd AS, Seger D, Vannucci S, Langley M, Abraham JL, King LE: **Mercury exposure and cutaneous disease.** *J Am Acad Dermatol* 2000, 43:81–90.

36. Glezos JD, Albrecht JE, Gair RD: **Pneumonitis after inhalation of mercury vapours.** *Can Respir J* 2006, 13:150–152.

37. Lorenzo Dus MJ, Viedma EC, Gutierrez JB, Bayo AL: **Pulmonary embolism caused by elemental mercury.** *Arch Bronconeumol* 2007, 43:585–587.

38. Brent J, Wallace KL, Burkhart KK, Phillips SD, Donovan JW: *Critical care toxicology diagnosis and management of the critically poisoned patient.* Philadelphia: ElesevierMosby; 2005.

39. Bates N: **Metallic and inorganic mercury poisoning.** *Emerg Nurse* 2003, 11:25–31.

40. Steinberg D: **The LDL modification hypothesis of atherogenesis: an update.** *J Lipid Res* 2009, 68:353–354.

41. Li D, Mehta JL: **Oxidized LDL, a critical factor in atherogenesis.** *Cardiovasc Res* 2005, 68:353–354.

42. Yoshizawa K, Rimm EB, Steven Morris J, Spate VL, Hsieh CC, Spiegelman D, Stampfer MJ, Willett WC: **Mercury and the risk of coronary heart disease in men.** *N Engl J Med* 2002, 347:1755–1760.

43. Houston MC: **Role of mercury toxicity in hypertension, cardiovascular disease, and stroke.** *J Clin Hypertens* 2011, 13:621–627.

44. Park JD, Zheng W: **Human exposure and health effects of Inorganic and elemental mercury.** *JPrev Med Publ Health* 2012, 45:344–352.

45. Verma S, Kumar R, Khadwal A, Singhi S: **Accidental inorganic mercury chloride poisoning in a 2-year old child.** *Indian J Pediatr* 2010, 77:1153–1155.

46. Li SJ, Zhang SH, Chen HP, Zeng CH, Zheng CX, Li LS, Liu ZH: **Mercury-induced membranous nephropathy: clinical and pathological features.** *Clin J Am Soc Nephrol* 2010, 5:439–444.

47. Guzzi GP, Fogazzi GB, Cantu M, Minoia C, Ronchi A, Pigatto PD, Severi G: **Dental amalgam, mercury toxicity, and renal autoimmunity.** *J Environ Pathol Toxicol Oncol* 2008, 27:147–155.

48. Koh C, Kwong KL, Wong SN: **Mercury poisoning: a rare but treatable cause of failure to thrive and developmental regression in an infant.** *Hong Kong Med J* 2009, 15:61–64.

49. Clarkson TW, Magos L, Myers GI: **The toxicology of mercury-current exposures and clinical manifest.** *N Engl J Med* 2003, 349:1731–1737.

50. Bernard S, Enayati A, Redwood L, Roger H, Binstock T: **Autism: a novel form of mercury poisoning.** *Med Hypotheses* 2001, 56:462–471.

51. Uchino M, Okajima T, Eto K, Kumamoto T, Mishima I, Ando M: **Neurologic features of chronic minamatadisease (organic mercury poisoning) certified at autopsy.** *Intern Med* 1995, 34:744–747.

52. Broussard LA, Hammett-Stabler LA, Winecker RE, Ropero-Miller JD: **The toxicology of mercury.** *Lab Med* 2002, 33:614–625.

53. Tang N, Li YM: **Neurotoxic effects in workers of the clinical thermometer manufacture plant.** *Int J Occup Med Environ Health* 2006, 19:198–201.

54. Florea AM, Busselberg D: **Occurrence, use and potential toxic effects of metals and metal compounds.** *BioMetals* 2006, 19:419–427.

55. Nuttall KL: **Interpreting mercury in blood and urine of individual patients.** *Ann Clin Lab Sci* 2004, 34:235–250.

56. Goldman LR, Shannon MW: **Technical report: mercury in the environment: implication for pediatricians.** *Pediatrics* 2001, 108:197–205.

57. Miklavcic A, Cuderman P, Mazej D, SnojTratnik J, Krsnik M, Planinsek P, Osredkar J, Horvat M: **Biomarkers of low-level mercury exposure through fish consumption in pregnant and lactating Slovenian women.** *Environ Res* 2011, 111:1201–1207.

58. Grandjean P, Budtz-Jorgensen E: **Total imprecision of exposure biomarkers: implications for calculating exposure limits.** *Am J Ind Med* 2007, 50:712–719.

59. Sakamoto M, Kaneoka T, Murata K, Nakai K, Satoh H, Akagi H: **Correlations between mercury concentrations in umbilical cord tissue and other biomarkers of fetal exposure to methylmercury in the Japanese population.** *Environ Res* 2007, 103:106–111.

60. Brockman JD, Raymond LJ, Ralston CR, Robertson JD, Bodkin N, Sharp N, Ralston NVC: **The nail as a noninvasive indicator of methylmercury exposures and mercury/selenium molar ratios in brain, kidney, and livers of long-evans rats.** *Biol Trace Elem Res* 2011, 144:812–820.

61. Linkov I, Kyle Satterstrom F, Corey LM: **Nanotoxicology and nanomedicine: making hard decisions.** *Nanomedicine* 2008, 4:167–171.

62. Surendiran A, Sandhiya S, Pradhan SC, Adithan C: **Novel applications of nanotechnology in medicine.** *Indian J Med Res* 2009, 130:689–701.

63. Zuo X, Wu H, Toh J, YauLi SF: **Mechanism of mercury detection based on interaction of single- strand DNA and hybridized DNA with gold nanoparticles.** *Talanta* 2010, 82:1642–1646.

64. Baptista P, Pereira E, Eaton P, Doria G, Miranda A, Gomes I, Quaresma P, Franco R: Gold nanoparticles for the development of clinical diagnosis method. *Anal Bioanal Chem* 2008, 391:943–950.

65. Ahmed MA, Hasan N, Mohiuddin S: Silver nanoparticles: green synthesis, characterization, and their usage in determination of mercury contamination in seafoods. *Hindawi Publ Corp ISRN Nanotechnol* 2014, 2014:5.

66. Lingxin C, Nan Q, Xiaokun W, Ling C, Huiyan Y, Jinhua L: Ultrasensitive surface-enhanced Raman scattering nanosensor for mercury ion detection based on functionalized silver nanoparticles. *RSC Adv* 2014, 2014:15055–15060.

67. Ramesh GV, Radhakrishnan TP: A universal sensor for mercury (Hg, HgI, HgII) based on silver nanoparticle-embedded polymer thin film. *ACS Appl Mater Interfaces* 2011, 3:988–994.

68. Deng L, Ouyang X, Jin J, Ma C, Jiang Y, Zheng J, Li J, Li Y, Tan W, Yang R: Exploiting the higher specificity of silver amalgamation: selective detection of mercury(II) by forming Ag/Hg amalgam. *Anal Chem* 2013, 85:8594–8600.

69. Lapus RM: Activated charcoal for pediatric poisonings: the universal antidote. *Curr Opin Pediatr* 2007, 19:216–222.

70. Mohammad-Khah A, Ansari R: Activated charcoal; preparation, characterization and applications: a review article. *Int J Chem Tech Res* 2009, 1:2745–2788.

71. Katzung BG, Masters SB, Trevor AJ: *Basic and clinical pharmacology.* McGrawHill: NewYork; 2009.

72. Yusef M, Neal R, Aykin N, Ercal N: High performance liquid chromatography analysis of D-penicillamine by derivatization with N-(1-pyrenyl) maleimide(NPM). *Biomed Chromatogr* 2000, 14:535–540.

73. Ford MD, Delaney KA, Ling LJ, Erickson T: *Clinical toxicology.* Philadelphia: W. B. Saunders Company; 2001.

74. Vilensky JA, Redman K: British anti-lewisite(dimercaprol): an amazing history. *Ann Emerg Med* 2003, 41:378–383.

75. Graeme KA, Pollack CV: Heavy metal toxicity, part I: arsenic and mercury. *J Emerg Med* 1998, 16:45–56.

76. Guzzi GP, LaPorta CAM: Molecular mechanisms triggered by mercury. *Toxicology* 2008, 244:1–12.

77. Rooney JPK: The role of thiols, dithiols, nutritional factors and interacting ligands in the toxicology of mercury. *Toxicology* 2007, 234:145–156.

78. Forman J, Moline J, Cernichiari E, Sayegh S, Torres C, Landrigan MM, Hudson J, Adel HN, Landrigan PJ: A cluster of pediatric metallic mercury exposure cases treated with meso-2,3-dimercaptosuccinic acid (DMSA). *Environ Health Perspect* 2000, 108:575–577.

79. Vamnes JS, Eide R, Isrenn R, Hol PJ, Gjerdet NR: Blood mercury following DMPS administration to subjects with and without dental amalgam. *Sci Total Environ* 2003, 308:63–71.

80. Pingree SD, Simmonds L, Woods JS: Effects of 2,3-dimercapto-1-propanesulfonic acid (DMPS) on tissue and urine mercury levels following prolonged methylmercury exposure in rats. *Toxicol Sci* 2001, 61:224–233.

81. Flora SJS, Pachauri V: Chelation in metal intoxication. *Int J Environ Res Publ Health* 2010, 7:2745–2788.

82. Miller AL: Imercaptosuccinic acid (DMSA), a non-toxic, water-soluble treatment for heavy metal toxicity. *Altern Med Rev* 1998, 3:199–207.

83. Flora SJS, Chouhan S, Kannon GM, Mittal M, Swarnker H: Combined administration of taurine and monoisoamyl DMSA protects arsenic induced oxidative injury in rats. *Oxid Med Cell Longev* 2008, 1:39–45.

84. Flora SJS, Bhadauria S, Pachauri V, Yadav A: Monoisoamyl 2,3-dimercaptosuccinic acid (MiADMSA) demonstrates higher efficacy by oral route in reversing arsenic toxicity: a pharmacokinetic approach. *Basic Clin Toxicol* 2012, 110:449–459.

85. Bhadauria S, Flora SJS: Arsenic induced inhibition of δ-aminolevulinate dehydratase activity in rat blood and its response to meso 2,3-dimercaptosuccinic acid and monoisoamyl DMSA. *Biomed Environ Sci* 2004, 17:101–108.

86. Flora SJS: Metal poisoning: threat and management. *Al Ameen J Med Sci* 2009, 2:4–26.

87. Bhadauria S, Flora SJS: Response of arsenic-induced oxidative stress, DNA damage, and metal imbalance to combined administration of DMSA and monoisoamyl-DMSA during chronic arsenic poisoning in rats. *Cell Biol Toxicol* 2007, 23:91–104.

88. Russi G, Marson P: Urgent plasma exchange: how, where and when. *Blood Transfus* 2011, 9:356–361.

89. Nenov VD, Marinov P, Sabeva J, Nenov DS: Current application of plasmapheresis in clinical toxicology. *Nephrol Dial Transplant* 2003, 18:v56–v58.

90. Dargan PI, Giles LJ, Wallace CI, Thomson AH, Beale RJ, Jones AL: Case report: severe mercuric sulphate poisoning treated with 2,3-dimercatopropane-1-sulphonate and haemodiafiltration. *Crit Care* 2003, 7:R1–R6.

91. Xue HB, Stumm W, Sigg L: The binding of heavy metals to algal surfaces. *Water Res* 1988, 22:917.

92. Sachdeva S, Sharma A: Azolla: role in phytoremediation of heavy metals. *Int J Eng Sci* 2012, 1:2277–9698.

93. Tsezos M: Biosorption of Radioactive Species. In *Biosorption of Heavy Metals.* Edited by Volesky B. Boston: CRC Press; 1990:45–50.

94. Omura Y: Beckman SL Role of mercury (Hg) in resistant infections & effective treatment of Chlamydia trachomatis and Herpes family viral infections (and potential treatment for cancer) by removing localized Hg deposits with Chinese parsley and delivering effective antibiotics using various drug uptake enhancement methods. *Acupunct Electrother Res* 1995, 20:195–229.

95. Omura Y, Shimotsuura Y, Fukuoka A, Fukuoka H, Nomoto T: Significant mercury deposits in internal organs following the removal of dental amalgam, & development of pre-cancer on the gingiva and the sides of the tongue and their represented organs as a result of inadvertent exposure to strong curing light (used to solidify synthetic dental filling material) & effective treatment: a clinical case report, along with organ representation areas for each tooth. *Acupunct Electrother Res* 1996, 21:133–160.

96. Nolan EM, Lippard SJ: The Application of Fluorescence Spectroscopy in the Mercury Ion Detection. *Chem Rev* 2008, 108:3443.

97. Pandy J, Khare R, Kamboj M, Khare S, Singh R: Potential of nanotechnology for the treatment of waste water. *Asian J Biochem Pharmaceut Res* 2011, 1:272–282.

98. Qu X, Alvarez PJJ, Li Q: Applications of nanotechnology in water and wastewater treatment. *Water Res* 2013, 47:3931–3946.

The effects of cichorium intybus extract on the maturation and activity of dendritic cells

Mohammad Hossein Karimi[1], Salimeh Ebrahimnezhad[1], Mandana Namayandeh[1] and Zahra Amirghofran[2*]

Abstract

Background: *Cichorium intybus* is a medicinal plant commonly used in traditional medicine for its benefits in immune-mediated disorders. There are several evidences showing that *C. intybus* can modulate immune responses. In the present study we have investigated the effects of the ethanolic root extract of this plant on the immune system by targeting dendritic cells (DCs). For this purpose, phenotypic and functional maturity of murine DCs after treatment with the extract was analyzed by flow cytometry and mixed lymphocyte reaction (MLR) assay.

Results: *C. intybus* did not change the expression of CD40, CD86 and MHC-II molecules as important co-stimulatory markers on DCs compared to the control, indicating that it could not promote DCs phenotypic maturation. Treatment of DCs with lower concentrations of the extract resulted in an increased production of IL-12 by these cells with no change in IL-10 release. The capacity of treated DCs to stimulate allogenic T cells proliferation and cytokines secretion was examined in the co-cuture of these cells with T cells in MLR. *C. intybus* at higher concentrations inhibited proliferation of allogenic T cells and in lower concentrations changed the level of cytokines such that IL-4 decreased and IFN-γ increased.

Conclusions: These results indicated that *C. intybus* extract at higher concentrations can inhibit T cell stimulating activity of DCs, whereas at lower concentrations can modulate cytokine secretion toward a Th1 pattern. These data may in part explain the traditional use of this plant in treatment of immune-mediated disorders.

Keywords: DCs, Cichorium intybus, Dendritic cells, Immunomodulation, T cell responses

Introduction

The use of herbal medicine is increasing in therapies of immune disorders, including autoimmune diseases and cancers in all over the world. *Cichorium intybus* (*C. intybus*) belonging to Asteraceae family, also known as chicory, grows as a wild plant and is a well-known herb with various biological activities. This plant is native to Europe and Asia and has been widely used in folk medicine for treatment of gallstones, appetite loss, gout, jaundice, skin swellings, rheumatism and liver inflammation [1,2]. The seed extract of *C. intybus* has shown high antioxidant activity, short- and long-term beneficial effects on diabetes [3] as well as ameliorating effects on non-alcoholic fatty liver disease [4]. Methanolic extract of *C. intybus* and its various fractions have revealed

wound healing effects. β-Sitosterol has been considered as a main component of chicory extract in wound healing [5]. The methanolic extract of the plant has demonstrated some anticancer and apoptosis inducing effects [5]. *C. intybus* could ameliorate the oxidative stress, hepatic injury and cellular damage induced by chemical compounds in rat [6,7]. In addition, this plant has shown anti-inflammatory activity by inhibiting TNF-α mediated inflammation and reducing cyclooxygenase (COX)-2 protein expression [1]. The ethanolic root extract of *C. intybus* has inhibited mitogen-activated human lymphocyte proliferation as well as allogenic T cell responses [8] which implies the ability of this plant to modulate immune responses.

Dendritic cells (DCs), as the most potent antigen presenting cells for naïve T cells, act as a link between the acquired and innate immune systems and are responsible for the initiation of the protective immune response as well as the induction of immune tolerance [9]. The function of these cells is affected by their maturation status, origin and phenotype [10]. These cells have the unique ability

---

* Correspondence: amirghz@sums.ac.ir
[2]Department of Immunology, Autoimmune Disease Research Center and Medicinal and Natural Products Chemistry Research Center, Shiraz University of Medical Sciences, Shiraz, Iran
Full list of author information is available at the end of the article

to stimulate and target naive T cells to either Th1 or Th2 cells [11]. They can also effectively down-regulate T-cell responses through the generation of T regulatory cells [12]. DCs in immature forms can effectively present antigen but because of low expression of co-stimulatory molecules such as CD86, CD40 and MHC II they cannot properly stimulate immune system [10]. T cells activation and proliferation are inhibited and suppressed with repeated stimulation by immature DCs. Maturation of DCs converts them to the cells that can stimulate immune system vigorously. Therefore inhibition of this process is a valuable strategy to modulate immune responses. In this regard, using DCs with low expression of co-stimulatory molecules can be considered as a beneficial approach in therapy of autoimmune disease and transplantation [13]. For this reason, considerable studies have been performed to use these cells as therapeutic targets for immunomodulatory effects of some pharmacological compounds.

Given the important role of DCs in immune response as well as immune regulation and the presence of data regarding the immunomodulatory effects of *C. intybus*, we hypothesized that this plant might have some modulatory effects on DCs. To the best of our knowledge, there is no study about the effect of *C. intybus* on DCs. Therefore in the present study we have investigated the effects of the root extract of this plant on the maturation and function of DCs through evaluation of the expression of DC maturation markers, their allostimulatory capacity and release of the main Th1 and Th2 cytokines.

Materials and methods
Animals
6- week-old male BALB/c and C57BL/6 mice were purchased from Razi Institute (Shiraz, Iran) and were kept under optimal conditions of hygiene and received standard mouse chow and water *ad libitum*. All experimental procedures on handling the animals were approved by the ethical committee of Shiraz University of Medical Sciences.

Purification of splenic DCs
In order to isolate DCs from spleen, the gradient media (Nycodenz, Axis Shields, Norway) was used as previously described [14]. Briefly, mice spleens were chopped and digested with 1 mg/ml collagenase D (Roche, Germany) and 0.02 mg/ml DNase (Roche) and meshed with 0.2 μm sieve. Cells were washed with RPMI 1640 culture medium (Sigma, St. Louis, MO, USA) containing 5 mM EDTA. The pellet was resuspended in culture medium with 10% fetal calf serum (FCS) and 5 mM EDTA. The cell suspension was layered on Nycodenz 12.5% (w/v), d = 1.068 and centrifuged at 1800 rpm and 4°C for 20 min. The interface layer was collected and washed two times and 1×10^4 cells cultured in 3 cm plate for 2 h at 37°C in a 5% CO_2 incubator. After that, non-adherent cells were discarded by washing

and adherent cells were used for tests. Purity of the adherent cells was determined with analysis for the expression of CD11c molecule by flow cytometry. The cells were routinely more than 90% CD11c positive.

Preparation of the ethanolic root extract of *C. intybus*
The roots of *C. intybus* were collected from Fars provinces at October and authenticated by Mr Iraj Mehregan, from Shiraz School of Pharmacy. A voucher specimen was deposited in the Herbarium of the School of Pharmacy. Samples were washed, dried and then 200 g of each shade dried powder was extracted in a percolator containing 70% ethanol. After 72 h, percolation was done and the extract solution was concentrated in a rotary evaporator (Heidolph, Germany). The dried extract was dissolved in dimethyl sulphoxide (DMSO) and then resuspended in RPMI 1640 medium to obtain 20 mg/ml solution.

Treatment of DCs with the extract
DCs were treated with *C. intybus* extract at final concentrations of 0.1, 1, 10 and 100 μg/ml in the cell culture plates. As negative control, cells were treated with the vehicle (DMSO) at the highest concentration used in the tests (0.1%) and as positive control, cells were treated with TNF-α (Sigma), the known DC maturation inducing cytokine, at concentration of 40 ng/ml.

MTT cell viability assay
In vitro cytotoxicity of the extract on DCs was tested by 3-(4, 5-dimethylthiazol-2-yl)-2, 5-diphenyltetrazolium bromide (MTT) colorimetric assay as described previously [15]. DCs were treated with different concentrations of the extract ranging from 0.1 to 100 μg/ml for 24 h, then 10 μl MTT (5 mg/ml, Sigma) was added to each well and cells were incubated for an additional 4 h at 37°C. The optical density (OD) of each well was measured at 570 with reference at 630 nm on an enzyme-linked immuosorbent assay (ELISA) plate reader. The viability was determined as the follows: (OD of extract-treated cells/OD of DMSO-treated cells) × 100.

Flow cytometry analysis
Isolated DCs were treated with non toxic concentrations of the extract for 18 h and were then analyzed for the expression of co-stimulatory molecules in a flow cytometer (FACSCalibur, Beckton Dickinson Biosciences, San Jose, CA). Cells were stained with phycoerythrin (PE)-conjugated anti-CD11c, fluorescence isothiocyanate (FITC)-conjugated anti-CD40, FITC-conjugated anti-CD86 and FITC-conjugated anti-MHC II antibody and appropriate conjugated isotypes all from Beckton Dickinson (BD) Pharminogen (San Diego, CA). Data were analyzed using Win MDI software (Scripps, La Jolla, CA). The ratio between the percentage of markers expression on

extract-treated DCs and DMSO-treated DCs was calculated. The mean florescent intensity (MFI) of the expression of markers on extract-treated DCs were also determined and compared with DMSO-treated DCs.

Allogeneic mixed lymphocyte reaction (MLR)

In order to evaluate the proliferative effect of extract-treated DCs on T lymphocytes, MLR assay was used. For this, T cells were purified from lymph nodes of C57BL/6 mice using nylon wool. The purity was determined using FITC-conjugated anti-CD3 antibody (BD Pharminogen) by flow cytometry. *C. intybus*-treated DCs were inactivated with mitomycin C (0.5 mg/ml) for 20 min, then cells were washed with phosphate buffered saline (PBS) for three times and resuspended in culture medium containing 10% FCS. For MLR assay, 10^4cells/well mitomycin-treated DCs, as stimulator cells, were added in a 96-well round-bottomed culture plate (Nunc, Denmark) in triplicates and co-cultured with 10^5 allogenic T cells, as responder cells, for 48 h. A triplicate wells containing DMSO-treated DCs plus allogenic T cells were used as negative control. T cell proliferation was measured by a 5-Bromo-20-deoxy-uridine (BrdU) cell proliferation assay kit (Roche, Germany) according to the manufacturer's instructions. Proliferation was determined as the follows: (OD of extract-treated culture/OD of DMSO-treated culture) × 100.

Cytokines assay

The supernatant of extract-treated DCs and MLR cultures were collected and used to measure IL-12, IFN-γ, IL-10 and IL-4 by ELISA kits according to the manufacturer's protocol (eBioscience, USA). The sensitivity of IL-4, IFN- γ, IL-10 and IL-12 kits were 4, 15, 30 and 15 pg/ml, respectively.

Statistics analysis

All data were representative of at least three or two independent experiments performed in triplicate and presented as mean ± standard deviation (SD). The differences between groups were analyzed by Student's *t*-test and oneway ANOVA using Graph-Pad Prism 5 software (Graph-Pad Software Inc, San Diego, CA). P vales less than 0.05 were considered significant.

Results

Effects of C. intybus on viability of DCs

In order to determine the effects of *C. intybus* on the viability of DCs, these cells were treated with different concentrations of the plant extract for 24 h and then MTT assay was performed. The results showed that this extract at concentration of 0.1, 1, 10 and 100 μg/ml had no cytotoxic effect on DCs (Figure 1), therefore these concentrations were used for the next experiments on DCs.

Effect of C. intybus on maturation of mouse splenic DCs

C. intybus-treated DCs were analyzed by flow cytometry for the expression of CD40, CD86 and MHC II co-stimulatory molecules. As data in Figure 2A shows, the extract did not significantly modulate the percentage expression of these molecules at concentration of 0.1 to 100 μg/ml (see Additional file 1: Figure S1 for dot plots). Although, an increasing concentrations of the extract has led to a decreasing MHC II fluorescence intensity of expression (p < 0.01), none of the molecules MFI was significantly different between the extract-treated cells and the corresponding control (Figure 2B).

Effect of C. intybus treated DCs on proliferation of T cells

In order to find the effects of the plant on DCs function, mouse splenic DCs were treated with concentrations of 0.1 to 100 μg/ml of the extract for 18 h and then cells were co-cultured with allogenic T cells in MLR assay. The proliferation of T lymphocytes was evaluated using BrdU incorporation assay. As results in Figure 3 show, ethanolic extract of *C. intybus* decreased the proliferation of T cells at higher concentrations. The proliferation of these cells decreased to 75.60 ± 2.5 and 79.80 ± 6.1 percent of control when DCs had been treated with 10 and 100 μg/ml of the extract, respectively (P < 0.05).

Effect of C. intybus-treated DCs on the production of cytokines

The effect of the extract on IL-4 and IFN- γ production in MLR is demonstrated in Figure 4A. A decreased IL-4 level in the supernatant of T cells co-cultured with DCs treated with lower concentrations of *C. intybus* in

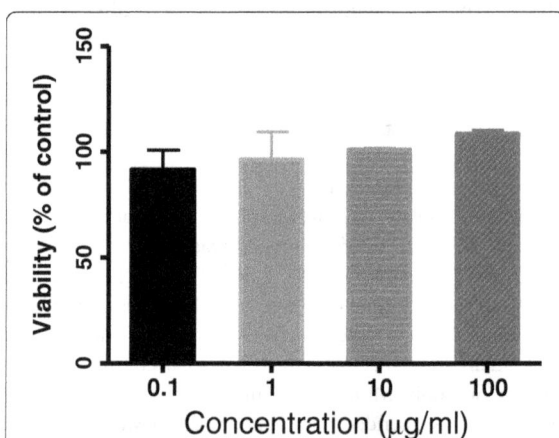

Figure 1 Cell viability assay of *C. intybus* ethanolic extract on DCs after 24 h treatment determined by MTT assay. Control was DCs treated with DMSO at the highest concentrations used in the tests (e.g., 0.1). The bars indicate mean ± standard deviation of three independent experiments performed in triplicate. The extract had no significant growth inhibitory effects on DCs.

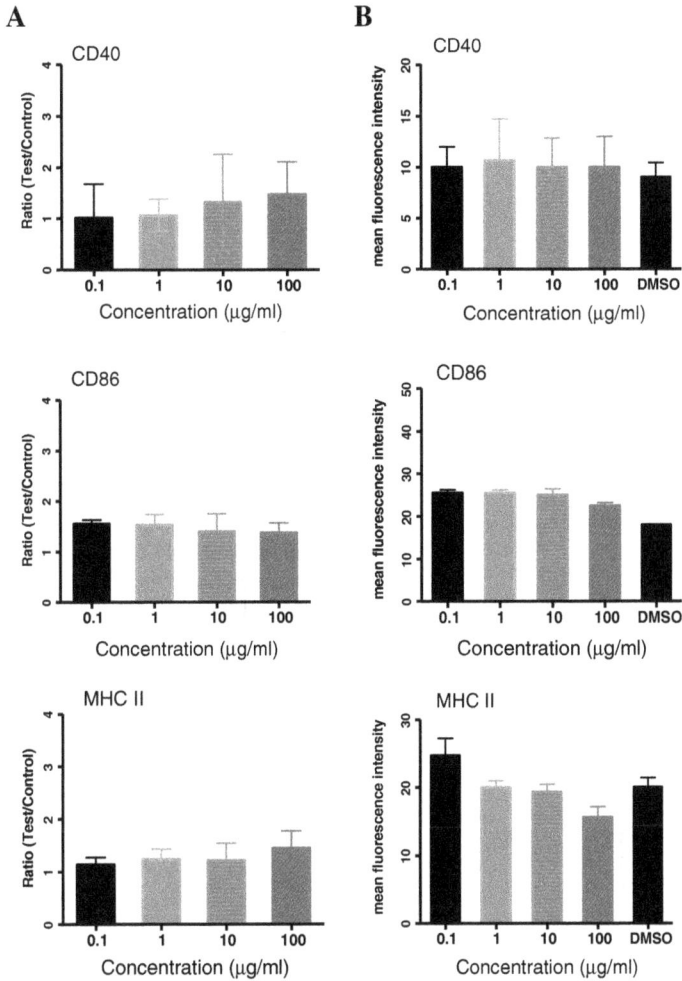

Figure 2 Effect of *C. intybus* ethanolic extract on phenotypic maturation of DCs. DCs were treated with the extract for 18 h and then the expression of CD40, CD86 and MHC II molecules was determined by flow cytometry. Negative control was DCs treated with DMSO. **A)** The bars indicate mean ± SD of the ratio between the percentage of markers expression on DCs treated with the extract and those treated with DMSO. **B)** The bars indicate mean ± SD of the mean fluorescence intensity (MFI) of the expression of markers. No significant difference in the ratio and MFI of the markers expression between extract-treated DCs and control cells was observed.

comparison with the control was observed (P < 0.05). The level of this cytokine was 12.98 ± 7.87 and 8 ± 2.51 pg/ml at concentrations of 0.1 and 10 µg/ml of the extract, respectively, compared to the control (32.04 ± 3.35 pg/ml). Conversely, *C. intybus* at concentration of 1 µg/ml significantly increased IFN-γ production in the supernatant of MLR culture in comparison with the control.

Effects of *C. intybus* on IL-12 and IL-10 production by DCs
The level of IL-12 and IL-10 in the supernatant of extract-treated DCs was measured. As the result in Figure 4B shows, IL-12 level was significantly higher at concentrations of 0.1 (280.6 ± 26.58 pg/ml) and 1 µg /ml of the extract (195.5 ± 16.88 pg/ml) than the negative control

(88.58 ± 23.87 pg/ml, P < 0.05). The level of IL-10 didn't show any significant differences in the supernatant of extract-treated and DMSO-treated DCs.

Discussion
In various studies the ability of plants and their derivatives to modulate DCs and induce changes in the expression of co-stimulatory molecules, cytokine secretion patterns and their T cell stimulating activity have been investigated [16,17]. DCs, the key cells of antigen presentation are considered as the important targets for immune response as well as immune regulation.

C. intybus has been widely used as a remedy for treatment of various inflammatory diseases. There are several

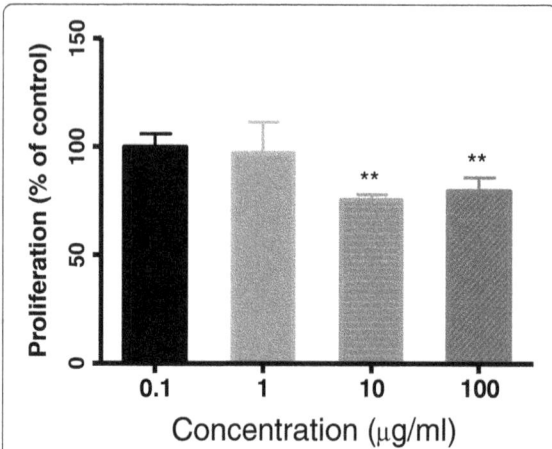

Figure 3 The effect of DCs treated with *C. intybus* extract on T cells proliferation in MLR assay. DCs were treated with the extract for 18 h and then co-cultured with allogenic T cells for 48 h. Control was DMSO-treated DCs plus T cells. Cell proliferation was measured by Brdu incorporation assay. The bars indicate mean ± SD of the cell proliferation in the presence of the extract as compared to the proliferation of controls taken to be 100%. DCs treated with 10 and 100 μg/ml of extract have decreased T cells proliferation (**P < 0.01).

reports about its pharmacological actions and anti-inflammatory effects [1,7]. The root extracts of this plant have shown anti-inflammatory properties in animal models of arthritis. Moreover, in a clinical trial, the safety and usefulness of a proprietary bioactive extract of its root in patients with osteoarthritis have been demonstrated [18]. A decrease observed in macrophage migration inhibitory factor (MIF) serum level in healthy volunteers consuming Chicory coffee [19] and an inhibition in the expression and activity of COX-2 by the ethyl acetate root extract in human colon carcinoma HT29 cells treated with the pro-inflammatory cytokine TNF-α are further evidences implying the effectiveness of this plant on modulation of immune mediators release [1].

As DCs have a critical role in inducing inflammation as well as immune responses, in the present study we arranged a set of experiments to examine the effect of the plant extract on maturation and function of splenic DCs. The phenotypic maturation of DCs was investigated via evaluation of the expression of CD40, CD86 and MHC-II molecules which are important co-stimulatory markers on DCs and have critical roles in antigen presentation and T cell activation. The extract revealed no significant effect on the expression of CD40 and CD86 molecules, showing that it could not promote DCs maturation. The expression

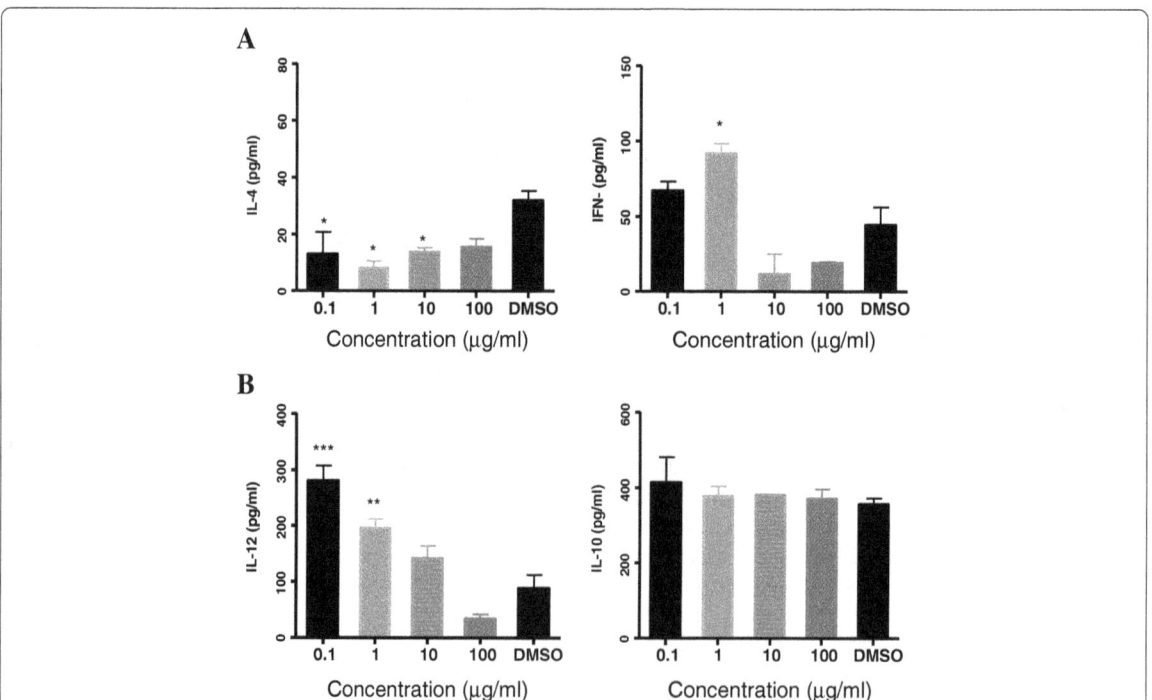

Figure 4 Effect of *C. intybus* extract on cytokine production. (A) The effect of the extract on IL-4 and IFN-γ production in MLR assay. Control was DMSO-treated DCs plus allogenic T cells. **(B)** The effect of the extract on IL-12 and IL-10 secretion by extract treated-DCs after 18 h. Control was DMSO-treated DCs. *P < 0.05, **P < 0.01, ***P < 0.001 shows significant difference with the negative control.

of MHC II antigen on DCs was not also significantly differ-ent with the control, however the intensity of expression of this molecule showed a significant decrease by increasing the concentration of the extract up to 100 μg/ml, indicating a dose-dependent trend to reduce the expression of this molecule on treated DCs as the extract concentration is increased. Any decrease in the expression of the co-stimulatory molecules like MHC II on DCs can be resulted in failure of such DCs to provide an effective response for T cells because these DCs are not only in an immature state but may also have acquired a tolerogenic feature. As result of our study showed, the extract at higher concentra-tions decreased the proliferation of T cells in allogenic response which is in line with the above results and suggests the ability of the extract to affect T cell signaling activity of DCs.

A major characteristic of DCs is synthesis and release of cytokines with modulatory functions during inflammation and T cell differentiation. Immune response is skewed to humoral or cellular immunity based on cytokines secreted by DCs. IL-12 is a cytokine expressed and released by DCs which can induce differentiation of T cells to Th1 and cellu-lar immunity, by contrast IL-10 is a Th1 inhibitory cytokine [20,21]. An elevated IL-12 secretion level by DCs at con-centrations of 0.1 and 1 μg/ml of the extract and no change in IL-10 release was observed in this study. As IL-4 and IFN-γ are landmark of deviation to Th1 or Th2, these cy-tokines were measured in the supernatant of MLR assay. The results indicated a decrease in IL-4 production versus an increase in IFN-γ secretion at concentrations of 0.1 and 1 μg/ml of the extract. In a normal immune response, splenic DCs expressing IL-12 in co-culture with T cells can induce production of IFN-γ and deviation to Th1 while neutralizing of IL-12 inhibit Th1 response and increase Th2 response [22]. Therefore, the increased IL-12 production by DCs when they were treated with low concentrations of the extract along with production of more IFN-γ and less IL-4 by T cells in MLR suggest the ability of *C. intybus* extract to deviate the cytokine pattern of T cells toward a Th1 re-sponse. Of note, the extract at concentration of 100 μg/ml has reduced both IL-12 secretion by treated DCs and IFN-γ release in MLR, which indicated the inhibitory effect of the extract at higher concentration on the im-mune response. It is reasonable to assume that the de-creasing trend observed in the expression of MHC II molecules on DCs, as mentioned before might be a reason for the diminished T cells proliferation and cy-tokines release observed at higher concentration of the extract. To confirm Th1 polarization in co-culture of T cells with *C. intybus* treated-DCs, study of the expression of T bet and GATA-3 as related transcription factors for Th1 and Th2 differentiation is recommended [23]. More-over, the difference between the effect of the extract at lower and higher concentrations may be attributed to the presence of various constituents in the extract with dif-ferent mode of actions. As we used ethanolic crude root extract of the plant, it would be necessary to iden-tify the compound/s responsible for the observed effects in future studies.

Conclusions

C. intybus extract at higher concentrations inhibited T cell stimulating activity of DCs. In contrast, at lower concentrations the extract increased IL-12 production by DCs and modulated cytokine release of T cells toward a Th1 pattern.

Based on these findings further in vivo studies to elu-cidate the effect of these compounds on the complex pathways of DC regulation via IFN-γ and IL-4 as well as their effects on other T cell subsets such as T regulatory cells may lead to the development of clinical applications exploiting these compounds for the treatment of various immune diseases.

Additional file

Additional file 1: Figure S1. Effect of *C. intybus* ethanolic extract on phenotypic maturation of DCs.

Competing interests
The authors declare that they have no competing interests.

Authors' contributions
ZA provided plant materials and with MHK designed and supervised the study and finalized the manuscript. SE carried out the experiments and prepared the draft of the manuscript. All authors read and approved the final manuscript.

Acknowledgement
We would like to thank the Research Vice-Chancellor of Shiraz University of Medical Sciences and Shiraz Transplant Research Center for financial support.

Author details
¹Transplant Research Center, Shiraz University of Medical Sciences, Shiraz, Iran. ²Department of Immunology, Autoimmune Disease Research Center and Medicinal and Natural Products Chemistry Research Center, Shiraz University of Medical Sciences, Shiraz, Iran.

References

1. Cavin C, Delannoy M, Malnoe A, Debefve E, Touché A, Courtois D, Schilter B: Inhibition of the expression and activity of cyclooxygenase-2 by chicory extract. *Biochem Biophys Res Commun* 2005, **18:**742–749.
2. Gazzani G, Daglia M, Papetti A, Gregotti C: In vitro and ex vivo anti- and prooxidant components of Cichorium intybus. *J Pharm Biomed Anal* 2000, **1:**127–133.
3. Ghamarian A, Abdollahi M, Su X, Amiri A, Ahadi A, Nowrouzi A: Effect of chicory seed extract on glucose tolerance test (GTT) and metabolic profile in early and late stage diabetic rats. *Daru* 2012, **15:**56.
4. Ziamajidi N, Khaghani S, Hassanzadeh G, Vardasbi S, Ahmadian S, Nowrouzi A, Ghaffari SM, Abdirad A: Amelioration by chicory seed extract of diabetes- and oleic acid-induced non-alcoholic fatty liver disease (NAFLD)/non-alcoholic steatohepatitis (NASH) via modulation of PPARα and SREBP-1. *Food Chem Toxicol* 2013, **58:**198–209.

5.   Suntar I, Kupeli Akkol E, Keles H, Yesilada E, Sarker SD, Baykal T:
     Comparative evaluation of traditional prescriptions from Cichorium
     intybus L. for wound healing: stepwise isolation of an active component
     by in vivo bioassay and its mode of activity. *J Ethnopharmacol* 2012,
     30:299–309.
6.   Hughes R, Rowland IR: **Stimulation of apoptosis by two prebiotic chicory
     fructans in the rat colon.** *Carcinogenesis* 2001, 22:43–437.
7.   Hassan HA, Yousef MI: **Ameliorating effect of chicory (Cichorium intybus L.)-
     supplemented diet against nitrosamine precursors-induced liver injury and
     oxidative stress in male rats.** *Food Chem Toxicol* 2010, 48:2163–2169.
8.   Amirghofran Z, Azadbakht M, Karimi MH: **Evaluation of the immunomodulatory
     effects of five herbal plants.** *J Ethnopharmacol* 2000, 72:167–172.
9.   Schuurhuis DH, Fu N, Ossendorp F, Melief CJ: **Ins and outs of dendritic
     cells.** *Int Arch Allergy Immunol* 2006, 140:53–72.
10. Reis e Sousa C: **Dendritic cells in a mature age.** *Nat Rev Immunol* 2006,
     6:476–483.
11. Gao Y, Nish SA, Jiang R, Hou L, Licona-Limón P, Weinstein JS, Zhao H,
     Medzhitov R: **Control of T helper 2 responses by transcription factor
     IRF4-dependent dendritic cells.** *Immunity* 2013, 17:722–732.
12. Min WP, Zhou D, Ichim TE, Strejan GH, Xia X, Yang J, Huang X, Garcia B,
     White D, Dutartre P, Jevnikar AM, Zhong R: **Inhibitory feedback loop
     between tolerogenic dendritic cells and regulatory T cells in transplant
     tolerance.** *J Immunol* 2003, 1:1304–1312.
13. Hubert P, Jacobs N, Caberg JH, Boniver J, Delvenne P: **The cross-talk between
     dendritic and regulatory T cells: good or evil?** *J Leukoc Biol* 2007, 82:781–794.
14. Amirghofran Z, Ahmadi H, Karimi M: **Immunomodulatory activity of the
     water extract of Thymus vulgaris, Thymus daenensis and Zataria
     multiflora on dendritic cells and T cells responses.** *J Immunoassay
     Immunochem* 2011, 33:388–402.
15. Amirghofran Z, Hashemzadeh R, Javidnia K, Golmoghaddam H, Esmaeilbeig
     A: **In vitro immunomodulatory effects of extracts from three plants of the
     Labiatae family and isolation of the active compound(s).** *J Immunotoxicol*
     2011, 8:265–273.
16. Yoshimura M, Akiyama H, Kondo K, Sakata K, Matsuoka H, Amakura Y,
     Teshima R, Yoshida T: **Immunological effects of oenothein B, an
     ellagitannin dimer, on dendritic cells.** *Int J Mol Sci* 2012, 14:46–56.
17. Bordbar N, Karimi MH, Amirghofran Z: **The effect of glycyrrhizin on
     maturation and T cell stimulating activity of dendritic cells.** *Cell Immunol*
     2012, 280:44–49.
18. Olsen NJ, Branch VK, Jonnala G, Seskar M, Cooper M: **Phase 1, placebo-controlled,
     dose escalation trial of chicory root extract in patients with osteoarthritis of
     the hip or knee.** *BMC Musculoskelet Disord* 2010, 11:156.
19. Schumacher E, Vigh E, Molnár V, Kenyeres P, Fehér G, Késmárky G, Tóth K,
     Garai J: **Thrombosis preventive potential of chicory coffee consumption:
     a clinical study.** *Phytother Res* 2011, 25:744–748.
20. Xia CQ, Peng R, Annamalai M, Clare-Salzler MJ: **Dendritic cells post-maturation
     are reprogrammed with heightened IFN-gamma and IL-10.** *Biochem Biophys
     Res Commun* 2007, 26:960–965.
21. Ho CY, Lau CB, Kim CF, Leung KN, Fung KP, Tse TF, Chan HH, Chow MS:
     **Differential effect of Coriolus versicolor (Yunzhi) extract on cytokine
     production by murine lymphocytes in vitro.** *Int Immunopharmacol* 2004,
     4:1549–1557.
22. Hibi M, Hachimura S, Ise W, Sato A, Yoshida T, Takayama T, Sasaki K, Senga
     T, Hashizume S, Totsuka M, Kaminogawa S: **Dendritic cells from spleen,
     mesenteric lymph node and peyer's patch can induce the production of
     both IL-4 and IFN-gamma from primary cultures of naive CD4(+) T cells
     in a dose-dependent manner.** *Cytotechnology* 2003, 43:49–55.
23. Kang H, Oh YJ, Choi HY, Ham IH, Bae HS, Kim SH, Ahn KS:
     **Immunomodulatory effect of Schizonepeta tenuifolia water extract on
     mouse Th1/Th2 cytokine production in-vivo and in-vitro.** *J Pharm
     Pharmacol* 2008, 60:901–907.

Synthesis and cytotoxic properties of novel (*E*)-3-benzylidene-7-methoxychroman-4-one derivatives

Saeedeh Noushini[1], Eskandar Alipour[1], Saeed Emami[2], Maliheh Safavi[3], Sussan Kabudanian Ardestani[3], Ahmad Reza Gohari[4], Abbas Shafiee[5] and Alireza Foroumadi[4,5*]

Abstract

Background and the purpose of the study: There has been increscent interest in the field of cancer chemotherapy by discovery and development of novel agents with high efficacy, low toxicity, and minimum side effects. In order to find new anticancer agents, we replaced the pyrazolone part of well-known cytotoxic agent SJ-172550 with 7-methoxychroman-4-one. Thus, a novel series of 3-benzylidene-4-chromanones were synthesized and tested in vitro against human cancer cell lines.

Methods: The title compounds were prepared by condensation of 7-methoxychroman-4-one with suitable aldehydes in appropriate alcohol in the presence of gaseous HCl. The antiproliferative activity of target compounds were evaluated against MDA-MB-231 (breast cancer), KB (nasopharyngeal epidermoid carcinoma) and SK-N-MC (human neuroblastoma) cell lines using MTT assay.

Results: Although the direct analog of SJ-172550 (compound **5d**) did not show any cytotoxic activity against tested cell lines, but 2-(2-chloro-6-methoxyphenoxy)acetic acid methyl ester analog **5c** showed some activity against MDA-MB-231 and SK-N-MC cells. Further modification of compound **5c** resulted in the 3-chloro-4,5-dimethoxybenzylidene derivative **5b** which demonstrated better cytotoxic profile against all tested cell lines (IC$_{50}$ values = 7.56–25.04 µg/ml).

Conclusion: The results demonstrated that the cytotoxic activity of compound **5b** against MDA-MB-231 and SK-N-MC cells is more than etoposide. Therefore, compound **5b** prototype could be considered as novel cytotoxic agent for further developing new anticancer chemotherapeutics.

Keywords: Synthesis, Chalcones, Cytotoxic activity, Cancer, Chroman-4-one

Introduction

Cancer has been known as one of the most impressive clinical problems in both developing and developed countries. In spite of improved diagnostic techniques and advances in prevention and chemotherapeutic management of cancer, the disease still afflicts millions of peoples in the world [1]. Cancer cells are defined by uncontrolled replications associated with self-sufficiency in growth signals, hyposensitivity to anti-growth signals, ongoing angiogenesis, metastasis, and evasion of apoptosis [2]. Anti-cancer agents cannot recognize cancer cells from normal cells, as a matter of fact, these agents usually act on metabolically active or rapidly proliferating cells [3]. Thus, there has been increscent interest in the field of cancer chemotherapy by discovery and development of novel agents with high efficacy, low toxicity, and minimum side effects.

During recent years, several researchers developed different chalcone-like compounds with anticancer activity through the introduction of heterocyclic scaffolds [4,5]. The chemical structure of chalcone is characterized by two aromatic rings connected by a three carbon, α,β-

* Correspondence: aforoumadi@yahoo.com
[4]Medicinal Plants Research Center, Tehran University of Medical Sciences, Tehran, Iran
[5]Department of Medicinal Chemistry, Faculty of Pharmacy and Pharmaceutical Sciences Research Center, Tehran University of Medical Sciences, Tehran, Iran
Full list of author information is available at the end of the article

unsaturated carbonyl system (1,3-diphenyl-2-propen-1-one) [6-8]. The highly significant advantage of chalcone derivatives as cytotoxic agents is the low propensity to interact with DNA; which omits the risk of mutagenesity as the common side effect of current chemotherapeutic agents [9].

Previously, Perjési et al. have reported cytotoxicity of 3-benzylidene-4-chromanones as rigid analogs of chalcones (Figure 1) [10]. Recently, high-throughput screening of drug libraries results in the identification of SJ-172550 that exhibited p53-dependent cytotoxic activity against cancer cell lines [11]. Structurally, SJ-172550 is characterized by having α,β-unsaturated carbonyl system attached to the 2-(2-chloro-6-ethoxyphenoxy)acetic acid methyl ester. Accordingly, in continuation of our research program to find novel anti-cancer agents [12-16] and considering the diverse biological activities of rigid chalcones [17], we have synthesized a series of 3-benzylidene-4-chromanones bearing 2-(2-chloro-6-alkoxyphenoxy) acetic acid esters. The related analogs of 3-benzylidene-4-chromanones were also prepared for more studying of structure-activity relationships (Figure 1).

Material and methods

Chemistry

All chemical reagents and solvents were provided from Merck AG (Darmstadt, Germany). The general procedures for the synthesis of 3-benzylidene-4-chromanones 5a–k, and aldehyde intermediates (compounds 7–9 and 11) are illustrated in Schemes 1 and 2, respectively. 7-Methoxychroman-4-one (4) was prepared as literature method [18,19]. Melting points of compounds were determined using Kofler hot stage apparatus and are

uncorrected. The IR spectra were recorded on a Shimadzu 470 spectrometer by using potassium bromide disks. The NMR spectra were obtained using a Bruker 400 MHz spectrometer (Bruker Bioscience, Billerica, MA, USA). Tetramethylsilane (TMS) was used as internal standard and chemical shifts (δ) are reported in ppm. Mass spectra were recorded on a Finnigan TSQ 70 spectrometer at 70 eV. Elemental analyses were carried out by using a HERAEUS CHN-O rapid elemental analyzer (Heraeus GmbH, Hanau, Germany) for C, H and N and the results are within ± 0.4% of the theoretical values.

Synthesis of 3-chloro-4-hydroxy-5-methoxybenzaldehyde (7a)

To a solution of vanillin (6a, 2.5 g, 16.4 mmol) in glacial acetic acid (15 ml) was slowly introduced a stream of chlorine gas over 30 min. White solid product was filtrated, washed with n-hexane (50 ml) to give compound 7a (1.9 g). The acetic acid filtrate was again treated with chlorine gas flow as above for 30 min to give 0.7 g of compound 7a [20]. A total of 2.6 g (85% yield) of white solid 7a was obtained and used in next step without purification. ^{1}H NMR (CDCl$_3$, 400 MHz) δ: 9.7 (s, 1H, CHO), 7.5 (d, J = 1.6 Hz, 1H, aromatic), 7.3 (d, J = 1.6 Hz, 1H, aromatic), 3.9 (s, 3H, OCH$_3$).

Synthesis of 3-chloro-5-ethoxy-4-hydroxybenzaldehyde (7b)

3-Ethoxy-4-hydroxybenzaldehyde (6b, 4 g, 5 mmol) was dissolved in a solution of glacial acetic acid (30 ml) and chloroform (10 ml) at 0°C and a stream of chlorine gas was slowly introduced over 15 min. Then, the solvents was evaporated and the residue was purified by silica gel column, eluting with a mixture of ethyl acetate/

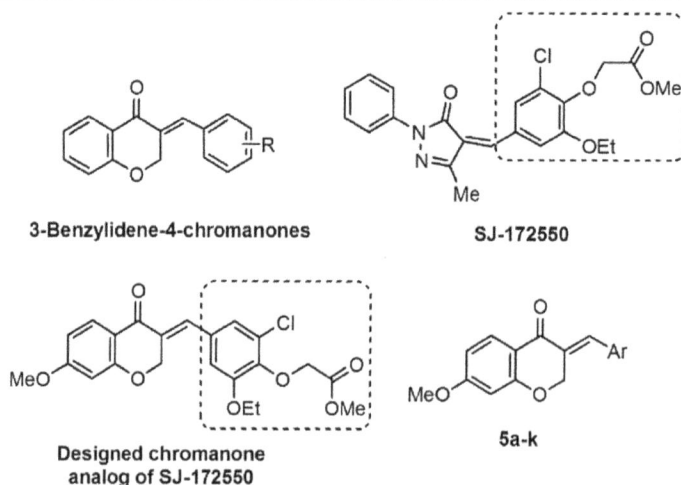

Figure 1 Structure of 3-benzylidene-4-chromanones as rigid analogs of chalcones exhibiting cytotoxic activity, structure of SJ-172550 as a lead compound that showed cytotoxic effects against tumour cell lines and designed compounds as cytotoxic agents.

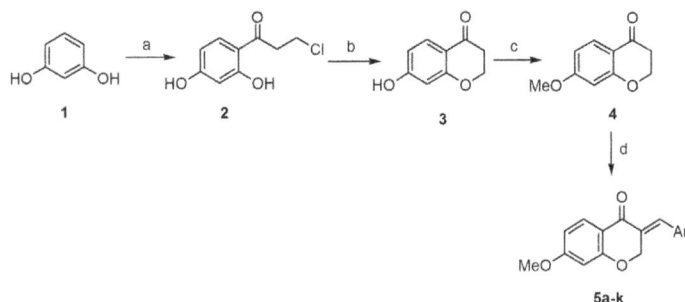

Scheme 1 General synthetic route to 3-benzylidene-4-chromanones 5a–k. *Reagents and conditions*: (a) 3-chloropropionic acid, CF$_3$SO$_3$H; (b) 2.0 M NaOH; (c) methyl iodide, K$_2$CO$_3$, DMF; (d) appropriate aldehyde, HCl (gas), ROH.

petroleum ether (40:60) to give compound **7b** in 65% yield. ^{1}H NMR (CDCl$_3$, 400 MHz) δ: 10.3 (s, 1H, CHO), 7.5 (br s, 1H, aromatic), 6.9 (br s, 1H, aromatic), 5.7 (s, 1H, OH), 4.2 (q, J = 7.2 Hz, 2H, CH$_2$), 1.5 (t, J = 7.2 Hz, 3H, CH$_3$).

Synthesis of methyl 2-(2-chloro-4-formyl-6-methoxyphenoxy)acetate (8a)

A mixture of 5-chlorovanillin (**7a**, 2 g, 10.7 mmol) and K$_2$CO$_3$ (1.5 g, 10.8 mmol) in ethyl methyl ketone (40 ml) was stirred under reflux. After 10 min, methyl bromoacetate (1.64 g, 10.8 mmol) was added, and the mixture was allowed to stir under reflux for another 4 h. After the reaction was completed, ethyl methyl ketone was removed, and the residue was extracted with EtOAc

(3 × 10 ml). The organic layer was dried over Na$_2$SO$_4$ and evaporated to give compound **8a** in 88.8% yield. ^{1}H NMR (CDCl$_3$, 400 MHz) δ: 9.8 (s, 1H, CHO), 7.4 (d, J = 1.6 Hz, 1H, aromatic), 7.3 (d, J = 1.6 Hz, 1H, aromatic), 4.8 (s, 2H, CH$_2$), 3.9 (s, 3H, OCH$_3$), 3.8 (s, 3H, OCH$_3$).

Synthesis of methyl 2-(2-chloro-6-ethoxy-4-formylphenoxy)acetate (8b)

To a solution of compound **7b** (200 mg, 1 mmol) in ethyl methyl ketone (4 ml), was added potassium carbonate (147 mg, 1 mmol) and methyl bromoacetate (153 mg, 1 mmol) successively. The mixture was stirred under reflux for 2 h, cooled to room temperature and the solvent was removed under reduced pressure. The residue was added to 5 ml of water and extracted three

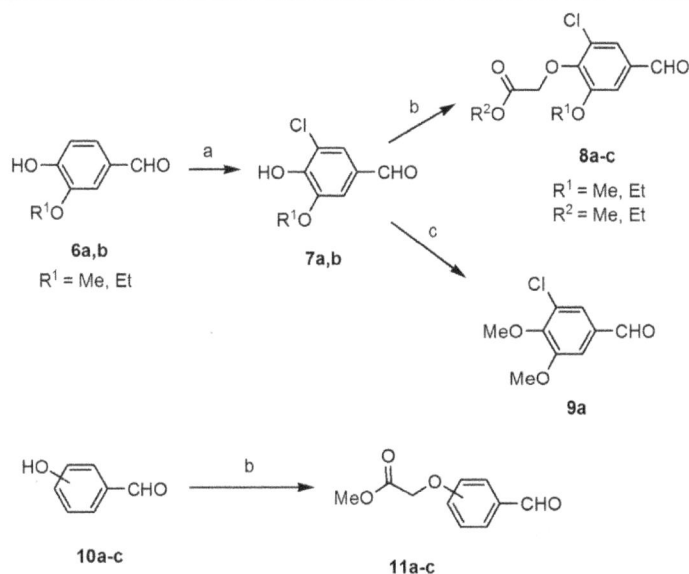

Scheme 2 Synthesis of aldehyde intermediates 7–9 and 11. *Reagents and conditions*: (a) Cl$_2$, CH$_3$COOH; (b) R^{2}OCOCH$_2$Br, K$_2$CO$_3$, CH$_3$COCH$_2$CH$_3$; (c) methyl iodide, K$_2$CO$_3$, DMF.

times with ethyl acetate (5 ml). The combined extracts was dried (Na_2SO_4), and concentrated to give **8b** as a white solid in 91% yield. ^{1}H NMR ($CDCl_3$, 400 MHz) δ: 10.3 (s, 1H, CHO), 7.3 (s, 1H, aromatic), 6.8 (s, 1H, aromatic), 4.7 (s, 2H, CH_2), 4.2 (q, $J = 7.2$ Hz, 2H, CH_2), 3.8 (s, 3H, OCH_3), 1.5 (t, $J = 7.2$ Hz, 3H, CH_3).

Synthesis of ethyl 2-(2-chloro-6-ethoxy-4-formylphenoxy) acetate (8c)

To a solution of compound **7b** (500 mg, 2.5 mmol) in ethyl methyl ketone (10 ml), was added potassium carbonate (370 mg, 2.5 mmol) and ethyl bromoacetate (2.5 - mmol) successively. The mixture was stirred under reflux for 3 h and then the solvent was removed under reduced pressure. The residue was added to 10 ml of water and extracted three times with ethyl acetate (10 ml). The combined extracts was dried (Na_2SO_4) and concentrated to give **8c** as a white solid in 88% yield. ^{1}H NMR ($CDCl_3$, 400 MHz) δ: 10.2 (s, 1H, CHO), 7.3 (s, 1H, aromatic), 6.9 (s, 1H, aromatic), 4.7 (s, 2H, CH_2), 4.25 (q, $J = 7.2$ Hz, 2H, CH_2), 1.5 (t, $J = 7.2$ Hz, 3H, CH_3), 1.3 (t, $J = 7.2$ Hz, 3H, CH_3).

Synthesis of 3-chloro-4,5-dimethoxybenzaldehyde (9a)

To a solution of 5-chlorovanillin (**7a**, 5 g, 26.8 mmol) in DMF (40 ml) was added potassium carbonate (3.7 g, 26.8 mmol) and iodomethane (4.56 g, 32.16 mmol) successively. The mixture was stirred at 80°C for 3 h, cooled to room temperature and poured to water (100 ml). The precipitated white solid was filtrated and washed with water to give 5.1 g of compound **9a** in 94.8 yield. ^{1}H NMR ($CDCl_3$, 400 MHz) δ: 9.85 (s, 1H, CHO), 7.5 (s, 1H, aromatic), 7.35 (s, 1H, aromatic), 3.97 (s, 3H, OCH_3), 3.94 (s, 3H, OCH_3).

General procedure for the preparation of compounds 11a-c

A mixture of hydroxybenzaldehyde **10a-c** (5 g, 40.95 mmol) and K_2CO_3 (6 g, 40.95 mmol) in ethyl methyl ketone (100 ml) was stirred under reflux. After 1 h, methyl bromoacetate was added, and the mixture was allowed to stir under reflux for another 3 h. After the reaction was completed, ethyl methyl ketone was removed, and the residue was extracted with EtOAc (3 × 20 ml). The organic layer was dried (Na_2SO_4) and evaporated to give methyl (formylphenoxy)acetate **11a-c** [21].

Methyl (2-formylphenoxy)acetate (11a)

This compound was obtained using general procedure as a pale yellow oil without further purification in 85% yield. IR (KBr, cm^{-1}): 1767 (C = O, ester), 1690 (C = O, aldehyde); ^{1}H NMR ($CDCl_3$, 400 MHz) δ: 10.56 (s, 1H, CHO), 7.87 (dd, $J = 5.6$ and 2 Hz, 1H, H_6-phenyl), 7.54 (t, $J = 7.6$ Hz, 1H, H_4-phenyl), 7.09 (t, $J = 7.6$ Hz, 1H, H_5-

phenyl), 6.86 (t, $J = 8.8$ Hz, 1H, H_3-phenyl), 4.7 (s, 2H, CH_2), 3.8 (s, 3H, OCH_3).

Methyl (3-formylphenoxy)acetate (11b)

This compound was obtained using general procedure as a pale yellow oil without further purification in 63% yield. IR (KBr, cm^{-1}): 1761 (C = O, ester), 1682 (C = O, aldehyde); ^{1}H NMR ($CDCl_3$, 400 MHz) δ: 10 (s, 1H, CHO), 7.51 (m, 2H, H_5, H_6-phenyl), 7.36 (s, 1H, H_2-phenyl), 7.25 (br s, 1H, H_4-phenyl), 4.71 (s, 2H, CH_2), 3.92 (s, 3H, OCH_3).

Methyl (4-formylphenoxy)acetate (11c)

This compound was obtained using general procedure as a pale yellow oil without further purification in 93% yield. IR (KBr, cm^{-1}): 1742 (C = O, ester), 1695 (C = O, aldehyde); ^{1}H NMR ($CDCl_3$, 400 MHz) δ: 9.9 (s, 1H, CHO), 7.9 (d, $J = 8$ Hz, 2H, aromatic), 7.0 (d, $J = 8$ Hz, 2H, aromatic), 4.73 (s, 2H, CH_2), 3.82 (s, 3H, CH_3O).

Synthesis of (E)-3-(3-chloro-4-hydroxy-5-methoxybenzylidene)-7-methoxychroman-4-one (5a)

A solution of 7-methoxychroman-4-one (**4**, 100 mg, 0.56 mmol), 5-chlorovanillin (**7a**, 105 mg, 0.56 mmol) in EtOH (2 ml) was stirred at room temperature for 5 min, while a stream of HCl gas was introduced. After 24 h at room temperature, the precipitation was filtrated, crystallized from EtOH to give **5a** as red solid in 52% yield. m.p. 171–173°C; IR (KBr, cm^{-1}): 3428 (OH), 1655 (C = O); ^{1}H NMR (DMSO-d_6, 400 MHz) δ: 7.8 (d, $J = 8.8$ Hz, 1H, H_5-chromanone), 7.6 (br s, 1H, CH-vinylic), 7.07 (d, $J = 1.5$ Hz, 1H, H_2-phenyl), 7.03 (d, $J = 1.6$ Hz, 1H, H_6-phenyl), 6.7 (dd, $J = 6.4$ and 2.4 Hz, 1H, H_6-chromanone), 6.5 (d, $J = 2.3$ Hz, 1H, H_8-chromanone), 5.4 (d, $J = 1.6$ Hz, 2H, H_2-chromanone), 3.89 (s, 3H, OCH_3), 3.83 (s, 3H, OCH_3); Anal. Calcd for $C_{18}H_{15}ClO_5$: C, 62.35; H, 4.36. Found: C, 62.04; H, 4.40.

Synthesis of (E)-3-(3-chloro-4,5-dimethoxybenzylidene)-7-methoxychroman-4-one (5b)

A solution of 7-methoxychroman-4-one (**4**, 500 mg, 2.8 mmol), 3-chloro-4,5-dimethoxybenzaldehyde (**9a**, 562 mg, 2.8 mmol) in EtOH (10 ml) was stirred at room temperature for 25 min, while a stream of HCl gas was introduced. After 24 h at room temperature, the precipitated solid was filtrated, crystallized from EtOH to afford compound **5b** as orange solid in 85% yield. m.p. 125–127°C; IR (KBr, cm^{-1}): 1670 (C = O); ^{1}H NMR ($CDCl_3$, 400 MHz) δ: 7.96 (d, $J = 8.8$ Hz, 1H, H_5-chromanone), 7.7 (br s, 1H, CH-vinylic), 6.8 (br s, 1H, H_2-phenyl), 6.7 (br s, 1H, H_6-phenyl), 6.6 (d, $J = 8$ Hz, 1H, H_6-chromanone), 6.4 (br s, 1H, H_8-chromanone), 5.3 (s, 2H, H_2-chromanone), 3.92 (s, 3H, OCH_3), 3.9 (s, 3H, OCH_3), 3.85 (s, 3H,

OCH$_3$); Anal. Calcd for C$_{19}$H$_{17}$ClO$_5$: C, 63.25; H, 4.75. Found: C, 62.88; H, 4.41.

Synthesis of (E)-methyl 2-(2-chloro-6-methoxy-4-((7-methoxy-4-oxo-2H-chromen-3(4H)-ylidene)methyl)phenoxy)acetate (5c)

A solution of 7-methoxychroman-4-one (**4**, 300 mg, 1.68 mmol), methyl 2-(2-chloro-4-formyl-6-methoxyphenoxy)acetate (**8a**, 435 mg, 1.68 mmol) in MeOH (6 ml) was stirred at room temperature for 20 min, while a stream of HCl gas was introduced. After 24 h at room temperature, the precipitation was filtrated, crystallized from MeOH to give compound **5c** as pink solid in 64% yield. m.p. 118–121°C; IR (KBr, cm^{-1}): 1767 (C = O), 1750 (C = O); ^{1}H NMR (CDCl$_3$, 400 MHz) δ: 7.9 (d, J = 9.2 Hz, 1H, H$_5$-chromanone), 7.7 (br s, 1H, CH-vinylic), 6.9 (s, 1H, H$_3$-phenyl), 6.7 (s, 1H, H$_5$-phenyl), 6.6 (d, J = 8.8 Hz, 1H, H$_6$-chromanone), 6.4 (br s, 1H, H$_8$-chromanone), 5.3 (s, 2H, OCH$_2$CO), 4.7 (s, 2H, H$_2$-chromanone), 3.87 (s, 3H, OCH$_3$), 3.85 (s, 3H, OCH$_3$), 3.83 (s, 3H, OCH$_3$); Anal. Calcd for C$_{21}$H$_{19}$ClO$_7$: C, 60.22; H, 4.57. Found: C, 60.36; H, 4.71.

Synthesis of (E)-methyl 2-(2-chloro-6-ethoxy-4-((7-methoxy-4-oxo-2H-chromen-3(4H)-ylidene)methyl)phenoxy)acetate (5d)

A solution of 7-methoxychroman-4-one (**4**, 200 mg, 1.12 - mmol), methyl 2-(2-chloro-6-ethoxy-4-formylphenoxy)acetate (**8b**, 288 mg, 1.12 mmol) in MeOH (4 ml) was stirred at room temperature for 25 min, while a stream of HCl gas was introduced. After 24 h at room temperature, the precipitated solid was filtrated, crystallized from MeOH to give pure compound **5d** as a pink solid in 52% yield. m.p. 151–153°C; IR (KBr, cm^{-1}): 1759 (C = O), 1737 (C = O); ^{1}H NMR (CDCl$_3$, 400 MHz) δ: 7.9 (d, J = 8.8 Hz, 1H, H$_5$-chromanone), 7.8 (br s, 1H, CH-vinylic), 6.9 (s, 1H, H$_3$-phenyl), 6.6 (br s, 2H, H$_6$-chromanone and H$_5$-phenyl), 6.4 (br s, 1H, H$_8$-chromanone), 5.1 (s, 2H, CH$_2$), 4.7 (s, 2H, H$_2$-chromanone), 4.1 (m, 2H, CH$_2$), 3.85 (s, 3H, OCH$_3$), 3.82 (s, 3H, OCH$_3$), 1.5 (t, J = 6.8 Hz, 3H, CH$_3$); Anal. Calcd for C$_{22}$H$_{21}$ClO$_7$: C, 61.05; H, 4.89. Found: C, 60.83; H, 5.03.

Synthesis of (E)-ethyl 2-(2-chloro-6-ethoxy-4-((7-methoxy-4-oxo-2H-chromen-3(4H)-ylidene)methyl)phenoxy)acetate (5e)

A solution of 7-methoxychroman-4-one (**4**, 50 mg, 0.28 mmol), ethyl 2-(2-chloro-6-ethoxy-4-formylphenoxy)acetate (**8c**, 76 mg, 0.28 mmol) in EtOH (2 ml) was stirred at room temperature for 15 min, while a stream of HCl gas was introduced. After 24 h at room temperature, the precipitation was filtrated, crystallized from EtOH to give compound **5e** as a white solid in 43% yield. m.p. 122–123°C; IR (KBr, cm^{-1}): 1748 (C = O); ^{1}H NMR (CDCl$_3$, 400 MHz) δ: 7.9 (d, J = 8.0, 1H, H$_5$-chromanone),

7.8 (br s, 1H, CH-vinylic), 6.9 (s, 1H, H$_3$-phenyl), 6.6 (br s, 2H, H$_6$-chromanone and H$_5$-phenyl), 6.4 (s, 1H, H$_8$-chromanone), 5.1 (s, 2H, H$_2$-chromanone), 4.6 (s, 2H, OCH$_2$CO), 4.2 (m, 2H, CH$_2$), 4.1 (m, 2H, CH$_2$), 3.85 (s, 3H, OCH$_3$), 1.4 (m, 3H, CH$_3$), 1.3 (s, 3H, CH$_3$); Anal. Calcd for C$_{23}$H$_{23}$ClO$_7$: C, 61.82; H, 5.19. Found: C, 62.01; H, 4.89.

Synthesis of (E)-methyl 2-(4-((7-methoxy-4-oxo-2H-chromen-3(4H)-ylidene)methyl)phenoxy)acetate (5f)

A solution of 7-methoxychroman-4-one (**4**, 100 mg, 0.56 mmol), methyl 2-(4-formylphenoxy)acetate (**11c**, 109 mg, 0.56 mmol) in anhydrous MeOH (2 ml) was stirred at room temperature for 25 min, while a stream of HCl gas was introduced. After 24 h at room temperature, the precipitation was filtrated, crystallized from methanol to afford pure compound **5f** as a red solid in 71% yield. m. p. 131–133°C; IR (KBr, cm^{-1}): 1760 (C = O), 1667 (C = O); ^{1}H NMR (CDCl$_3$, 400 MHz) δ: 7.8 (d, J = 8.4 Hz, 1H, H$_5$-chromanone), 7.6 (s, 1H, CH-vinylic), 7.41 (d, J = 8.8 Hz, 2H, H$_2$- and H$_6$-phenyl), 7.05 (d, J = 8.4 Hz, 2H, H$_3$- and H$_5$-phenyl), 6.7 (d, J = 8.2 Hz, 1H, H$_6$-chromanone), 6.5 (s, 1H, H$_8$-chromanone), 5.4 (s, 2H, OCH$_2$CO), 4.8 (s, 2H, H$_2$-chromanone), 3.8 (s, 3H, OCH$_3$), 3.7 (s, 3H, OCH$_3$); MS, m/z: 354, 295, 281, 265, 253, 151, 131, 115, 77, 63, 45. Anal. Calcd for C$_{20}$H$_{18}$O$_6$: C, 67.79; H, 5.12; Found: C, 68.00; H, 4.98.

Synthesis of (E)-ethyl 2-(4-((7-methoxy-4-oxo-2H-chromen-3(4H)-ylidene)methyl)phenoxy)acetate (5g)

A solution of 7-methoxychroman-4-one (**4**, 100 mg, 0.56 mmol), methyl 2-(4-formylphenoxy)acetate (**11c**, 109 mg, 0.56 mmol) in anhydrous EtOH (2 ml) was stirred at room temperature for 20 min, while a stream of HCl gas was introduced. After 24 h at room temperature, the precipitation was filtrated, crystallized from ethanol to give compound **5 g** as a red solid in 71% yield. m.p. 133–135°C; IR (KBr, cm^{-1}): 1760 (C = O), 1659 (C = O); ^{1}H NMR (DMSO-d_6, 400 MHz) δ: 7.8 (d, J = 8.4 Hz, 1H, H$_5$-chromanone), 7.6 (s, 1H, CH-vinylic), 7.41 (d, J = 8.8 Hz, 2H, H$_2$- and H$_6$-phenyl), 7.05 (d, J = 8.4 Hz, 2H, H$_3$- and H$_5$-phenyl), 6.7 (d, J = 8.2 Hz, 1H, H$_6$-chromanone), 6.5 (s, 1H, H$_8$-chromanone), 5.4 (s, 2H, OCH$_2$CO), 4.8 (s, 2H, H$_2$-chromanone), 3.8 (s, 3H, OCH$_3$), 3.7 (s, 3H, OCH$_3$); MS, m/z: 368, 281, 253, 164, 151, 131, 115, 77. Anal. Calcd for C$_{21}$H$_{20}$O$_6$: C, 68.47; H, 5.47. Found: C, 68.27; H, 5.51.

Synthesis of (E)-propyl 2-(4-((7-methoxy-4-oxo-2H-chromen-3(4H)-ylidene)methyl)phenoxy)acetate (5h)

A solution of 7-methoxychroman-4-one (**4**, 300 mg, 1.68 mmol), methyl 2-(4-formylphenoxy)acetate (**11c**, 327 mg, 1.68 mmol) in n-PrOH (6 ml) was stirred at room temperature for 15 min, while a stream of HCl gas was introduced. After 24 h at room temperature, the precipitation was filtrated, crystallized from PrOH to give compound **5 h** as a pink solid in 47% yield. m.p. 102–105°C; IR (KBr, cm^{-1}): 1758 (C = O), 1660 (C = O); ^{1}H NMR (DMSO-d_6, 400 MHz) δ: 7.8 (d, J = 8.4 Hz, 1H, H$_5$-chromanone), 7.6 (s, 1H, CH-vinylic), 7.4 (d, J = 8.0 Hz, 2H, H$_2$- and H$_6$-phenyl), 7.0 (d, J = 8.4 Hz, 2H, H$_3$- and H$_5$-phenyl), 6.7 (d, J = 8.0 Hz, 1H, H$_6$-chromanone), 6.5 (s, 1H, H$_8$-chromanone), 5.4 (s, 2H, OCH$_2$CO), 4.89 (s, 2H, H$_2$-chromanone), 4.09 (t, J = 6.4 Hz, 2H, OCH$_2$), 3.8 (s, 3H,OCH$_3$), 1.6 (m, 2H, CH$_2$), 0.87 (t, J = 7.2 Hz, 3H, CH$_3$); MS, m/z: 382, 354, 295, 281, 265, 151, 131, 115, 77, 69, 57, 43. Anal. Calcd for C$_{22}$H$_{22}$O$_6$: C, 69.10; H, 5.80. Found: C, 68.90; H, 6.07.

Synthesis of (E)-butyl 2-(4-((7-methoxy-4-oxo-2H-chromen-3 (4H)-ylidene)methyl)phenoxy)acetate (5i)

A solution of 7-methoxychroman-4-one (**4**, 100 mg, 0.56 mmol), methyl 2-(4-formylphenoxy)acetate (**11c**, 109 mg, 0.56 mmol) in *n*-BuOH (2 ml) was stirred at room temperature for 10 min, while a stream of HCl gas was introduced. After 24 h at room temperature, the precipitation was filtrated, crystallized from *n*-BuOH to afford compound **5i** as a pink solid in 36% yield. m.p. 85–87°C; IR (KBr, cm^{-1}): 1766 (C = O), 1664 (C = O); ^{1}H NMR (DMSO-d_6, 400 MHz) δ: 7.8 (d, J = 8.8 Hz, 1H, H$_5$-chromanone), 7.6 (br s, 1H, CH-vinylic), 7.4 (d, J = 8.0 Hz, 2H, H$_2$- and H$_6$-phenyl), 7.0 (d, J = 8.4 Hz, 2H, H$_3$- and H$_5$-phenyl), 6.7 (d, J = 7.6 Hz, 1H, H$_6$-chromanone), 6.5 (br s, 1H, H$_8$-chromanone), 5.4 (s, 2H, OCH$_2$CO), 4.8 (s, 2H, H$_2$-chromanone), 4.1 (t, J = 7.6 Hz, 2H, OCH$_2$), 3.8 (s, 3H, OCH$_3$), 1.5 (m, 2H, CH$_2$), 1.3 (m, 2H, CH$_2$), 0.8 (t, J = 7.6 Hz, 3H, CH$_3$); MS, m/z: 396, 281, 265, 253, 167, 149, 131, 115, 107, 81, 57, 41. Anal. Calcd for C$_{23}$H$_{24}$O$_6$: C, 69.68; H, 6.10. Found: C, 69.80; H, 6.37.

Synthesis of (E)-methyl 2-(2-((7-methoxy-4-oxo-2H-chromen-3(4H)-ylidene)methyl)phenoxy)acetate (5j)

A solution of 7-methoxychroman-4-one (**4**, 100 mg, 0.56 mmol), methyl 2-(2-formylphenoxy)acetate (**11a**, 109 mg, 0.56 mmol) in anhydrous MeOH (2 ml) was stirred at room temperature for 35 min, while a stream of HCl gas was introduced. After 24 h at room temperature, the precipitation was filtrated, crystallized from methanol to give compound **5j** as yellow viscous oil in 32% yield. IR (KBr, cm^{-1}): 1755 (C = O), 1664 (C = O); ^{1}H NMR (CDCl$_3$, 400 MHz) δ: 7.98 (br s, 1H, H$_5$-chromanone), 7.96 (s, 1H, CH-vinylic), 7.35 (d, J = 7.6 Hz, 1H, H$_3$-phenyl), 7.07 (m, 2H, H$_4$- and H$_5$-phenyl), 6.81 (d, J = 8 Hz, 1H, H$_6$-phenyl), 6.62 (d, J = 7.6 Hz, 1H, H$_6$-chromanone), 6.4 (s, 1H, H$_8$-chromanone), 5.22 (s, 2H, OCH$_2$CO), 4.7 (s, 2H, H$_2$-chromanone), 3.8 (s, 3H, OCH$_3$), 3.79 (s, 3H, OCH$_3$); MS, m/z: 354, 295, 281, 265, 151, 131, 77, 67, 57, 43.

Anal. Calcd for C$_{20}$H$_{18}$O$_6$: C, 67.79; H, 5.12. Found: C, 68.02; H, 4.98.

Synthesis of (E)-methyl 2-(3-((7-methoxy-4-oxo-2H-chromen-3(4H)-ylidene)methyl)phenoxy)acetate (5k)

A solution of 7-methoxychroman-4-one (**4**, 100 mg, 0.56 mmol), methyl 2-(3-formylphenoxy)acetate (**11b**, 109 mg, 0.56 mmol) in anhydrous MeOH (2 ml) was stirred at room temperature for 30 min, while a stream of HCl gas was introduced. After 24 h at room temperature, the precipitation was filtrated, crystallized from methanol to give compound **5 k** as a pink solid in 79% yield. m.p. 111–114°C; IR (KBr, cm^{-1}): 1758 (C = O), 1670 (C = O); ^{1}H NMR (DMSO-d_6, 400 MHz) δ: 7.8 (d, J = 8.8 Hz, 1H, H$_5$-chromanone), 7.7 (s, 1H, CH-vinylic), 7.4 (t, J = 6.8 Hz, 1H, H$_6$-phenyl), 7.0 (m, 3H, H$_2$ and H$_4$- and H$_5$-phenyl), 6.7 (dd, J = 6.8 and 2.0 Hz, 1H, H$_6$-chromanone), 6.5 (d, J = 2.0 Hz, 1H, H$_8$-chromanone), 5.4 (s, 2H, OCH$_2$CO), 4.9 (s, 2H, H$_2$-chromanone), 3.8 (s, 3H, OCH$_3$), 3.7 (s, 3H, OCH$_3$); MS, m/z: 354, 281, 178, 167, 150, 122, 107, 79, 69, 57, 43. Anal. Calcd for C$_{20}$H$_{18}$O$_6$: C, 67.79; H, 5.12. Found: C, 67.65; H, 5.33.

Cytotoxicity assay

The in-vitro cytotoxic activity of each synthesized compounds **5a-k** was assessed using MTT colorimetric assay according to the literature method [22]. Each set of experiments was independently performed three times. For each compound, the concentration causing 50% cell growth inhibition (IC$_{50}$) compared with the control was calculated from concentration-response curves by regression analysis.

Results and discussion
Chemistry

Reaction sequence employed for the synthesis of (*E*)-3-benzylidene-7-methoxychroman-4-one derivatives **5a-k** is shown in Scheme 1. The reaction of resorcinol **1** with 3-chloropropionic acid in the presence of trifluoromethane sulfonic acid furnished 2′,4′-dihydroxy-3-chloropropiophenone (**2**) which was cyclized using 2 M NaOH to give 7-hydroxy-4-chromanone (**3**). Compound **4** was obtained by reacting intermediate **3** with iodomethane in the presence of potassium carbonate in DMF. Condensation of 7-methoxychroman-4-one (**4**) with suitable aldehydes **7–9** and **11** in appropriate alcohol in the presence of gaseous HCl gave the target compounds **5a-k**.

The corresponding aldehydes **7–9** and **11** were prepared as shown in Scheme 2. Chlorination of 3-alkoxy-4-hydroxybenzaldehyde **6a,b** using acetic acid as a solvent gave 3-chloro-4-hydroxy-5-alkoxybenzaldehyde **7a,b** which was reacted with suitable alkyl bromoacetate in the presence of potassium carbonate to give compounds

Table 1 Cytotoxic activity (IC$_{50}$, µg/ml) of compounds 5a-k against different cell lines in comparison with etoposide

Compounds	Ar	MDA-MB-231	KB	SK-N-MC
5a		19.70 ± 3.07	36.85 ± 2.97	12.60 ± 8.45
5b		7.56 ± 2.23	25.04 ± 10.60	9.64 ± 2.71
5c		20.03 ± 4.27	>100	58.04 ± 21.08
5d		>100	>100	>100
5e		>100	>100	>100
5f		16.47 ± 1.47	>100	>100
5g		16.32 ± 2.67	>100	>100
5h		18.87 ± 0.43	>100	>100
5i		7.10 ± 2.99	>100	>100

Table 1 Cytotoxic activity (IC$_{50}$, µg/ml) of compounds 5a-k against different cell lines in comparison with etoposide
(Continued)

5j		14.23 ± 4.37	>100	>100
5k		10.53 ± 0.86	>100	>100
Etoposide		21.2 ± 2.12	18.93 ± 1.78	14.04 ± 1.05

8a-c. On the other hand, *O*-methylation of compound 7a afforded dimethoxybenzaldehyde derivative 9a. Methyl (formylphenoxy)acetate 11a-c was synthesized by heating compounds 10a-c with methyl bromoacetate and potassium carbonate in ethyl methyl ketone.

In vitro cytotoxic activity

The cytotoxic activity of synthesized compounds 5a-k was evaluated against three cell lines namely MDA-MB-231 (breast cancer), KB (nasopharyngeal epidermoid carcinoma) and SK-N-MC (human neuroblastoma) cells. The results of cytotoxic assay were mentioned as IC$_{50}$ (µg/ml) of compounds in comparison with reference drug etoposide in Table 1.

In the case of MDA-MB-231 cell line, the IC$_{50}$ values of all compounds were ≤20 µg/ml with the exception of compounds 5d and 5e. Furthermore, compounds 5b and 5i exhibited the highest cytotoxic activity against this cell line (IC$_{50}$ < 10 µg/ml). Compound 5b was also the most potent derivative against KB cell line with IC$_{50}$ value of 25.04 µg/ml. Beside compound 5b, compound 5a exhibited good activity against KB cells, but remaining compounds 5c-k showed no activity against this cell line (IC$_{50}$ >100 µg/ml). Against SK-N-MC cells, compound 5b followed by compounds 5a and 5c showed significant inhibitory activity with IC$_{50}$ values of 9.64, 12.6 and 58.04 µg/ml, respectively.

Overall, it is clear that among the test compounds described in this study, the 3-chloro-4,5-dimethoxy-benzylidene derivative 5b demonstrated better cytotoxic profile against all tested cell lines (IC$_{50}$ values = 7.56–25.04 µg/ml). Generally, the comparison of IC$_{50}$ values of compound 5b with those of etoposide demonstrated that the cytotoxic activity of compound 5b against MDA-MB-231 and SK-N-MC cells is more than etoposide.

In this work, as part of an ongoing program to find new cytotoxic agents, we have focused our attention on modification of the 3-benzylidene-4-chromanones and introducing new functionality on the benzylidene moiety.

Thus, we designed novel 3-benzylidene-4-chromanones that possessed a 2-(2-chloro-6-alkoxyphenoxy)acetic acid ester. These modifications were made on the basis of SJ-172550, a new cytotoxic agent possessing 2-(2-chloro-6-ethoxyphenoxy)acetic acid methyl ester attached to the pyrazolone ring. Surprisingly, compound 5d, the chromanone analog of SJ-172550 showed no activity against tested cell lines. Also, the ethyl ester counterpart of 5d (compound 5e) was inactive against tumor cell lines. However, the 2-(2-chloro-6-methoxyphenoxy)acetic acid methyl ester analog 5c was active against MDA-MB-231 and SK-N-MC cells. We have briefly investigated the SAR of compounds by simplification of the functionality on the benzylidene part of the basic molecule.

As can be deduced from the cytotoxic data of compounds 5f-k which characterized by the lack of 2-chloro-6-alkoxy functionality, the cytotoxic activity against MDA-MB-231 can be served by the simple phenoxyacetic acid ester derivatives. However, the lack of 2-chloro-6-alkoxy functionality results in the lack of activity against KB and SK-N-MC cells. Among the compounds 5f-k, butyl ester derivative 5i showed the highest activity against MDA-MB-231 being 3-fold more potent than standard drug etoposide.

To determine the effect of acetic acid ester substitution in compound 5c, we prepared both the 4-hydroxy derivative 5a and 4-methoxy analog 5b. When compared to 5c, both compounds had similar or better in vitro activities against tested cell lines.

The cytotoxic activities of regio-isomeric compounds 5f, 5j and 5 k against MDA-MB-231cells revealed that changing the position of oxyesteric group has led to non-significant changes in activities. As seen from data, in poly-substituted compounds changing of methoxy group on phenyl ring to ethoxy group (for example 5d versus 5c) dramatically decreased the cytotoxic potency in MDA-MB-231 and SK-N-MC cells.

In summary, in the pursuit for finding new cytotoxic agents, we replaced the pyrazolone part of well-known cytotoxic agent SJ-172550 with 7-methoxychroman-4-one. Although the direct analog of SJ-172550 (compound **5d**) did not show any cytotoxic activity against tested cell lines, but 2-(2-chloro-6-methoxyphenoxy) acetic acid methyl ester analog **5c** showed some activity against MDA-MB-231 and SK-N-MC cells. Further modification of compound **5c** resulted in the 3-chloro-4,5-dimethoxybenzylidene derivative **5b** which demonstrated better cytotoxic profile against all tested cell lines (IC$_{50}$ values = 7.56–25.04 µg/ml).

It is worthwhile to mention that, since we have originally designed the target compounds based on p53-dependent cytotoxic agent SJ-172550, it was better using the latter compound as standard drug in our cytotoxic assay. However, our primary cytotoxic experiments on the closest compound to SJ-172550 (compound **5d**) in a side-by-side comparison manner with etoposide revealed that compound **5d** had no activity against cancer cell lines. On the other hand, simplified compounds **5a** and **5b** with more dissimilarity respect to the SJ-172550 showed better profile of cytotoxicity. Based on these results, it seems that a different mechanism is responsible for potential cytotoxic activity of compound **5b** prototype.

We employed MTT cell viability assay as a standard and well-documented in vitro method for evaluation of the cytotoxic potential of designed compounds. Although these types of in vitro models are beneficial and promising as early screening tools for finding new lead compounds, but these models are associated with some limitations [23]. Thus, for efficacy and safety evaluation of lead compounds, conducting a method based on animal model is necessary in the next steps of study.

In conclusion, the results demonstrated that the cytotoxic activity of 3-(3-chloro-4,5-dimethoxybenzylidene)-7-methoxychroman-4-one (**5b**) against MDA-MB-231 and SK-N-MC cells is more than standard drug etoposide. Therefore, compound **5b** prototype bearing 3-chloro-4,5-dimethoxybenzylidene moiety could be considered as novel lead compound for further developing new anticancer chemotherapeutics. Although, compound **5b** showed promising activity in vitro, but to identify a promising anticancer drug candidate that has good pharmacokinetic and toxicological profiles, the in vivo ADME-Tox studies of compound **5b** prototype should be conducted.

Competing interests
The authors declare that they have no competing interests.

Authors' contributions
SN: Synthesis of target compounds. EA: Supervision of the synthetic part. SE: Collaboration in design and identifying of the structures of target compounds, manuscript preparation. MS: Performed the cytotoxic tests. SKA: Supervision of the cytotoxic tests. ARG: Collaboration in identifying the structures of target compounds. AS: Collaboration in identifying the structures of target compounds. AF: Design of target compounds and supervision of the synthetic and pharmacological parts. All authors read and approved the final manuscript.

Acknowledgements
This work was financially supported by grants from Tehran University of Medical Sciences and Iran National Science Foundation (INSF).

Author details
[1]Department of Chemistry, Islamic Azad University, Tehran-North Branch, Zafar St, Tehran, Iran. [2]Department of Medicinal Chemistry and Pharmaceutical Sciences Research Center, Faculty of Pharmacy, Mazandaran University of Medical Sciences, Sari, Iran. [3]Institute of Biochemistry and Biophysics, University of Tehran, Tehran, Iran. [4]Medicinal Plants Research Center, Tehran University of Medical Sciences, Tehran, Iran. [5]Department of Medicinal Chemistry, Faculty of Pharmacy and Pharmaceutical Sciences Research Center, Tehran University of Medical Sciences, Tehran, Iran.

References
1. Chen YL, Lin SZ, Chang JY, Cheng YL, Tsai NM, Chen SP, Chang WL, Harn HJ: In vitro and in vivo studies of a novel potential anticancer agent of isochaihulactone on human lung cancer A549 cells. *Biochem Pharmacol* 2006, 72:308–319.
2. Hanahan D, Weinberg RA: The hallmarks of cancer. *Cell* 2000, 100:57–70.
3. Ananda Kumar CS, Nanjunda Swamy S, Thimmegowda NR, Benaka Prasad SB, Yip GW, Rangappa KS: Synthesis and evaluation of 1-benzhydryl-sulfonyl-piperazine derivatives as inhibitors of MDA-MB-231 human breast cancer cell proliferation. *Med Chem Res* 2007, 16:179–187.
4. Reddy MV, Su C-R, Chiou W-F, Liu Y-N, Chen RY-H, Bastow KF, Lee K-H, Wu T-S: Design, synthesis, and biological evaluation of Mannich bases of heterocyclic chalcone analogs as cytotoxic agents. *Bioorg Med Chem* 2008, 16:7358–7370.
5. Firoozpour L, Edraki N, Nakhjiri M, Emami S, Safavi M, Ardestani SK, Khoshneviszadeh M, Shafiee A, Foroumadi A: Cytotoxic activity evaluation and QSAR study of chromene-based chalcones. *Arch Pharm Res* 2012, 35:2117–2125.
6. Patil CB, Mahajan SK, Katti SA: Chalcone: A versatile molecule. *J Pharm Sci Res* 2009, 1:11–22.
7. Nowakowska Z: A review of anti-infective and anti-inflammatory chalcones. *Eur J Med Chem* 2007, 42:125–137.
8. Akihisa T, Tokuda H, Hasegawa D, Ukiya M, Kimura Y, Enjo F, Suzuki T, Nishino H: Chalcones and other compounds from the exudates of and their cancer chemopreventive effects. *J Nat Prod* 2006, 69:38–42.
9. Dimmock JR, Elias DW, Beazely MA, Kandepu NM: Bioactivities of chalcones. *Curr Med Chem* 1999, 6:1125–1149.
10. Perjési P, Das U, De Clercq E, Balzarini J, Kawase M, Sakagami H, Stables JP, Lorand T, Rozmer Z, Dimmock JR: Design, synthesis and antiproliferative activity of some 3-benzylidene-2,3-dihydro-1-benzopyran-4-ones which display selective toxicity for malignant cells. *Eur J Med Chem* 2008, 43:839–845.
11. Reed D, Shen Y, Shelat AA, Arnold LA, Ferreira AM, Zhu F, et al: Identification and characterization of the first small molecule inhibitor of MDMX. *J Biol Chem* 2010, 285:10786–10796.
12. Nakhjiri M, Safavi M, Alipour E, Emami S, Atash AF, Jafari-Zavareh M, Ardestani SK, Khoshneviszadeh M, Foroumadi A, Shafiee A: Asymmetrical 2,6-bis(benzylidene)cyclohexanones: Synthesis, cytotoxic activity and QSAR study. *Eur J Med Chem* 2012, 50:113–123.
13. Mahmoodi M, Aliabadi A, Emami S, Safavi M, Rajabalian S, Mohagheghi MA, Khoshzaban A, Samzadeh-Kermani A, Lamei N, Shafiee A, Foroumadi A: Synthesis and in-vitro cytotoxicity of poly-functionalized 4-(2-arylthiazol-4-yl)-4H-chromenes. *Arch Pharm* 2010, 7:411–416.
14. Fallah-Tafti A, Tiwari R, Shirazi AN, Akbarzadeh T, Mandal D, Shafiee A, Parang K, Foroumadi A: 4-Aryl-4H-chromene-3-carbonitrile derivatives: evaluation of Src kinase inhibitory and anticancer activities. *Med Chem* 2011, 7:466–472.
15. Bazl R, Ganjali M, Saboury A, Foroumadi A, Nourozi P, Amanlou M: A new strategy based on pharmacophore-based virtual screening in adenosine deaminase inhibitors detection and in-vitro study. *DARU J Pharmaceut Sci* 2012, 20:64. doi:10.1186/2008-2231-20-64.
16. Rafinejad A, Fallah-Tafti A, Tiwari R, Nasrolahi Shirazi A, Mandal D, Shafiee A, Parang K, Foroumadi A, Akbarzadeh T: 4-Aryl-4H-naphthopyrans

derivatives: One-pot synthesis, evaluation of Src kinase inhibitory and anti-proliferative activities. *DARU J Pharmaceut Sci* 2012, **20**:100.

17. Nadri H, Pirali-Hamedani M, Moradi A, Sakhteman A, Vahidi A, Sheibani V, Asadipour A, Hosseinzadeh N, Abdollahi M, Shafiee A, Foroumadi A: **5,6-Dimethoxybenzofuran-3-one derivatives: a novel series of dual Acetylcholinesterase/Butyrylcholinesterase inhibitors bearing benzyl pyridinium moiety.** *DARU J Pharmaceut Sci* 2013, **21**:15. doi:10.1186/2008-2231-21-15.

18. Foroumadi A, Samzadeh-kermani A, Emami S, Dehghan G, Sorkhi M, Arabsorkhi F, Heidari MR, Abdollahi M, Shafiee A: **Synthesis and antioxidant properties of substituted 3-benzylidene-7-alkoxychroman-4-ones.** *Bioorg Med Chem Lett* 2007, **17**:6764–6769.

19. Ayati A, Falahati M, Irannejad H, Emami S: **Synthesis, in vitro antifungal evaluation and in silico study of 3-azolyl-4-chromanone phenylhydrazones.** *DARU J Pharmaceut Sci* 2012, **20**:46. doi:10.1186/2008-2231-20-46.

20. Hua DH, Huang X, Chen Y, Battina SK, Tamura M, Noh SK, Koo SI, Namatame I, Tomoda H, Perchellet EM, Perchellet JP: **Total syntheses of (+)-chloropuupehenone and (+)-chloropuupehenol and their analogues and evaluation of their bioactivities.** *J Org Chem* 2004, **69**:6065–6078.

21. Cheng M-F, Fang J-M: **Liquid-phase combinatorial synthesis of 1,4-benzodiazepine-2,5-diones as the candidates of endothelin receptor antagonism.** *J Comb Chem* 2004, **6**:99–104.

22. Mosmann T: **Rapid colorimetric assay for cellular growth and survival: application to proliferation and cytotoxicity assays.** *J Immunol Methods* 1983, **65**:55–63.

23. Shetab-Boushehri SV, Abdollahi M: **Current concerns on the validity of in vitro models that use transformed neoplastic cells in pharmacology and toxicology.** *Int J Pharmacol* 2012, **8**:594–595.

Angiogenic effect of the aqueous extract of *Cynodon dactylon* on human umbilical vein endothelial cells and granulation tissue in rat

Hamid Soraya[1*], Milad Moloudizargari[2], Shahin Aghajanshakeri[2], Soheil Javaherypour[2], Aram Mokarizadeh[3], Sanaz Hamedeyazdan[4], Hadi Esmaeli Gouvarchin Ghaleh[5], Peyman Mikaili[1] and Alireza Garjani[6]

Abstract

Background: *Cynodon dactylon*, a valuable medicinal plant, is widely used in Iranian folk medicine for the treatment of various cardiovascular diseases such as heart failure and atherosclerosis. Moreover, its anti-diabetic, anti-cancer and anti-microbial properties have been also reported. Concerning the critical role of angiogenesis in the incidence and progression of tumors and also its protective role in cardiovascular diseases, we investigated the effects of the aqueous extract prepared from the rhizomes of *C. dactylon* on vascular endothelial growth factor (VEGF) expressions in Human Umbilical Vein Endothelial Cells (HUVECs) and also on angiogenesis in carrageenan induced air-pouch model in rats.

Methods: In the air-pouch model, carrageenan was injected into an air-pouch on the back of the rats and following an IV injection of carmine red dye on day 6, granulation tissue was processed for the assessment of the dye content. Furthermore, in an *in vitro* study, angiogenic property of the extract was assessed through its effect on VEGF expression in HUVECs.

Results: Oral administration of 400 mg/kg/day of the extract significantly increased angiogenesis ($p < 0.05$) and markedly decreased neutrophil ($p < 0.05$) and total leukocyte infiltration ($p < 0.001$) into the granulation tissues. Moreover, the extract increased the expression of total VEGF in HUVECs at a concentration of (100 µl/ml).

Conclusion: The present study showed that the aqueous extract of *C. dactylon* promotes angiogenesis probably through stimulating VEGF expression.

Keywords: Cynodon dactylon, Angiogenesis, Air pouch, HUVECs, VEGF

Background

Recently, medicinal plants have been largely considered as the harmless alternate to synthetic drugs, especially due to their more safety and less side effects as compared to the chemical drugs. *Cynodon dactylon*, also known as Bermuda grass, is a perennial grass native to the warm temperate and tropical regions [1]. In North West of Iran, *C. dactylon* is known as "Chayer" and the aqueous extract of its rhizomes is widely used in the treatment of cardiovascular disorders such as atherosclerosis and heart failure due to its hypolipidemic and cardiac tonic effects [2,3].

However, despite the presence of several reports on the anti-diabetic, anti-microbial [4], hypolipidemic [5], hepato-protective [6], anti-emetic and anti-inflammatory [7] properties of *C. dactylon*, the probable role of angiogenesis as the mechanism involved in cardioprotective effect of the plant has remained largely elusive.

Angiogenesis, the formation of new blood vessels from pre-existing capillaries, plays an important role in many physiologic and also pathologic processes including cancer, ischemic heart diseases and chronic inflammation [8,9]. Moreover, since the therapeutic interference with angiogenesis offers a valuable tool for clinical application in several pathological conditions, much attention has been paid on medications or compounds that alter the gene expression profile of vascular endothelial cell growth

* Correspondence: soraya.h@umsu.ac.ir
[1]Department of Pharmacology, Faculty of Pharmacy, Urmia University of Medical Sciences, Urmia, Iran
Full list of author information is available at the end of the article

factor (VEGF) and fibroblast growth factors (FGFs) as two key pro-angiogenic molecules [10]. In some cases such as heart failure or cardiac ischemia-reperfusion, stimulation of angiogenesis is beneficial and can be considered as a target to improve the disease condition, however in several other diseases such as cancer, atherosclerosis, rheumatoid arthritis and diabetic retinopathy, excessive angiogenesis is part of the pathology and progression of the disease [9-11]. Therefore, stimulation or inhibition of angiogenesis to reach therapeutic purpose is dependent on the type of the disease.

Marappan and Subramaniyan [12] assessed anti-tumor effects of the methanolic extract of *C. dactylon* leaves against ascetic lymphoma (ELA) in Swiss albino mice. The results showed that the plant possesses significant anti-tumor effects [12]. Another study by Krishramoorthy and Ashwini [13] also reported anti-cancer effects of *C. dactylon* in Swiss albino mice. The hydroalcoholic extract from rhizomes of *C. dactylon* has been shown to have strong protective effect on right heart failure in rats, in part by improving cardiac function and increasing the contractile force [2]. In another study this effect was also attributed to its anti-arrhythmic activity [14]. The plant also increased heart beat rate in a study on zebrafish with a potency greater than that of betamethasone [15].

As stated above, *C. dactylon* has been proven to be an effective cardiovascular agent by several studies; however almost none of the studies have precisely investigated the underlying mechanisms through which this plant exerts its effects on the cardiovascular system. The authors speculate that such beneficial effects of *C. dactylon* might be at least partly associated with its probable effects on angiogenesis. Since there have been no studies conducted so far on the possible effects of *C. dactylon* on angiogenesis, the present study was carried out to investigate the possible angiogenic activity of the plant in human umbilical vein endothelial cells (HUVECs) and also in an air-pouch model in rats.

Materials and methods
Extract preparation
C. dactylon was purchased from a traditional herbal market and the genus and species was authenticated at the Herbarium of Botany, Faculty of Pharmacy, Urmia, Iran. The rhizomes of the plant were dried in shade and coarsely ground to powder using an automatic grinder. 200 g of the powder was mixed in 2 L of distilled water and placed on a magnet stirrer at a temperature of 50°C for three days. The mixture was then filtered three times using the Wattman's paper. The solution was finally evaporated to dryness for 12 hrs at 70°C. The total amount of the crude extract obtained was 34 g. The extract was diluted with water in order to be given orally by gavage needle.

Preliminary phytochemical screening
Qualitative phytochemical analysis of *C. dactylon* aqueous extract was conducted following the standard procedures as described by Harborne [16], Sofowora [17] and Trease and Evans [18].

Alkaloids
Crude extract was mixed with 2 ml of 1% HCl and heated gently. Mayer's reagent was then added to the mixture. Turbidity of the resulting precipitate is as evidence for the presence of alkaloids.

Anthocyanins
2 ml of aqueous extract was added to 2 ml of 2 N HCl and NH_3. Manifestation of pink-red turning blue-violet indicates the presence of anthocyanins.

Coumarins
3 ml of 10% NaOH was added to 2 ml of aqueous extract, formation of yellow color indicates the presence of coumarins.

Flavonoids
Crude extract was mixed with few fragments of magnesium ribbon and concentrated HCl was added drop wise. Appearance of pink scarlet color after few minutes indicates the presence of flavonoids (Shinoda test).

Saponins
Crude extract was mixed with 5 ml of distilled water in a test tube and shaken vigorously to obtain a stable persistent froth. The frothing is then mixed with 3 drops of olive oil and for the formation of emulsion which indicates the presence of saponins.

Tannins
Crude extract was mixed with 2 ml of 2% solution of $FeCl_3$. Observed blue-green or black coloration indicates the presence of tannins.

Assay for in vitro antioxidant activity
The free radical scavenging capacity of the extract was measured from the bleaching of the purple-colored methanolic solution of 2,2-diphenyl-1-picrylhydrazyl)DPPH), a routinely practiced material for the assessment of antiradical properties of different compounds [19]. The stock concentration of the *C. dactylon* aqueous extract (1 mg/mL) was prepared followed by dilution to reach for concentrations 5×10^{-1}, 2.5×10^{-1}, 1.25×10^{-1}, 6.25×10^{-2}, 3.13×10^{-2} and 1.56×10^{-2} mg/mL of the extract. The acquired concentrations in the same volumes of 2 mL were added to 2 mL of a 0.08 % of DPPH solution [20-22]. Later than a 30 min of incubation at 30°C, the absorbance of each solution was read against a blank sample at 517 nm (Shimadzu

2100 spectrophotometer - Japan). The average absorption value was noted for each sample after the test was carried out in triplicate. Besides, as the positive control the same procedure was gone over with quercetin. The inhibition percentage of DPPH free radicals of by the aqueous extract was calculated as follows:

$$R\,(\%) \;=\; 100 \;\times\; [(A\;blank - A\;sample)/A\;blank]$$

Herein, "A blank" stands for the absorbance value of the control reaction and "A sample" is the absorbance value for each sample. Additionally, RC_{50} value, the concentration of the extract reducing 50% of the DPPH free radicals, was calculated from the graph of inhibition percentages versus concentrations of *C. dactylon* extract in mg/mL.

Assay for total phenolics content
Total phenolic constituents of the *C. dactylon* aqueous extract was verified by assigning Folin-Ciocalteu reagent and gallic acid as the standard compound for phenolics, the same procedure as given in the literature [23-26]. Briefly, 0.5 mL of the extract was mixed with 5 mL of Folin-Ciocalteu reagent (10% v/v in distilled water) with 4 mL of 1 M aqueous Na_2CO_3 after 5 min and the mixture was allowed to stand for 15 min with intermittent shaking. The absorbance of the blue color produced by the reaction was measured using a UV/visible spectrophotometer (Shimadzu 2100 - Japan) at 765 nm. The standard curve was prepared using 25–300 µg/mL solutions of gallic acid in methanol: water (50:50, v/v). Eventually, the value for total phenol content of the *C. dactylon* extract was represented in terms of gallic acid equivalent which is a common reference compound.

Animals
Albino Wistar rats (220-250 g) were used in this study. Rats were housed at constant temperature ($20 \pm 1.8°c$) and relative humidity ($50 \pm 10\%$) in standard polypropylene cages, eight per cage, under a 12 L:12D schedule and were allowed food and water freely. This study was performed in accordance with the Guide for the Care and Use of Laboratory Animals of Urmia University of Medical Sciences, Urmia-Iran.

In vivo angiogenesis assay
Rats were divided into 5 groups consisting 8 rats each. Rats in group 1 (carrageenan) received intra-pouch injection of carrageenan and normal saline as vehicle (0.5 ml) was given orally. Rats in group 2 received intra-pouch injection of carrageenan and intraperitoneal injection of dexamethasone. Rats in group 3 to 5 received intra-pouch injection of carrageenan and cynodon dactylon extract was given orally at doses 100, 200 and 400 mg/kg/day. For

analyzing the effects of the aqueous extract of *C. dactylon* on *in vivo* angiogenesis, the air-pouch model described by Gosh *et al.* [8] was used with minor modifications. Briefly, rats (n = 8) were lightly anesthetized with diethyl ether, the back was shaved and then swabbed with 70% ethanol. Subsequently, 8 ml of sterile air was injected subcutaneously on the back of the animals to make an air-pouch oval in shape. Twenty four hours later, 4 ml of a 1% (w/v) solution of carrageenan (Sigma Co; USA) in saline was injected into the air-pouch under light diethyl ether anesthesia. The carrageenan solution had been sterilized by autoclaving at 121°C for 15 min and supplemented with penicillin G potassium and streptomycin sulfate (JaberEbne – e- Hayyan, Iran) (0.1 mg/ml of the solution) after cooling to 40–45°C. The aqueous extract of *C. dactylon* was administered orally at doses of 100, 200 and 400 mg/kg/day and dexamethasone as a standard anti-inflammatory agent (10 mg/kg/day) was injected intraperitoneally, a day before and for 6 days after carrageenan injection.

Determination of angiogenesis in granulation tissue
Six days after carrageenan injection, measurement of the angiogenesis in the granulation tissue was carried out using carmine dye, as an indicator of angiogenesis, according to the methods described by *Gosh et al.* [8] with slight modification. Briefly, the rats were anesthetized by intraperitoneal injection of a mixture of ketamine (60 mg/kg) and xylazine (10 mg/kg). Then 3 ml of 5% (w/v) carmine dye (Sigma Co; USA) in 5% (w/v) gelatin (Sigma Co; USA) in saline at 37°C was injected into the jugular vein of each rat. The carcasses were chilled on ice for 3 hrs and then the entire granulation tissue was dissected and weighted. After being washed with PBS (PH 7.4) the whole granulation tissue was homogenized in two volumes of 0.5 mM sodium hydroxide using a T25 basic homogenizer (IKA labortechnik, Gremany) for 4 min at $10000\,g$ on an ice bed. The tissue homogenate was centrifuged at $3000\,g$ and 4°C for 45 min and 500 µl of the supernatant was diluted 2-fold with 0.5 mM sodium hydroxide and centrifuged again. Then 100 µl of the supernatant was diluted with 900 µl of 0.5 mM sodium hydroxide and the carmine dye content was assessed spectrophotometrically at a wavelength of 490 nm. For histopathological visualization of the granulation tissues, the tissues were fixed in 10% (v/v) formalin in PBS for 48 hrs at 4°C. The samples were dehydrated by continuous immersion in 70% (v/v) ethanol for 48 hrs, 90% (v/v) ethanol for 48 hrs, and pure ethanol for 48 hrs. After dehydration, the samples were cleared by their immersion in the cedarwood oil (Sigma Co; USA) for 14 days. Retention of carmine dye within the vascular bed was observed with a light microscope (40× magnification).

Determination of pouch fluid accumulation, granulation tissue weight, total leukocyte infiltration along with lymphocyte and neutrophil percentage in the pouch exudates

Six days after the carrageenan injection, total pouch fluid was collected, the volume was measured and the entire granulation tissue was dissected and weighted. The total leukocyte count was determined in a neubauer chamber and the differential cell count was determined by microscopic counting of Gimsa stained slides.

In vitro angiogenesis assay

The expression changes in cytoplasmic and surface levels of VEGF in PBS or extract treated HUVECs were determined using a PAS flow cytometer (Partec GmbH, Germany). Briefly, human umbilical vein endothelial cells (HUVECs) were cultured at 37°C and 5% CO2 in low-glucose Dulbecco's Modified Eagle's Medium (LG-DMEM) supplemented by Supplement Mix (PromoCell) and10% fetal bovine serum (FBS). At second passage cells were treated with PBS (100 μl/ml) and *C. dactylon* extract (100 μl/ml). After 12 hrs using trypsin/EDTA (Ethylenediaminetetraacetic acid) solution (0.25%), cells were detached and then washed twice in PBS. The collected cells were permeablized with 0.1% PBS-Tween for 20 min. After incubation in 1× PBS/10% normal goat serum/0.3 M glycine to block non-specific interactions, unconjugated rabbit anti human VEGF antibody (abcam) was added. Subsequently, staining was performed using secondary goat anti-rabbit IgG PE antibody. The total 20000 events for each sample were acquired. Flow max software was used for data analysis.

Statistical analysis

Data were presented as mean ± standard error of the mean (SEM) and were analysed using one-way-ANOVA to make comparisons between the groups. If the ANOVA analysis indicated significant differences, Student–Newman–Keuls post test was performed to compare the mean values between the treatment groups and the control group. Differences between groups were considered significant at $P < 0.05$.

Results

Phytochemical analysis

Phytochemical compounds such as alkaloids, anthocyanins, coumarins, flavonoids, saponins, tannins and phenolic compounds were screened in the *C. dactylon* aqueous extract. Availability of these compounds, important secondary metabolites, has been tabulated in Table 1. Among

the selected compounds alkaloids, coumarins, saponins and some phenolics, were present in the plant which could be responsible for the medicinal values of the respective plant. Moreover, the amount of total phenolic compounds in the *C. dactylon* aqueous extract established through Folin Ciocalteu method was calculated as gallic acid equivalent. The equation [Sample absorbance = 0.0067 × gallic acid (μg) + 0.0132, (R^2: 0.987)] achieved by the standard gallic acid graph was applied in calculation of the phenolic compounds concentration. Subsequently, the content for *C. dactylon* total phenolics showed the value 39.82 mg of gallic acid equivalent in g of plant extract (Table 1). The findings of the antioxidant activity for *C. dactylon* aqueous extract, accomplished by the DPPH method, revealed sensible values *in vitro*. Regarding the results for the DPPH radical scavenging antioxidant assay, *C. dactylon* extract exhibited pleasant antioxidant activity with RC_{50} values of 0.70 mg/ml for the extract and 3 μg/mL for the control quercetin (Table 1). Quantitative phytochemical analysis revealed that the plant contained phenolic compounds a class of phytochemicals that could be responsible for the antioxidant and free radical scavenging effect of the plant material.

Effects of the aqueous extract of C. dactylon on angiogenesis in granulation tissue

Six days after the injection of carrageenan solution into the air-pouch, a dissectible granulation tissue was formed in the subcutaneous tissue. Following intravenous injection of carmine red dye to the anaesthetized animals, the dye was accumulated in the granulation tissue and the amount of the dye was assessed as an index of angiogenesis. As shown in Figure 1, oral administration of the aqueous extract of *C. dactylon* (400 mg/kg) produced a significant ($P < 0.05$) increase in angiogenesis. In agreement with these findings, vascular network formation was also stimulated by *C. dactylon* as shown in Figure 1 (upper trace; right).

Effects of the aqueous extract of C. dactylon on pouch fluid volume, leukocyte Infiltration and granulation tissue weight

The treatment of rats with oral administration of the aqueous extract of *C. dactylon* at doses of 100, 200 and 400 mg/kg which was started one day before the intra-pouch injection of carrageenan and continued for 6 days, dose dependently reduced neutrophil (p < 0.05) and total leukocyte (p < 0.001) recruitment whereas increased lymphocyte recruitment into the exudates (Table 2). In contrast, administration of *C. dactylon* dose dependently

Table 1 Phytochemical analysis, DPPH radical scavenging capacity and total phenols content of *C. dactylon* aqueous rhizomes extract

	Alkaloids	Anthocyanins	Coumarins	Flavonoids	Saponins	Tannins	Total phenols	DPPH (IC_{50})
C. dactylon extract	+	-	+	-	++	-	39.82 mg/g	0.70 mg/ml

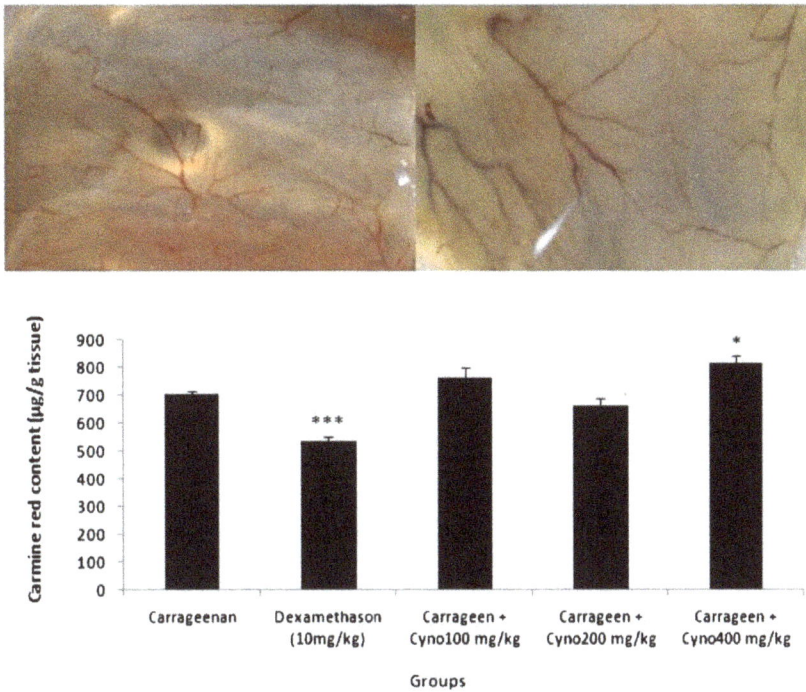

Figure 1 Upper trace: Effects of the aqueous extract of *C. dactylon* (400 mg/kg) on angiogenesis in granulation tissue versus positive control (carrageenan; left) in the air pouch model of angiogenesis in rats. Lower trace: The effect of oral administration of aqueous extract of *C. dactylon* on carmine dye content (as an index of angiogenesis) in granulation tissue in the air pouch model of angiogenesis in rats. Cyno: Cynodon dactylon, Carrageen: Carrageenan. Data represented as mean ± SEM. N = 6. *$P < 0.05$ and ***$P < 0.001$ *vs* control group (Carrageenan).

increased pouch fluid volume and granulation tissue weight in comparison to the carrageenan group (Figure 2). Dexamethasone was used as a positive control which significantly reduced total leukocyte accumulation in the exudate, pouch fluid volume and granulation tissue weight compared to the carrageenan group (Table 2, Figure 2).

Effects of the aqueous extract of C. Dactylon on VEGF expression in human umbilical vein endothelial cells (HUVEC)

The results obtained from flow cytometric analysis showed the increased expression of total VEGF (both in cytoplasmic and surface levels) in HUVECs treated with the aqueous extract of *C. dactylon* as compared to those

treated with PBS. Three experiments were performed and 12% increase in expression of VEGF was detected in extract-treated cells as compared to the PBS-treated ones (Figure 3).

Discussion

Overall, as far as we know, the long history of use and prevailing reputation of many types of natural resources, particularly higher plant species, among the nations are impressive. More recently, herbal medicines have been identified as sources of various phytochemicals, many of which possess different countless activities. Accordingly, *C. dactylon* signifying to have medicinally valuable secondary metabolite types of phytochemicals like alkaloids,

Table 2 Effect of the aqueous extract of *C. dactylon* on leukocytes recruitment into the pouch exudate

	Carrageenan	Dexamethasone	Carrageen + Cyno 100 mg/kg	Carrageen + Cyno 200 mg/kg	Carrageen + Cyno 400 mg/kg
Neutrophil percentage	20 ± 1	12 ± 0.33*	22 ± 1.2	17 ± 3	13 ± 2*
Lymphocyte percentage	58 ± 2.8	50 ± 1.8	57 ± .32	59 ± 4.4	67 ± 3.7
Total leukocyte (10^5)	895 ± 6.4	498 ± 15.2***	635 ± 14.3***	629 ± 33***	523 ± 19.1***

Data represented as mean ± SEM. N = 6. *$P < 0.05$ and *** $P < 0.001$ *vs* control group (Carrageenan) using one way ANOVA with Student-Newman-Keuls *post-hoc* test. Carrageen: Carrageenan; Cyno: Cynodon dactylon.

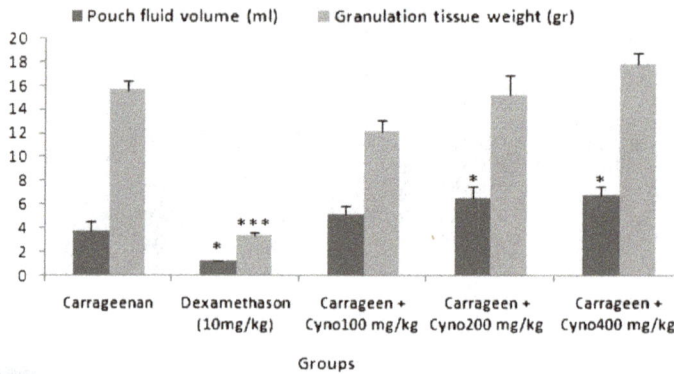

Figure 2 Effect of the aqueous extract of *C. dactylon* at various doses on pouch fluid volume and granulation tissue weight 6 days after carrageenan injection. Cyno: Cynodon dactylon, Carrageen: Carrageenan. Data represented as mean ± SEM. N = 6–8. *p < 0.05 and ***p < 0.001 versus the carrageenan group.

coumarins, saponins and some types of phenolics might have a role in angiogenesis.

Nonetheless, further research is required to meet the challenges of isolation and structural elucidation of the major active compounds in the plant for identifying an efficient natural medicine which is reliant on a better understanding of the association between chemical constituents and biological properties of natural resources. In this time of increasing requisite for effective, affordable health promotion and treatment strategies for our growing populations and enlarging health problems, the history and reputation of herbal medicines must be examined in a rigorous and scientific way which may be translated into clinical benefit.

C. dactylon has been widely used in the traditional medicine of Iran and other countries for the treatment of several cardiovascular conditions such as heart failure [2], and arrhythmias [14]. Moreover, various pharmacological

effects of the plant have been proven in several studies [27]. Examples of these effects include analgesic and anti-pyretic [28], negative ionotropic and negative chronotropic effects [29], anti-arthritic, and anti-inflammatory activities [30]. Although promotion of angiogenesis has been a therapeutic strategy in the treatment of cardiovascular diseases such as ischemic heart disease; however, it can be part of the pathogenesis of several other diseases such as cancer [9,10].

The present study was carried out to evaluate the possible effects of *C. dactylon* on angiogenesis which thought to mediate the part of beneficial effects of the plant in cardiovascular conditions. Accordingly, the possible angiogenic effect of the plant was assessed in both Carrageenan-induced air-pouch model as an *in vivo* and human umbilical vein endothelial cells as an *in vitro* models. The results demonstrated that the constituents present in the aquatic extract of the plant have the potential to increase angiogenesis probably

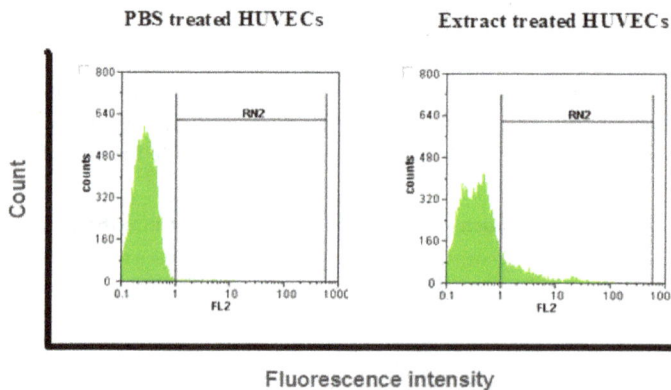

Figure 3 The expression change of VEGF in HUVECs by flow cytometric procedure. The expression level of VEGF in PBS treated cells set as control and the expression changes following treatment with *C. dactylon* extract compared to it. The increased expression of VEGF in extract treated HUVECs has been shown as compared to the PBS treated ones. Histograms are representative of three separate experiments.

through up-regulation of VEGF-gene expression. Other angiogenesis parameters including exudate volume and granulation tissue weight were increased dose dependently following the administration of the extract. These results were accompanied with the decreased total leukocyte and neutrophil infiltration into the air-pouch. Since decreasing total leukocyte and neutrophil count indicates the anti-inflammatory effect of *C. dactylon* the obtained results were parallel to the findings of the previous studies [7]. However, the extract of *C. dactylon* exerts an anti-inflammatory effect against acute inflammation, while increasing angiogenesis. It has been already shown that simultaneous administration of two different substances may upregulate the angiogenic responses, while downregulating the inflammatory responses [31]. The same effect can be also attributed to different constituents present in the aqueous extract of the plant.

In vitro study on the effect of *C. dactylon* on the expression of VEGF in human umbilical vein endothelial cells revealed that there might be a positive correlation between the angiogenic effect of the plant and its ability to increase VEGF expression. This might be the possible underlying mechanism through which the plant exerts its effect. It has been also shown in several studies that the extract of *C. dactylon* possesses significant anti-tumor activities [32,33]. As noted earlier, angiogenesis plays a central role in the pathogenesis of neoplastic diseases [34], however the exact mechanism(s) responsible for such effect of the plant is not yet clearly understood. In the mentioned studies, the sole reversal effects of the plant against undesired consequences of tumors [12] and its anti-oxidant properties [16] have been partly attributed to this effect of the plant without adequate evaluation of other mechanisms affecting tumor growth. For instance, none of these studies have evaluated the *in vivo* angiogenesis changes of the tumors affected by the administration of the extract. Based on the findings of the present study which indicate the potential of the plant to promote angiogenesis at high doses, it has to be taken into consideration that the plant might contain unsafe agents which may aid in the growth of the tumor through increasing the tumor angiogenesis. This is probably the first study that reveals an unsafe aspect of this plant in contrast to its beneficial properties previously shown in anti-cancer studies.

Conclusion

To the best of our knowledge, this is the first study showing the angiogenic property of the aquatic extract of *C. dactylon*. Based on these findings, *C. dactylon* is suggested as a potential source of angiogenic compounds, the effects of which might be attributable to its increasing effect on the expression of VEGF, a growth factor mainly involved in angiogenesis. Accordingly, this plant can be used in the development of novel herbal medicines for the

amelioration of the consequences of conditions such as ischemic heart disease, and other cardiovascular complications. Our findings are in contrast with the results of previously conducted studies on the anti-tumor effects of *C. dactylon*, indicating that in addition to its beneficial effect as an anti-cancer source, it might be a toxic agent due to increasing tumor angiogenesis. Therefore, critical care should be taken on the safety of the plant to be introduced as an anti-tumor agent. Indeed, further studies are required to clarify the precise underlying mechanisms and to identify the safe aspects of the plant to be employed as a therapeutic source.

Competing interests
The authors declare that they have no competing interests.

Authors' contributions
HS: Supervising and directing the project, carried out the data analysis and interpretations and prepared the manuscript. MM: Carried out angiogenesis experiments. SA: Accompanied Milad Moloudizargari in angiogenesis experiments. SJ: Animal grouping and handling. AM: Carried out flow cytometric procedure and interpretation. SH: Performed phytochemical analysis. HE-G: Carried out inflammation studies. PM: Prepared the plant material and the extract. AG: Contributed in data analysis, interpretation and preparation of the manuscript. All authors read and approved the final manuscript.

Acknowledgments
The present study was supported by a grant from the Research Vice Chancellors of Urmia University of Medical Sciences, Urmia, Iran.

Author details
[1]Department of Pharmacology, Faculty of Pharmacy, Urmia University of Medical Sciences, Urmia, Iran. [2]Student of Veterinary Medicine, Faculty of Veterinary Medicine, Urmia University, Urmia, Iran. [3]Department of Immunology, Faculty of Medicine, and Cellular & Molecular Research Center, Kurdistan University of Medical Sciences, Sanandaj, Iran. [4]Department of Pharmacognosy, Faculty of Pharmacy, Tabriz University of Medical Sciences, Tabriz, Iran. [5]Department of Microbiology, Faculty of Veterinary Medicine, Urmia University, Urmia, Iran. [6]Department of Pharmacology & Toxicology, Faculty of Pharmacy, Tabriz University of Medical Sciences, Tabriz, Iran.

References
1.	Ashokkumar K, Selvaraj K, Muthukrishnan SD. *Cynodon dactylon* (L.) Pers.: An updated review of its phytochemistry and pharmacology. J Med Plants Res. 2013;7:3477–83.
2.	Garjani A, Afrooziyan A, Nazemiyeh H, Najafi M, Kharazmkia A, Maleki-Dizaji N. Protective effects of hydroalcoholic extract from rhizomes of *Cynodon dactylon* (L.) Pers. on compensated right heart failure in rats. BMC Complement Altern Med. 2009;9:28.
3.	Kaup SR, Arunkumar N, Bernhardt LK, Vasavi RG, Shetty SS, Pai SR, et al. Antihyperlipedemic activity of *Cynodon dactylon* extract in high-cholesterol diet fed Wistar rats. Genomic Medicine, Biomarkers, and Health Sciences. 2011;3:98–102.
4.	Singh SK, Kesari AN, Gupta RK, Jaiswal D, Watal G. Assessment of antidiabetic potential of *Cynodon dactylon* extract in streptozotocin diabetic rats. J Ethnopharmacol. 2007;114:174–9.
5.	Singh SK, Rai PK, Jaiswal D, Watal G. Evidence-based Critical Evaluation of Glycemic Potential of *Cynodon dactylon*. Evid Based Complement Alternat Med. 2008;5:415–20.
6.	Singh SK, Rai PK, Jaiswal D, Rai DK, Sharma B, Watal G. Protective effect of *Cynodon dactylon* against STZ induced hepatic injury in rats. J Ecophysiol Occup Hlth. 2008;8:195–9.
7.	Garg VK, Paliwal SK. Anti-inflammatory activity of aqueous extract of *Cynodon dactylon*. Int J pharmacol. 2011;7:370–5.

8. Ghosh AK, Hirasawa N, Niki H, Ohuchi K. Cyclooxygenase-2-mediated angiogenesis in carrageenin-induced granulation tissue in rats. J Pharmacol Exp Ther. 2000;295:802–9.

9. Khurana R, Simons M, Martin JF, Zachary IC. Role of angiogenesis in cardiovascular disease: a critical appraisal. Circulation. 2005;112:1813–24.

10. Griffioen AW, Molema G. Angiogenesis: potentials for pharmacologic intervention in the treatment of cancer, cardiovascular diseases, and chronic inflammation. Pharmacol Rev. 2000;52:237–68.

11. Folkman J. Angiogenesis in cancer, vascular, rheumatoid and other disease. Nat Med. 1995;1:27–31.

12. Marappan S, Subramaniyan A. Antitumor activity of methanolic extract of Cynodon dactylon leaves against Ehrlich ascites induced carcinoma in mice. J Adv Scient Res. 2012;3:105–8.

13. Krishnamoorthy M, Ashwini P. Anticancer activity of Cynodon dactylon L. extract on Ehrlich ascites carcinoma. J Environ Res Dev. 2011;5:551–7.

14. Najafi M, Ghavimi H, Gharakhani A, Garjani A. Effects of hydroalcoholic extract of Cynodon dactylon (L.) pers. on ischemia/reperfusion-induced arrhythmias. DARU J Pharm Sci. 2008;16:233–8.

15. Kannan RR, Vincent SG. Cynodon dactylon and Sida acuta extracts impact on the function of the cardiovascular system in zebrafish embryos. J Biomed Res. 2012;26:90–7.

16. Harbone JB. Phytochemical methods. London: Chapman and Hall, Ltd; 1973. p. 49–188.

17. Sofowora A. Medicinal plants and traditional medicine in Africa. Ibadan, Nigeria: Spectrum Books; 1993. p. 191–289.

18. Trease GE, Evans WC. Pharmacognosy. 11th ed. London: Bailliere Tindall; 1989. p. 45–50.

19. Mishra K, Ojha H, Chaudhury NK. Estimation of antiradical properties of antioxidants using DPPH radical dot assay: A critical review and results. Food Chem. 2012;130:1036–43.

20. Nahar L, Russell W, Middleton M, Shoeb M, Sarker S. Antioxidant phenylacetic acid derivatives from the seeds of Ilex aquifolium. Acta Pharm. 2005;55:187–93.

21. Fathiazad F, Matlobi A, Khorrami A, Hamedeyazdan S, Soraya H, Hammami M, et al. Phytochemical screening and evaluation of cardioprotective activity of ethanolic extract of Ocimum basilicum L. (basil) against isoproterenol induced myocardial infarction in rats. DARU J Pharm Sci. 2012;20:87.

22. Hamedeyazdan S, Sharifi S, Nazemiyeh H, Fathiazad F. Evaluating antiproliferative and antioxidant activity of Marrubium crassidens. Adv Pharm Bull. 2014;4(Suppl1):459–64.

23. Folin O, Denis W. On phosphotungstic-phosphomolybdic compounds as color reagents. J Biol Chem. 1912;12:239–43.

24. Singleton VL, Orthofer R, Lamuela-Raventos RM. Analysis of total phenols and other oxidation substrates and antioxidants by means of folin-ciocalteu reagent. Methods Enzymol. 1999;299:152–78.

25. McDonald S, Prenzler PD, Autolovich M, Robards K. Phenolic content and antioxidant activity of olive extracts. Food Chem. 2001;73:73–84.

26. Ebrahimzadeh MA, Pourmorad F, Hafezi S. Antioxidant activities of Iranian corn silk. Turk J Biol. 2008;32:43–9.

27. Nagori BP, Solanki R. Cynodon dactylon (L.) Pers.: a valuable medicinal plant. Res J Med Plant. 2011;5:508–14.

28. Garg VK, Khosa RL. Analgesic and anti-pyretic activity of aqueous extract of Cynodon dactylon. Pharmacologyonline. 2008;3:12–8.

29. Shabi MM, Raj CD, Sasikala C, Gayathri K, Joseph J. Negative Inotropic and Chronotropic Effects of Phenolic Fraction from Cynodon dactylon (linn) on Isolated Perfused Frog Heart. J Sci Res. 2012;4:657–63.

30. Sindhu G, Ratheesh M, Shyni GL, Helen A. Inhibitory effects of Cynodon dactylon L. on inflammation and oxidative stress in adjuvant treated rats. Immunopharmacol Immunotoxicol. 2009;31:647–53.

31. Zachman AL, Crowder SW, Ortiz O, Zienkiewicz KJ, Bronikowski CM, Yu SS, et al. Pro-angiogenic and anti-inflammatory regulation by functional peptides loaded in polymeric implants for soft tissue regeneration. Tissue Eng Part A. 2013;19:437–47.

32. Kanimozhi D, Bai VR. In vitro anticancer activity of ethanolic extract of Cynodon dactylon against HT-29 cell line. Int J Curr Sci. 2013;5:74–81.

33. Khlifi D, Hayouni EA, Valentin A, Cazaux S, Moukarzel B, Hamdi M, et al. LC–MS analysis, anticancer, antioxidant and antimalarial activities of Cynodon dactylon L. extracts. Ind Crop Prod. 2013;45:240–7.

34. Soraya H, Esfahanian N, Shakiba Y, Ghazi-Khansari M, Nikbin B, Hafezzadeh H, et al. Anti-angiogenic Effects of Metformin, an AMPK Activator, on Human Umbilical Vein Endothelial Cells and on Granulation Tissue in Rat. Iran J Basic Med Sci. 2012;15:1202–9.

Doxorubicin-conjugated PLA-PEG-Folate based polymeric micelle for tumor-targeted delivery: Synthesis and *in vitro* evaluation

Zahra Hami[1], Mohsen Amini[2], Mahmoud Ghazi-Khansari[3], Seyed Mehdi Rezayat[1,3,4] and Kambiz Gilani[5*]

Abstract

Background: Selective delivery of anticancer agents to target areas in the body is desirable to minimize the side effects while maximizing the therapeutic efficacy. Anthracycline antibiotics such as doxorubicin (DOX) are widely used for treatment of a wide variety of solid tumors.
This study evaluated the potential of a polymeric micellar formulation of doxorubicin as a nanocarrier system for targeted therapy of a folate-receptor positive human ovarian cancer cell in line.

Results: DOX-conjugated targeting and non-targeting micelles prepared by the dialysis method were about 188 and 182 nm in diameter, respectively and their critical micelle concentration was 9.55 µg/ml. The DOX-conjugated micelles exhibited a potent cytotoxicity against SKOV3 human ovarian cancer cells. Moreover, the targeting micelles showed higher cytotoxicity than that of non-targeting ones (IC_{50} = 4.65 µg/ml vs 13.51 µg/ml).

Conclusion: The prepared micelle is expected to increase the efficacy of DOX against cancer cells and reduce its side effects.

Keywords: Doxorubicin, Folate, Micelle, PLA-PEG block copolymer

Background

Anthracycline antibiotics such as doxorubicin are widely used for treatment of a wide variety of solid tumors and hematological malignancies [1-3], but their clinical use is limited by their low water solubility, severe side effects such as cardiotoxicity and inherent drug resistance [4,5]. Drug delivery systems such as polymeric nanocarriers [6,7], liposomes [8] and dendrimers [9] can improve the antitumour efficacy and reduce toxicity of free DOX. Micelles that consist of hydrophilic shell and hydrophobic core are spherical nanoparticulate carriers with unique properties such as high solubility, high stability, appropriate size (20–200 nm) and long circulation in blood [10,11]. The use of polymeric micelles as carriers of anticancer drugs has been reported in previous studies [12-16].

Selective delivery of anticancer agents to target areas in the body is desirable to minimize the side effects

* Correspondence: gilani@tums.ac.ir
[5]Aerosol Research Laboratory, Department of Pharmaceutics, School of Pharmacy, Tehran University of Medical Sciences, Tehran, Iran
Full list of author information is available at the end of the article

while maximizing the therapeutic efficacy. Non-specific drug delivery often causes adverse effects on normal cells. Folate (FOL) has several advantages over various targeting ligands such as transferrin, peptides and antibodies. FOL has a small size, non-immunogenicity, low molecular weight and stability [17]. Therefore, micellar delivery systems have further been modified with target-specific ligands (FOL) to enhance tumor specificity and improve the tumor uptake by folate receptor-mediated endocytosis. Many approaches have also been described to prepare pH-sensitive micelles that can release the encapsulated drugs in acidic environment of tumors. Bae et al. have reported the pH-sensitive polymeric micelles based on poly (ethylene glycol)-poly(aspartate hydrazone-adriamycin) for DOX delivery that can release the drug in response to acidic pH at endosomes (pH 5.0–6.0) and lysosomes (pH 4.0–5.0). The micelles showed high antitumor activity in C-26 bearing mice [18]. Folate-poly (ethylene glycol)-poly (aspartate hydrazone-adriamycin) micelles For active intracellular drug delivery was also prepared. The micelles showed good antitumor effect in KB cell line [17]. In another study, Liua and co-workers prepared a targeting micelle based on poly(N-isopropy-lacrylamide-co-N,Ndimethylacrylamide-co-2-aminoethyl methacrylate)-b-poly (10-undecenoic acid) block copoly-mer and showed that the micelles was able to target the KB cells and release the drug in acidic pH of the tumor. The micelles significantly enhanced KB cell growth inhibition [19].

Covalent conjugation of anticancer drugs to their nano-particulate carrier is more advantageous than physical encapsulation of drugs because it helps to stabilize the drug and prevent premature drug release into the blood circulation to assure drug delivery into the cancerous cells. Therefore, in this study, a folate functionalized PLA-PEG block copolymer was synthesized and doxorubicin was conjugated to the block copolymer via a pH-sensitive hydrazone bond. The prepared micelle was characterized for the structure of prepared block copolymer, average size and critical micelle concentration (CMC). The *in vitro* cytotoxicity of the folate targeting micelle against SKOV3 human ovarian cancer cells was evaluated using the 3-[4,5-dimethylthiazol-2-yl]-2,5-diphenyltet-razolium bromide (MTT) assay and compared with the folate-free micelle. Epithelial cancer cell lines such as SKOV3 demonstrate overexpression of folate receptors (FRs) [20]. MTT is a tetrazolium salt, which is reduced within the mitochondria in metabolically active viable cells. The resulting formazan crystals are impermeable to the cell membranes and accumulate only in uninjured cells [21], therefore this assay provides a measure of mitochondrial function following exposure to the test compound.

Material and methods
Instrumentation
The IR spectra were recorded on a Nicollet FT-IR Magna 550 spectrometer, Madison, USA. The ^{1}H NMR spectrum was recorded on a Bruker DRX (Avance 500) spectrom-eter, Rheinstetten, Germany, 500 MHz. A double beam UV-Visible spectrophotometer (model 2100, Shimadzu, Japan) was utilized for spectrophotometric measure-ments. Dynamic light scattering (DLS) (Zetasizer Nano-ZS, Malvern Instruments Ltd., UK) was used to determine the dynamic diameter, size distribution and zeta potential of the micelles.

Materials
Doxorubicin was purchased from RPG Life Sciences limited (Mumbai, India). L-lactide, poly(ethylene glycol) (PEG) with MW 4000 g/mol, Hydrazine, N-hydroxysuccinimide (NHS), dicyclohexylcarbodiimde (DCC), 1-ethyl-3-(3-dimethylaminopropyl) carbodiimide (EDC), stannous octoate, folate and MTT were obtained from Sigma (St Louis, MO, USA). *p*-Nitrophenyl chloroformate (p-NPC), acetonitrile, toluene, dichloromethane and

acetone (analytical grade) were purchased from Merck (Darmstadt, Germany). RPMI 1640 medium and peni-cillin/streptomycin solution were obtained from Gibco Invitrogen (Carlsbad, CA, USA). All other chemicals were of analytical grade.

Preparation of folate-conjugated PLA-PEG block copolymer by ring opening polymerization
Preparation of PLA-PEG block copolymer containing ter-minal carboxylate group was started with the synthesis of monocarboxylated PEG according to the method described by WH Jo et al. [22] with some modifications and followed by ring-opening polymerization of the lactide in the presence of carboxylated PEG [23]. Briefly, vacuum-dried lactide (16 g) and carboxylated PEG (3 g) were allowed to react in anhydrous toluene in the presence of and tin (II) 2-ethylhexanoate (200 mg) as a catalyst at the refluxing temperature of toluene. The PLA-PEG copolymer was extracted by chloroform after evaporation of the reaction solvent. The prepared PLA-PEG–COOH (1 g) was activated by adding EDC (50 mg) and NHS (40 mg) in dimethyl sulfoxide (DMSO, 10 ml) 5 h at room temperature. To prepare the folate-functionalized copoly-mer, folate-NH$_2$ was synthesized from reaction of folic acid (250 mg) and triethylamine (TEA, 0.5 ml) in the presence of NHS and EDC in methanol. After 2 h, 1 ml of ethylene diamine was added and the reaction continued overnight at room temperature. The prepared folate-NH$_2$ was added to the activated copolymer in DMSO and the reaction continued for additional 48 h. The mixture was then dialyzed against deionized water to remove unreacted folate-NH$_2$. The formation of monocarboxylated PEG and PLA-PEG copolymer was confirmed by infrared (IR) spectroscopy. The conjugation of folate to the co-polymer was also confirmed by ^{1}H NMR spectroscopy. The total amount of folate conjugated to copolymer was determined by UV spectroscopy at 365 nm.

Preparation of doxorubicin-conjugated PLA-PEG block copolymer and micelle formation
Conjugation of Hydrazone Derivative of doxorubicin (Hyd-DOX) to the activated PLA-PEG-FOL block copolymer was carried out according to previously described method with some modifications [14]. The terminal PLA in copoly-mer was activated by adding *p*-NPC (340 mg) and dry pyri-dine (230 mg) to PLA-PEG-FOL (3 g) in dry methylene chloride at 0°C, followed by reaction at room temperature under nitrogen atmosphere. The conjugation of DOX-Hyd to freeze-dried activated block copolymer was performed in dry tetrahydrofurane under nitrogen atmosphere for 36 h. In the final step, dialysis method was employed to prepare the micelles. The folate-free micelles were also prepared in a similar way. The doxorubicin content in the copolymer was measured by UV spectroscopy at 490 nm.

Particle size and zeta potential measurements by dynamic light scattering (DLS)

Particle size, polydispersity index (PDI) and zeta potential of blank and DOX-conjugated polymeric micelles were measured using a Zetasizer (Nano-ZS, Malvern Instruments Ltd., UK). All measurements were performed in triplicate.

Determination of the critical micelle concentration (CMC)

The CMC of prepared micelles was estimated by fluorescence spectroscopy using pyrene as a fluorescent probe [24]. Briefly, 10 ml of DOX-conjugated copolymer aqueous solutions with different concentrations (0.05 µg/ml to 500 µg/ml) were added to the volumetric flasks containing solvent-dried pyrene (10^{-7} M). The solutions were sonicated at 40°C for 30 minutes, followed by stirring for 24 h at room temperature. The excitation wavelength was set at 334 nm and the intensity ratios of I_{383} to I_{372} were plotted as a function of concentration of the block copolymer solutions. The CMC of DOX-conjugated micelle was taken from the copolymer concentration at which the relative fluorescence intensity ratio began to increase.

In vitro cytotoxicity studies

SKOV3 human ovarian cancer cells were cultured in RPMI-1640 medium supplemented with 10% fetal bovine serum (FBS) and 1% penicillin-streptomycin at 37°C in a humidified incubator with 5% CO2. The cytotoxic activity of free DOX and chemically conjugated DOX in targeting (DOX-Hyd-PLA-PEG-FOL) and non-targeting micelles against SKOV3 cells was measured using MTT assay. The cells were seeded in 96-well plates at 10,000 cells per well and incubated for 24 h before test. Free DOX and DOX-conjugated targeting and non-targeting PLA-PEG micelles were dissolved and diluted in the growth medium to give different concentrations of DOX (equivalent DOX concentrations;

10^{-2} - 10^5 ng/ml). The blank micelle concentrations (0.01-100 µg/ml) in RPMI 1640 were also prepared. The old media in the plates were replaced with 100 µl of the media containing the test compounds. After 72 h incubation, 20 µl of MTT solution (5 mg/ml) was added to each well and the plates were then maintained in incubator for an additional 4 h. The media containing MTT were then removed and the purple formazan crystals were dissolved in 100 µl of DMSO. The absorbance of the formazan crystals was read with a Synergy HT Microplate Reader (Bio-Tek Instruments, Winooski, VT) at 570 nm. The IC50 values (The concentration of the test compounds at which 50% cell growth is inhibited) were calculated by using GraphPad Prism Software (Version 5.04, GraphPad Software, San Diego California, USA).

Data analysis

All experiments were carried out three times and results were expressed as mean ± SD. All data analyses were performed using GraphPad Prism version 5.04. The significance level was set at $p < 0.05$.

Results and discussion

Preparation of doxorubicin-conjugated PLA-PEG-Folate micelle

The synthesis pathway of DOX-Hyd-PLA-PEG-FOL is illustrated in Figure 1. PEG with two different end groups was first synthesized for the conjugation of folic acid to the carboxylate terminal group. The polymerization of lactide was then carried out in the presence of monocarboxylated PEG which PLA was conjugated to the hydroxyl terminal group of PEG. Spectral data of the prepared compounds are shown in Table 1. The structure of monocarboxylated PEG and PLA-PEG copolymer were confirmed by the IR spectrum (Figure 2). The peak at 1708 cm^{-1} in Figure 2(a) indicates the presence of carbonyl group of -COOH in the structure of carboxylated

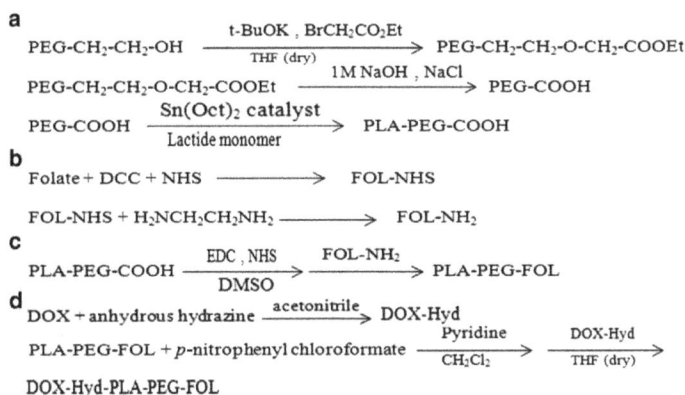

Figure 1 Synthesis scheme of DOX-conjugated PLA-PEG diblock copolymer. Synthesis of PLA-PEG-COOH (**a**), Folate-NH$_2$ (**b**), PLA-PEG-FOL (**c**) and DOX-PLA-PEG-FOL (**d**).

Table 1 Spectral data of the prepared compounds

Compounds	IR (KBr) Vmax in cm^{-1}	^{1}H-NMR (CDCl$_3$) δ in ppm
PEG-COOH	1708 (C=O)	
PLA-PEG-COOH	1755 (C=O in PLA), 1091(C-O-C in PEG), 1635 (C=O in PEG)	3.6 (-OCH$_2$CH$_2$- in PEG), 1.6 (CH$_3$ in PLA), 5.2 (CH in PLA)
p-NPC-PLA-PEG-FOL		7.1, 8.1, 1(FOL),
		7.5, 8.4 (p-NPC)

PEG. In the IR spectrum of PLA-PEG copolymer (Figure 2 (b)), the characteristic sharp peak at 1755 cm^{-1} is attributed to the carbonyl (C = O) group in the PLA block of PLA-PEG-COOH. Besides, the peaks related to the C-O-C stretching and C = O of COOH in PEG appeared at 1091 and 1635 cm^{-1}, respectively. The IR spectrum strongly indicates the ring opening polymerization of lactide and formation of PLA-PEG block copolymer. The^{1}H-NMR spectrum (Figure 3) of prepared PLA-PEG copolymer was used to estimate the average molecular weight of the copolymer by comparing the peak ratio of the methylene protons of PEG (–OCH$_2$CH$_2$–: δ 3.6 ppm) with the peak ratio of methine protons of PLA (CH:δ 5.2 ppm). The molecular weight of PEG was 4000 g/mol, therefore the molecular weight of PLA-PEG copolymer was approximately 30,000. From these results, the degree of polymerization (DP) of lactate, n, is 373. In the next step, folate-NH$_2$ was synthesized, as shown in Figure 1 and its conjugation to carboxylate-terminal group of PEG was

carried out after activation of block copolymer. The effect of reaction solvent and temperature was evaluated in the synthesis of folate-NH$_2$ and the best results were achieved at room temperature in methanol solvent. The conjugation of folate to the copolymer was confirmed by ^{1}H NMR spectroscopy. The ^{1}H NMR spectrum (Figure 3) shows the corresponding peaks of folate (small peaks at 7.1 ppm, 8.1 ppm and approximately 1 ppm) and p-nitrophenyl chloroformate (small peaks at 7.5 ppm and 8.4 ppm). The molar percent of folate in the copolymer is 66.8% measured by UV absorbance at 365 nm. The spectrum also shows the characteristic peaks of PEG (CH$_2$: 3.6 ppm) and PLA (CH$_3$: 1.6 ppm and CH: 5.2 ppm). To provide controlled release of doxorubicin, hydrazine was used as an acid-sensitive linker for DOX conjugation to the PLA backbone. Compared to the published method by Etrych et al. [25], the conjugation method was carried out in mild reaction conditions with a less time consuming and less costly reaction. The drug-conjugated micelle was prepared

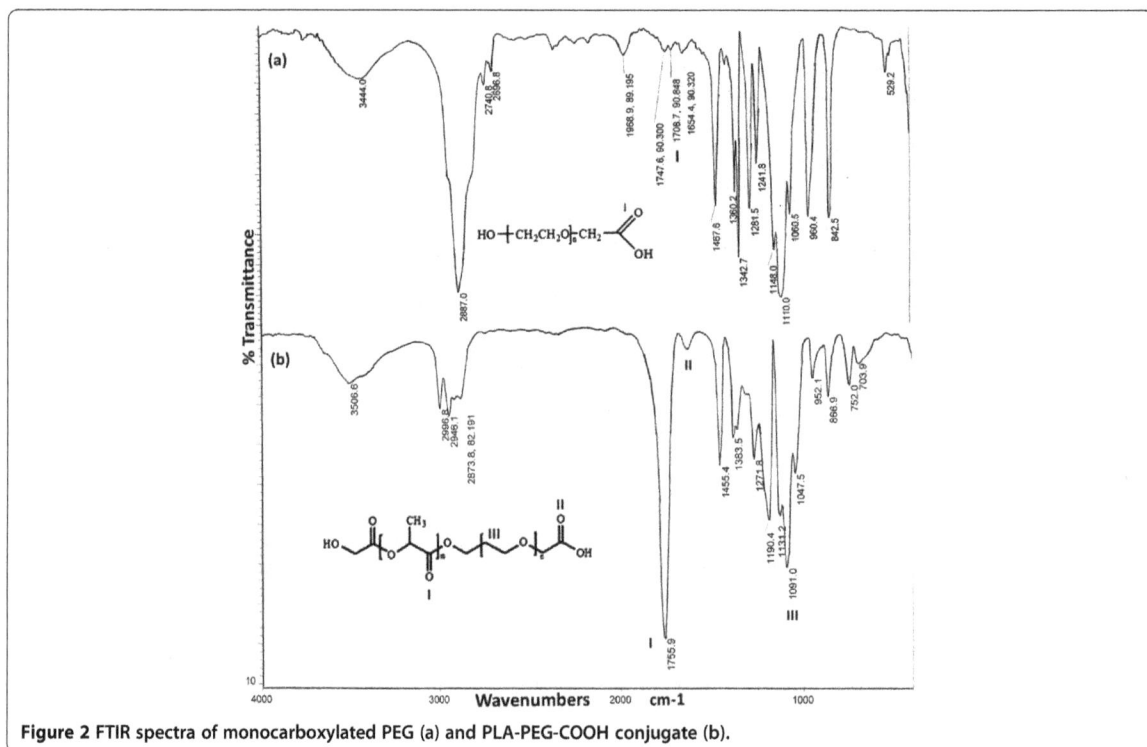

Figure 2 FTIR spectra of monocarboxylated PEG (a) and PLA-PEG-COOH conjugate (b).

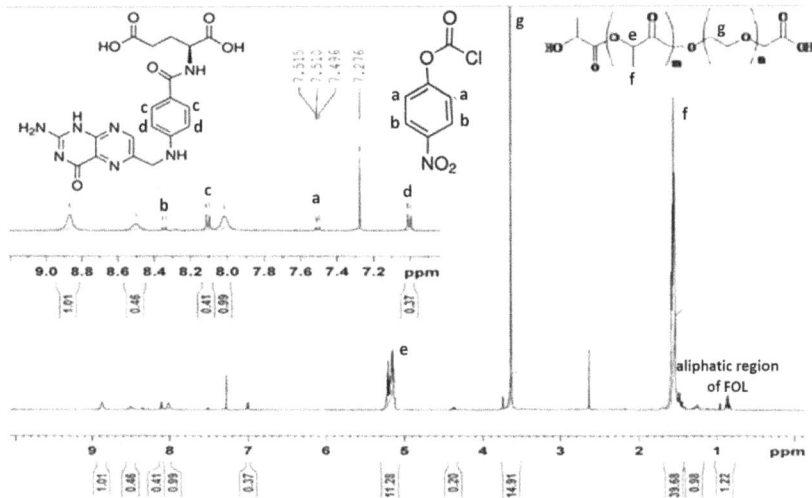

Figure 3 ^{1}H NMR spectrum of p-nitrophenyl chloroformate-PLA-PEG-FOL (500 MHz, CDCl$_3$).

using dialysis method. The amount of DOX attached onto the copolymer was 39.6% (molar percent) determined by UV absorbance at 480 nm.

Particle size distribution

The average diameter and zeta potential data of the blank, DOX-conjugated targeting and non-targeting polymeric micelles in deionized water measured using DLS technique are listed in Table 2. The mean diameters of the drug-free PLA-PEG-FOL micelles and the drug-conjugated targeting and non-targeting micelles were 176.71, 188.43 and 182.19 nm, respectively. In addition, the polydispersity index values indicate that the formed micelles had narrow size distribution. The particle size values were comparable to those obtained for other block copolymeric micelles with similar molecular weights [26]. In general, the size of nanoparticles affects their in vivo bio distribution. The size cut-off of tumor vasculature is about 200–700 nm [27]. The average size of both blank and DOX-conjugated micelles was smaller than 200 nm; therefore they are acceptable for drug delivery in cancer treatment. As presented in Table 2, the zeta potential values of micelles with folate ligand are more negative than that of non-targeting micelles which is due to the negative charged carboxyl groups of the folate ligand [28].

The negative charge enhances the dispersion stability of the micelles. Since the particle size and surface chemistry determine the fate of the micelles in blood circulation, the polymeric micelles prepared in this study may be appropriate for in vivo applications in cancer therapy.

The CMC of DOX-conjugated PLA-PEG block copolymer

The formation of micelles was studied using the CMC of DOX-Hyd-PLA-PEG-FOL determined by a fluorescence spectrophotometer measurement in the presence of pyrene as a fluorescent probe. The intensity ratio of the third band to the first band of the pyrene emission spectra (I_{383}/I_{372}) was used to evaluate the polarity of the pyrene environment [29]. The CMC of DOX-Hyd-PLA-PEG-FOL was 9.55 µg/ml as derived from Figure 4. Depending on the copolymer length, the CMC values of PLA-PEG copolymer reported in similar studies are 1–100 µg/ml [30,31]. The low CMC value reported in our study indicates that pyrene is located in a hydrophobic environment which is due to the relatively high molecular weight of the PLA backbone in the copolymer. Micelles with low CMC value exhibit a relative stability upon dilution in vivo [32], which is true in the case of prepared DOX-Hyd-PLA-PEG-FOL micelles.

Table 2 Particle size, polydispersity index and zeta potential of blank and DOX-conjugated micelles prepared by the dialysis method

Zeta potential (mV)	Polydispersity	Particle size (nm)	Micelles
−12.47 ± 2.92	0.25 ± 0.06	176.71 ± 12.61	Blank micelles
−10.24 ± 1.57	0.28 ± 0.04	188.43 ± 8.96	DOX-Hyd-PLA-PEG-FOL micelles
−7.12 ± 1.23	0.16 ± 0.05	182.19 ± 6.38	DOX-Hyd-PLA-PEG micelles

Values are presented as mean ± SD (n = 3).

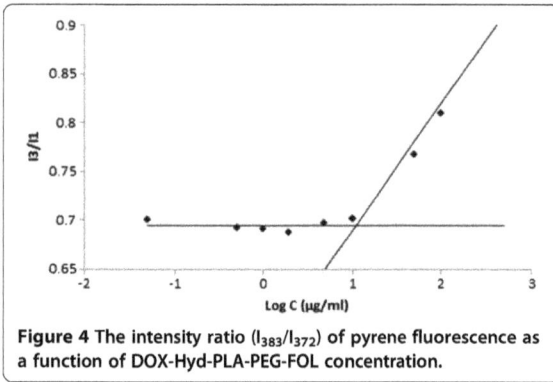

Figure 4 The intensity ratio (I_{383}/I_{372}) of pyrene fluorescence as a function of DOX-Hyd-PLA-PEG-FOL concentration.

In vitro cytotoxicity studies

Figure 5 compared *in vitro* cytotoxicity of free DOX, DOX-Hyd-PLA-PEG-FOL micelles and DOX-Hyd-PLA-PEG micelles against SKOV3 cells as determined by the MTT assay. All three test compounds decreased the viability of the cells in a dose-dependent manner. The IC_{50} value of DOX, the concentration of DOX at which 50% cell growth is inhibited, was 0.08, 4.65 and 13.51 µg/ml for free DOX, DOX-conjugated targeting and non-targeting micelles, respectively. DOX-conjugated targeting micelles exhibited higher cytotoxicity than that of non-targeting ones (IC_{50} = 4.65 µg/ml vs 13.51 µg/ml). The overexpression of FRs on the surface of SKOV3 cells [33] enhanced the uptake of the DOX-Hyd-PLA-PEG-FOL micelles via FR-mediated endocytosis and resulted in 3-fold higher cytotoxicity. Free DOX also showed higher cytotoxic activity compared to DOX-conjugated targeting and non-targeting micelles. The higher cytotoxicity of free DOX seems to be due to the rapid diffusion of this small molecule into the cells, while the DOX-conjugated micelles are internalized into the cells via the endocytosis

process. Moreover, the prepared micelles released DOX in a sustained and controlled manner using the acid labile hydrazone linkage (data not shown). Some other nanoparticulate delivery systems with sustained drug release also exhibited a less cytotoxic activity compared to the corresponding free drug [34-37]. It should be noted that the blank micelles did not show any cytotoxicity against SKOV3 cells (data not shown). The DOX-conjugated targeting micelles exhibited a potent cytotoxicity against SKOV3 cells, therefore the DOX-Hyd-PLA-PEG-FOL micelles can provide an effective treatment for ovarian cancer.

Conclusions

Doxorubicin-conjugated PLA-PEG-folate micelles with the hydrazone linkage were prepared with active targeting capability. This formulation showed a superior cytotoxicity compared to non-targeting ones against a folate-receptor positive cell line. The prepared DOX-conjugated micelles with folate ligand, appropriate size and low CMC value have a great potential for *in vivo* applications in cancer therapy.

Competing interests
The authors declare that they have no competing interests.

Authors' contributions
ZH: Carried out synthesis studies of block copolymer, micelle preparation and characterization, In vitro cytotoxicity studies and drafted the manuscript. MA: Supervisor and participated in polymer synthesis studies and carried out the interpretation of the NMR data. MGK: Supervisor and participated in design and interpretation of in vitro cytotoxicity studies. SMR: Supervisor and participated in the design of the study. KG: Supervisor, conceived of the study, and participated in its design and coordination and helped to draft the manuscript. All authors read and approved the final manuscript.

Acknowledgements
This work was financially supported by grant from Research Council of Tehran University of Medical Sciences grant No.90-02-87-11816.

Author details
[1]Department of Medical Nanotechnology, School of Advanced Technologies in Medicine, Tehran University of Medical Sciences, Tehran, Iran. [2]Department of Medicinal Chemistry, Faculty of Pharmacy and Drug Design & Development Research Center, Tehran University of Medical Sciences, Tehran, Iran. [3]Department of Pharmacology, School of Medicine, Tehran University of Medical Sciences, Tehran, Iran. [4]Department of Toxicology & Pharmacology, Faculty of Pharmacy, Pharmaceutical Sciences Branch, Islamic Azad University (IAUPS), Tehran, Iran. [5]Aerosol Research Laboratory, Department of Pharmaceutics, School of Pharmacy, Tehran University of Medical Sciences, Tehran, Iran.

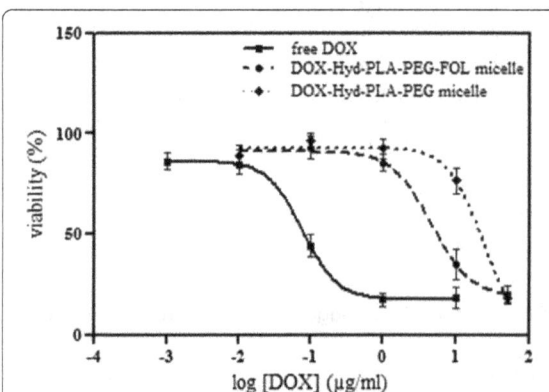

Figure 5 *In vitro* cytotoxicity of free DOX and DOX-conjugated targeting/non-targeting micelles against SKOV3 cell line after 72 h measured with the MTT assay. Cell viability is expressed as mean ± S.D.

References
1. Sharpe M, Easthope SE, Keating GM, Lamb HM: Spotlight on polyethylene glycol-liposomal doxorubicin in solid and hematological malignancies and AIDS-related Kaposi's Sarcoma. *Am J Cancer* 2003, 2:67–72.
2. Primeau AJ, Rendon A, Hedley D, Lilge L, Tannock IF: The distribution of the anticancer drug doxorubicin in relation to blood vessels in solid tumors. *Clin Cancer Res* 2005, 11:8782–8788.
3. Bisht S, Maitra A: Dextran–doxorubicin/chitosan nanoparticles for solid tumor therapy. *Wiley Interdiscip Rev Nanomed Nanobiotechnol* 2009, 1:415–425.

4. Horenstein MS, Vander Heide RS, L_Ecuyer TJ: **Molecular basis of anthracycline-induced cardiotoxicity and its prevention.** *Mol Genet Metab* 2000, **71:**436–444.

5. Orhan B: **Doxorubicin cardiotoxicity: growing importance.** *J Clin Oncol* 1999, **17:**2294–2296.

6. Minko T, Kopečková P, Kopeček J: **Efficacy of the chemotherapeutic action of HPMA copolymer-bound doxorubicin in a solid tumor model of ovarian carcinoma.** *Int J Cancer* 2000, **86:**108–117.

7. Dufresne MH, Garrec DL, Sant V, Leroux JC, Ranger M: **Preparation and characterization of water-soluble pH-sensitive nanocarriers for drug delivery.** *Int J Pharm* 2004, **277:**81–90.

8. Ishida T, Kirchmeier MJ, Moase EH, Zalipsky S, Allen TM: **Targeted delivery and triggered release of liposomal doxorubicin enhances cytotoxicity against human B lymphoma cells.** *Biochim Biophys Acta* 2001, **1515:**144–158.

9. Lai PS, Lou PJ, Peng CL, Pai CL, Yen WN, Huang MY, Young TH, Shieh MJ: **Doxorubicin delivery by polyamidoamine dendrimer conjugation and photochemical internalization for cancer therapy.** *J Control Release* 2007, **122:**39–46.

10. Kataoka K, Harada A, Nagasaki Y: **Block copolymer micelles for drug delivery: design, characterization and biological significance.** *Adv Drug Delivery Rev* 2012, **64:**37–48.

11. Hrubý M, Koňák Č, Ulbrich K: **Polymeric micellar pH-sensitive drug delivery system for doxorubicin.** *J Control Release* 2005, **103:**137–148.

12. Nakanishi T, Fukushima S, Okamoto K, Suzuki M, Matsumura Y, Yokoyama M, Okano T, Sakurai Y, Kataoka K: **Development of the polymer micelle carrier system for doxorubicin.** *J Control Release* 2001, **74:**295–302.

13. Kohori F, Yokoyama M, Sakai K, Okano T: **Process design for efficient and controlled drug incorporation into polymeric micelle carrier systems.** *J Control Release* 2002, **78:**155–163.

14. Yoo HS, Park TG: **Biodegradable polymeric micelles composed of doxorubicin conjugated PLGA–PEG block copolymer.** *J Control Release* 2001, **70:**63–70.

15. Rapoport N, Marin A, Luo Y, Prestwich GD, Muniruzzaman MD: **Intracellular uptake and trafficking of pluronic micelles in drug-sensitive and MDR cells: effect on the intracellular drug localization.** *J Pharm Sci* 2002, **91:**157–170.

16. Lee SC, Kim C, Kwon IC, Chung H, Jeong SY: **Polymeric micelles of poly(2-ethyl-2-oxazoline)-block-poly(q-caprolactone) copolymer as a carrier for paclitaxel.** *J Control Release* 2003, **89:**437–446.

17. Bae Y, Jang WD, Nishiyama N, Fukushima S, Kataoka K: **Multifunctional polymeric micelles with folate-mediated cancer cell targeting and pH-triggered drug releasing properties for active intracellular drug delivery.** *Mol Bio Syst* 2005, **1:**242–250.

18. Bae Y, Nishiyama N, Fukushima S, Koyama H, Yasuhiro M, Kataoka K: **Preparation and biological characterization of polymeric micelle drug carriers with intracellular pH-triggered drug release property: tumor permeability, controlled subcellular drug distribution, and enhanced *in vivo* antitumor efficacy.** *Bioconjug Chem* 2005, **16:**122–130.

19. Liua SQ, Wiradharma N, Gao SJ, Tong YW, Yang YY: **Biofunctional micelles self-assembled from a folate-conjugated block copolymer for targeted intracellular delivery of anticancer drugs.** *Biomaterials* 2007, **28:**1423–1433.

20. Konda SD, Aref M, Wang S, Brechbiel M, Wiener EC: **Specific targeting of folate–dendrimer MRI contrast agents to the high affinity folate receptor expressed in ovarian tumor xenografts.** *Magn Reson Mater Phys Biol Med* 2001, **12:**104–113.

21. Knockaert L, Descatoire V, Vadrot N, Fromenty B, Robin MA: **Mitochondrial CYP2E1 is sufficient to mediate oxidative stress and cytotoxicity induced by ethanol and acetaminophen.** *Toxicol In Vitro* 2011, **25:**475–484.

22. Kim GM, Bae YH, Jo WH: **pH-induced micelle formation of poly (histidine-co- phenylalanine)-block-poly (ethylene glycol) in aqueous media.** *Macromol Biosci* 2005, **5:**1118–1124.

23. Li S, Vert M: **Synthesis, characterization, and stereocomplex-induced gelation of block copolymers prepared by ring-opening polymerization of L (D)-lactide in the presence of poly (ethylene glycol).** *Macromolecules* 2003, **36:**8008–8014.

24. Basu Ray G, Chakraborty I, Moulik SP: **Pyrene absorption can be a convenient method for probing critical micellar concentration (cmc) and indexing micellar polarity.** *J Colloid Interface Sci* 2006, **294:**248–254.

25. Ts E, Šírová M, Starovoytova L, Říhová B, Ulbrich K: **HPMA copolymer conjugates of paclitaxel and docetaxel with pH-controlled drug release.** *Mol Pharm* 2010, **7:**1015–1026.

26. Hsiue GH, Wang CH, Lo CL, Wang CH, Li JP, Yang JL: **Environmental-sensitive micelles based on poly (2-ethyl-2-oxazoline)-b-poly (l-lactide) diblock copolymer for application in drug delivery.** *Int J Pharm* 2006, **317:**69–75.

27. Hobbs SK, Monsky WL, Yuan F, Roberts WG, Griffith L, Torchilin VP, Jain RK: **Regulation of transport pathways in tumor vessels: role of tumor type and microenvironment.** *Proc Natl Acad Sci U S A* 1998, **95:**4607–4612.

28. Guo W, Lee RJ: **Efficient gene delivery via non-covalent complexes of folic acid and polyethylenimine.** *J Control Release* 2001, **77:**131–138.

29. Wu Y, Li M, Gao H: **Polymeric micelle composed of PLA and chitosan as a drug carrier.** *Polymers* 2008, **2008**(16):11–18.

30. Liggins RT, Burt HM: **Polyether-polyester diblock copolymers for the preparation of paclitaxel loaded polymeric micelle formulations.** *Adv Drug Deliv Rev* 2002, **54:**191–202.

31. Yasugi K, Nagasaki Y, Kato M, Kataoka K: **Preparation and characterization of polymer micelles from poly(ethylene glycol)-poly(D, L-lactide) block copolymers as potential drug carrier.** *J Control Release* 1999, **2:**89–100.

32. Kabanov AV, Batrakova EV, Alakhov VY: **Pluronic block copolymers as novel polymer therapeutics for drug and gene delivery.** *J Control Release* 2002, **82:**189–212.

33. Bhattacharya R, Patra CR, Earl A, Wang S, Katarya A, Lu L, Kizhakkedathu JN, Yaszemski MJ, Greipp PR, Mukhopadhyay D: **Attaching folic acid on gold nanoparticles using noncovalent interaction via different polyethylene glycol backbones and targeting of cancer cells.** *Nanomedicine* 2007, **3:**224–238.

34. Alani AW, Bae Y, Rao DA, Kwon GS: **Polymeric micelles for the pH-dependent controlled, continuous low dose release of paclitaxel.** *Biomaterials* 2010, **31:**1765–1772.

35. Xiong XB, Mahmud A, Uludağ H, Lavasanifar A: **Multifunctional polymeric micelles for enhanced intracellular delivery of doxorubicin to metastatic cancer cells.** *Pharm Res* 2008, **25:**2555–2566.

36. Kim JO, Kabanov AV, Bronich TK: **Polymer micelles with cross-linked polyanion core for delivery of a cationic drug doxorubicin.** *J Control Release* 2009, **138:**197–204.

37. Shuai X, Ai H, Nasongkla N, Kim S, Gao J: **Micellar carriers based on block copolymers of poly (ε-caprolactone) and poly (ethylene glycol) for doxorubicin delivery.** *J Control Release* 2004, **98:**415–426.

New aspects of *Saccharomyces cerevisiae* as a novel carrier for berberine

Roshanak Salari[1], BiBi Sedigheh Fazly Bazzaz[1,2], Omid Rajabi[1,3] and Zahra Khashyarmanesh[1*]

Abstract

Background: Berberine was encapsulated in yeast cells of *Saccharomyces cerevisiae* as novel carriers to be used in different food and drug industries. The microcapsules were characterized by differential scanning calorimetry (DSC), fourier transform infra red spectroscopy (FT-IR) and fluorescence microscopy. The encapsulation factors such as plasmolysis of yeast cells which affects the % encapsulation yield were studied.

Results: Fluorescence microscopy showed the yeast cells became fluorescent after encapsulation process. DSC diagram was representing of new peak for microcapsule which was not the same as berberine and the empty yeast cells peaks, separately. FTIR spectrums of microcapsules and yeast cells were almost the same. The plasmolysed and non plasmolysed microcapsules were loaded with berberine up to about $40.2 \pm 0.2\%$ w/w.

Conclusion: Analytical methods proved that berberine was encapsulated in the yeast cells. Fluorescence microscopy and FTIR results showed the entrance of berberine inside the yeasts. DSC diagram indicated the appearance of new peak which is due to the synthesis of new product. Although plasmolysis caused changes in yeast cell structure and properties, it did not enhance berberine loading in the cells. The results confirmed that *Saccharomyces cerevisiae* could be an efficient and safe carrier for active materials.

Keywords: Berberine, Encapsulation, *Saccharomyces cerevisiae* yeast cells

Background

Microencapsulation is a process that nowadays developed in many industries. Encapsulation has a lot of advantages. The encapsulated compound can be released in a controlled way in different systems. Besides, it stabilizes the active materials against oxygen or other molecules by wall material as a physical barrier [1]. The stability and release properties of microcapsules are dependent on cell wall properties [2,3]. However, the new or novel coatings are needed due to the cost and legal limits in the food industries [4].

Saccharomyces cerevisiae yeast cell can be mentioned as an ideal carrier due to its food-grade and low cost characteristics. Unlike other carriers, it does not depend on active ingredients for its synthesis. We could culture this kind of carriers as much as needed without any excess expenses. Besides, its membrane phospholipids act like liposome structure and have been used for encapsulation of different molecules, hydrophobic and hydrophilic, like resveratrol [5-8].

It possesses the external thick cell wall which composes of a beta glucan network and a small amount of chitin associated with a mannoprotein layer [9]. These cell wall properties make *S. cerevisiae* such a kind of sustained release drug delivery system. The mechanical characteristics of the yeasts structure allow them to load different molecules.

Barberry (*Berberis vulgaris* L. family Berberidaceae) grows in Asia and Europe. The plant is famous worldwide for its medicinal properties [10]. Berberine is the most significant alkaloid of this plant which is responsible for its beneficial effects. Berberine is mostly accumulated in the root. Berberine as an isoquinoline alkaloid is a member of protoberberines class [11]. Berberine shows a lot of pharmacological effects [12].

Berberine shows antiplatelet effects and it is also used in treatment of congestive heart failure (CHF) [13-16]. Extracts are used to cure various inflammatory diseases such as lumbago and rheumatism and to reduce fever [17]. The reports represented immunosuppressive effect

* Correspondence: khashaiarmaneshz@mums.ac.ir
[1]Department of Drug and Food Control, School of Pharmacy, Mashhad University of Medical Sciences, Mashhad, Iran
Full list of author information is available at the end of the article

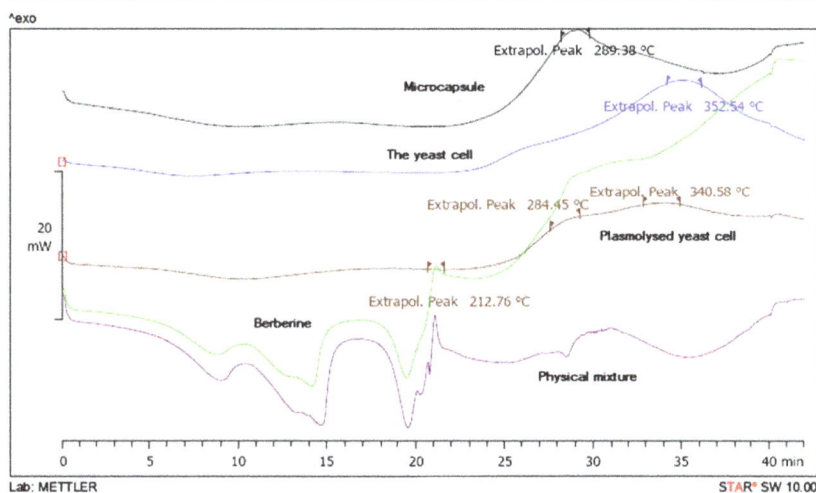

Figure 1 DSC thermograms of microcapsules, *Saccharomyces cerevisiae* yeast cell, berberine, plasmolysed yeast cells and physical mixture of berberine and yeast cells.

of berberine in the tubulointerstitial nephritis model. Peng et al. showed the antianxiety properties of berberine [11]. Berberine can be mentioned as an expectorant due to its ability to increase mucin release [18].

Berberine has been used to treat infectious diarrhea and gastroenteritis in China in the past [19]. Berberine is defined as an effective drug to cure acute diarrhea which is due to *Escherichia coli* or *Vibrio cholerae* [20,21]. Berberine shows significant antibacterial and antifungal activity against broad spectrum of microorganisms [22-28].

Berberine's poor water solubility and susceptibility to environmental conditions prevent its application in many industries. The goal of this study was to evaluate the new aspect of yeast cells of *S. cerevisiae* as an encapsulation carrier for berberine. Moreover, the berberine microcapsules were studied by different analytical methods such as fluorescence microscopy, (DSC) and (FT-IR).

Methods
Preparation of plasmolysed yeast cells, non plasmolysed yeast cells and berberine microcapsules
The yeast cells (commercially Bakers *S. cerevisiae)* were cultured in soybean casein digest broth medium (Himedia, India) for 10 hours [29] in shaker incubator (20 rpm) (JTSL 20, Iran). The medium was centrifuged and the yeast cells were washed for three times with deionised water. The final cells were classified in two groups. First group as non plasmolysed cells was directly freeze dried. The second one as plasmolysed cells was plasmolysed in different concentration of sodium chloride solutions. The yeast cells suspensions were provided in three different flasks. Each flask contained 10%, 20%, 30% w/w NaCl solutions, respectively. Then the

flasks were stirred at 200 rpm for 72 h. The plasmolysed cells were centrifuged and washed three times with deionised water to remove impurities. At last, they have been freeze-dried. The freeze-dried plasmolysed and non plasmolysed yeast cells were studied as carriers [30].

Two kinds of freeze dried cells (plasmolysed and non plasmolysed) (100 mg) were suspended in two flasks containing 50 ml berberine solutions (500 mM). Berberine hydrochloride was obtained from China (XI AN Rongsheng biotechnology CO., LTD). The flasks were stirred at 200 rpm for 72 h and then centrifuged (6000 rpm, 20 min). The precipitants were washed three times to remove the free berberine. Then the berberine loaded microcapsules were freeze dried.

Analytical methods for confirmation of berberine encapsulation
Three methods were performed for confirmation of encapsulation process including fluorescence microscopy (color CCTV camera, model No.MV-CP470/G), fourier-transform Infrared Spectroscopy (FT-IR) (model. Spectrum two) and differential scanning calorimetry (DSC) (Mettler Toledo).

Fluorescence microscopy images were obtained from empty freeze-dried yeast cells and the yeast cells which encapsulated berberine. Besides Fluorescence microscopy, DSC and FT-IR studies were carried out to confirm the encapsulation of berberine in yeast cells.

In DSC studies, five types of freeze-dried samples were studied: empty yeast cells, berberine powder, physical mixture of berberine and empty cells, cells loaded with berberine (microcapsules) and plasmolysed empty yeast cells. To prepare a DSC sample, a definite amount of

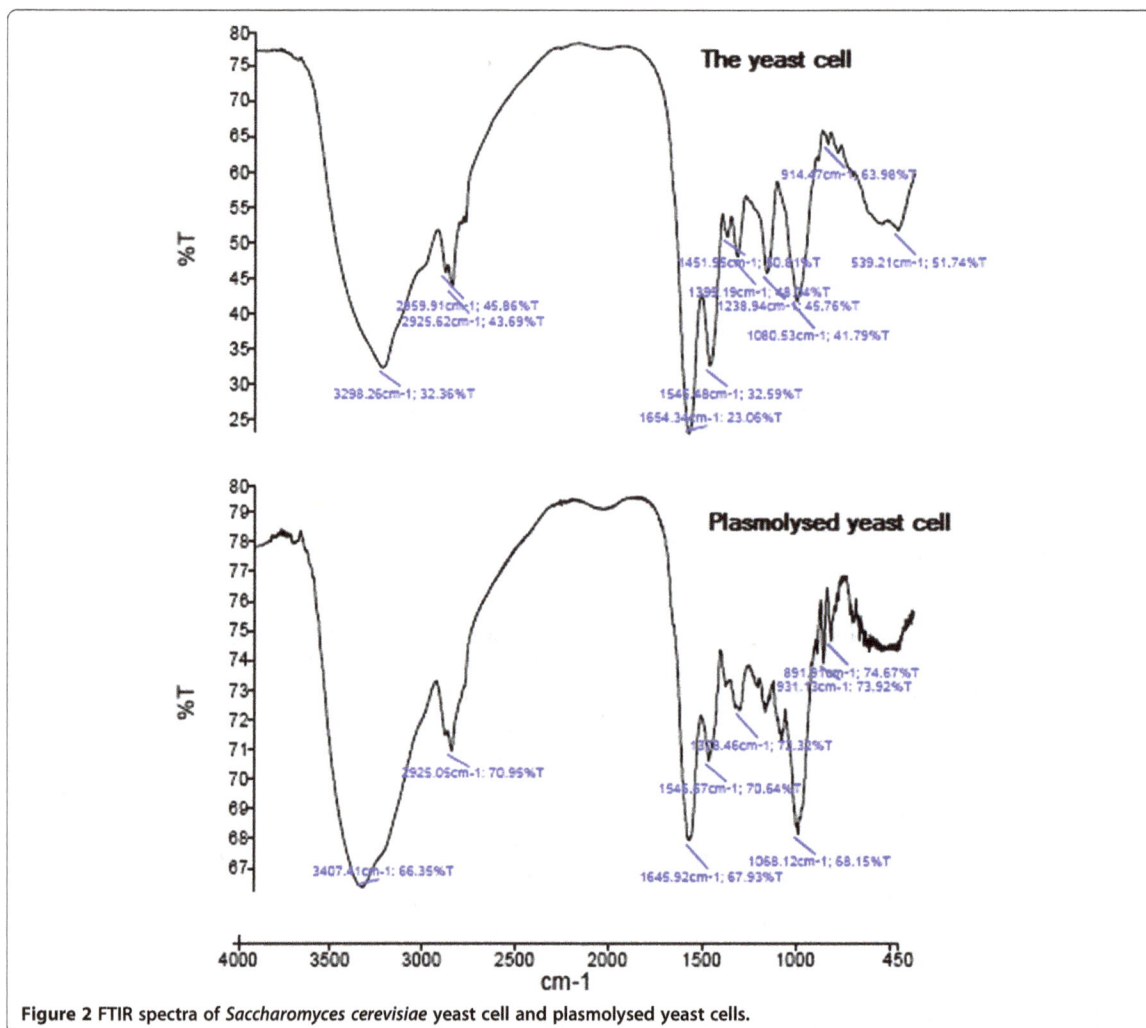

Figure 2 FTIR spectra of *Saccharomyces cerevisiae* yeast cell and plasmolysed yeast cells.

each sample was placed in 50 µl closed aluminium pans. The scan rate was 10°C/min between 0 and 400°C. The IR spectra (KBr disc method) of all the above mentioned samples were also obtained using an FT-IR spectrophotometer [8,10].

To determine the encapsulation yield (% EY), berberine was extracted from two kinds of microcapsules. In extraction process, each sample (50 mg) was suspended in deionised water and ethanol by ratio of 1:4. Then the suspensions were stirred for 48 h in room temperature. Each cell suspension was then centrifuged. Berberine in the supernatant was then quantified by UV/Visible spectroscopy. Then the (% EY) was calculated [28]:

$$(\%EY) = Mass\ of\ encapsulated\ berberine$$
$$\div\ Mass\ of\ the\ resulted\ microcapsule \times 100$$

Results and discussion
Analytical studies of freeze-dried plasmolysed and non plasmolysed yeast cells

The DSC thermograms are showed in Figure 1. DSC thermograms indicate the heat capacity changes of a product based on temperature or time. Besides, we can prove the formation of a new product by omitting or obtaining of new peaks. The DSC thermogram shows an exothermic peak with maximum occurrence at 352°C for freeze-dried non plasmolysed yeast (Figure 1). This peak is originated from the phase transition temperature (Tm) of yeasts' phospholipid bilayer and at 352°C the hydrocarbon tail melted [30]. Tm is influenced by membrane structure so the DSC thermogram of the freeze-dried yeasts cells that had been plasmolysed in 20% w/w NaCl solution showed exothermic peaks with maximum occurrence at 284 and 340°C. It confirms that plasmolysis process causes

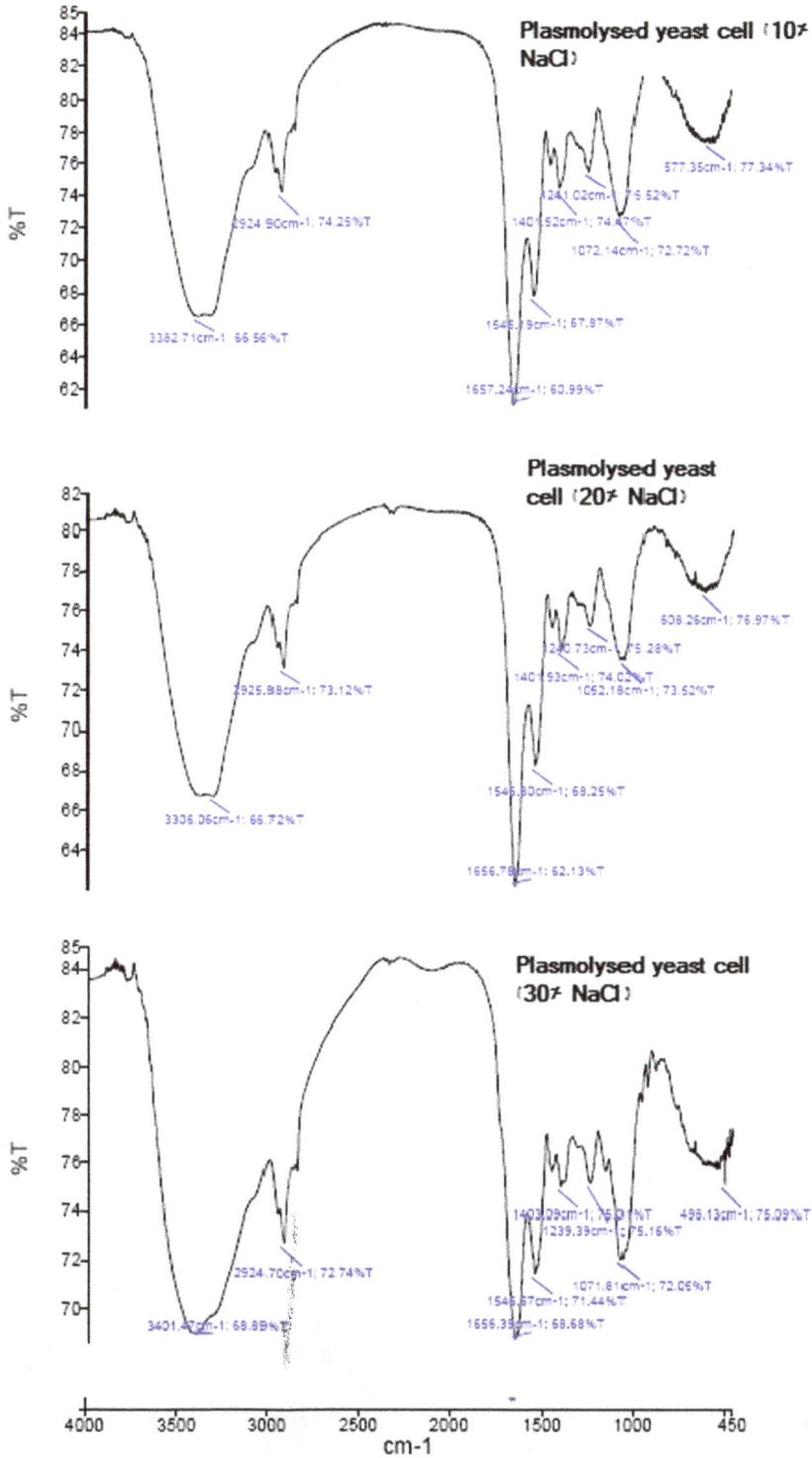

Figure 3 FTIR spectra of 10%, 20% and 30% plasmolysed *Saccharomyces cerevisiae* yeast cells.

changes in lipid composition of membrane and shows different maximum occurrence in comparison with non plasmolysed yeast cells [31]. Tm also depends on different parameters such as strain of *S. cerevisiae*, so we observed different Tm in different studies.

FT-IR was also used to study changes in the cells structure as a result of yeast cell plasmolysis. The IR spectra of both plasmolysed and non plasmolysed freeze-dried yeast cells are shown in Figure 2. The spectra of different plasmolysed yeast cells with 10%, 20% and 30% w/w NaCl solutions (Figure 3) show no significant differences among each other but in comparison with the spectra of non plasmolysed yeast cells (Figure 2), we could see characteristic changes that they represent the effects of plasmolysis on cell wall or membrane compositions such as proteins, carbohydrates, lipids and even nucleic acids.

The contributions of hydroxyl vibrations of carbohydrates and NH vibrations of proteins can be observed in a band at 3750–3000 cm^{-1} in IR spectra [31].

Region 3050–2700 cm^{-1} shows us the information about lipid composition of yeast cells. Plasmolysed yeast cells indicated a minor increase of their absorption intensities due to the changes in the length of membrane lipid chains in comparison with non plasmolysed yeast cells absorption peaks in 2959 and 2925 cm^{-1} (Figure 2) [32]. These two peaks are due to the vibrations of methyl and methylene groups. Plasmolysis effects on cell wall and membrane proteins could be seen in different regions. According to protein degradation by plasmolysis, we faced some changes in peak intensities in the region 1700–1550 cm^{-1}. After plasmolysis, some changes happened in the absorption bands at 1659 and 1553 cm^{-1}, which referred to protein amide I and amide II and carbon-nitrogen vibrations of yeast cells due to the shift of the degradated proteins to an unfolded state. Degradation of one part of yeast proteins in the cell membrane and the cell wall could be detected in the band region from 1530 to 1385 cm^{-1}.

Plasmolysis caused the cell wall polysaccharides degradation which could be detected by changes in the IR region from 1156 to 768 cm^{-1} (Figure 2).

Hypophosphite vibrations are originated from nucleic acid molecules, so we could find the effect of plasmolysis on nucleic acids degradation as the 1240 cm^{-1}. Nucleic acid molecules are placed inside the cell so the presence of their IR spectra are indicative of cells which are not completely emptied by plasmolysis (Figure 2).

Finally the results show us that plasmolysis causes disorganisation to the cell plasma membrane and thickness of cell wall but higher concentrations of NaCl solutions showed no additional disruptions in the yeast cell.

Plasmolysis enhances the intracellular space so it improves the capacity of carriers for encapsulation process [33]. Nowadays, yeast cells plasmolysis with NaCl [7] were mainly used for the encapsulation of different active materials.

The results indicated that the %encapsulation yield values were statistically similar ($p > 0.05$) amongst plasmolysed and non plasmolysed cells which confirms other researches results [30]. The average %encapsulation yield was 40.2±0.2%. No differences were observed in the %encapsulation yield amongst plasmolysed yeast cells when exposed to 10%, 20% or 30% w/w NaCl.

Analytical studies for confirmation of berberine encapsulation

In the fluorescence micrographs, empty yeast cells could not emit fluorescence (Figure 4b). But the yeast cells loaded with berberine emitted fluorescence due to the presence of berberine which shows fluorescence properties (Figure 4a). This event proved the interaction of berberine with yeast cells. Further analyses were carried out using DSC and FT-IR to find out the effect of plasmolysis on cells structure.

Figure 1 showed the DSC thermograms of non-plasmolysed yeast cells, berberine, physical mixture of berberine and

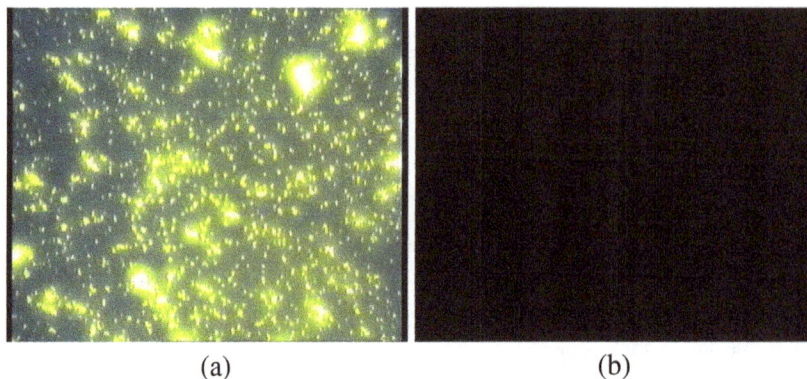

Figure 4 Fluorescence micrographs of berberine yeast microcapsules (a) and empty *Saccharomyces cerevisiae* yeast cells (b).

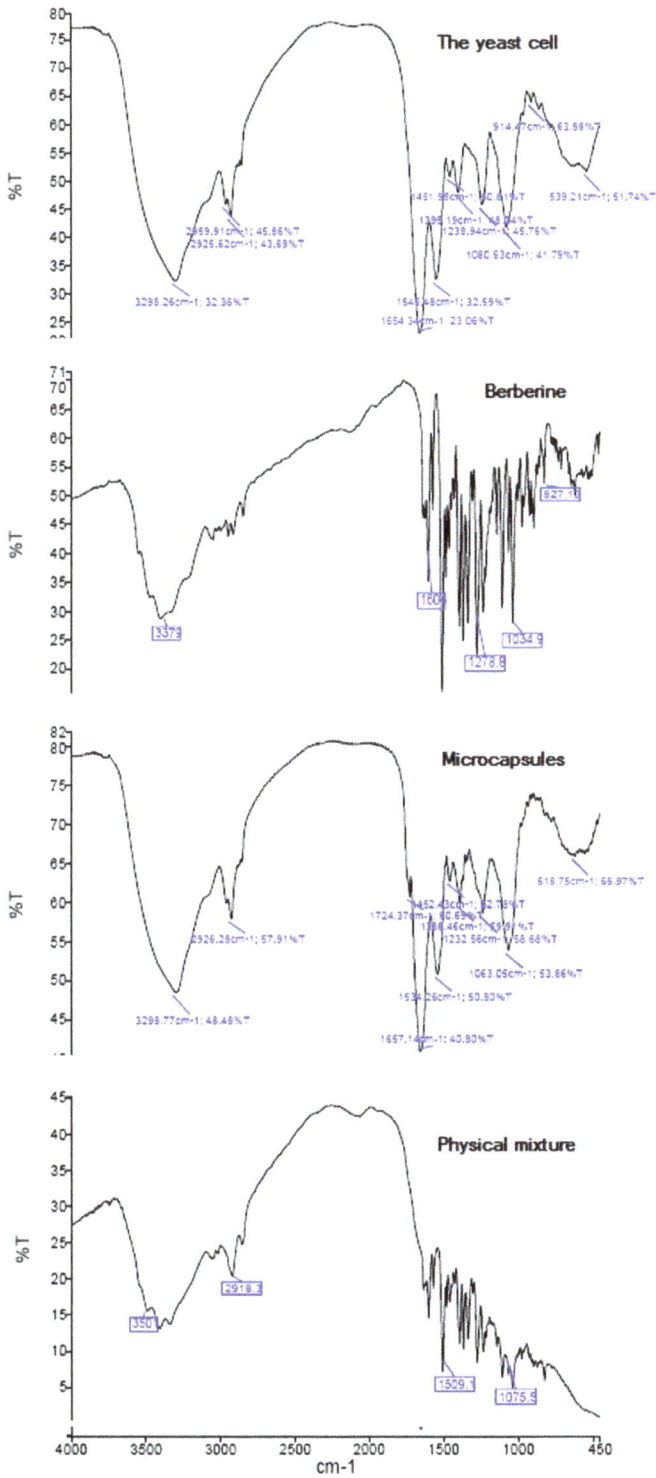

Figure 5 FTIR spectra of *Saccharomyces cerevisiae* yeast cells, berberine, berberine microcapsules and physical mixture.

yeast cells as well as berberine microcapsules and plasmo-lysed yeast cells.

The new peak that appeared at 289°C which differed from the peak of empty yeast cells and physical mixture showed that the new product was produced. This Tm variation was due to decrease of Van der Waals interactions happened to membrane as a result of berberine's integration. On the other hand, berberine influenced the bilayer organization by interaction of its polar groups with membrane polar groups. So the membrane became more fluid and Tm of microcapsules was lowered in comparison with empty yeast cells.

The samples were studied with FTIR spectroscopy too and their spectra are showed in Figure 5. The interaction of berberine with yeast cell would alter the intensity of yeast cell absorption bands and causes shifts of characteristic bands.

The characteristic absorption bands of berberine are shown in Figure 5. The IR spectra of empty yeast cells are explained before. The 3298 and 1654 cm^{-1} bands are due to the phenolic and carbonyl groups, respectively. The absorption peak at 1545 cm^{-1} shows us the carbonyl and carbon-carbon vibration. The peak at 1451 cm^{-1} refered to carbon-hydrogen vibration. The absorption peak at 1238 cm^{-1} is indicative of phenolic vibration. The methoxy groups are responsible for the 1080 cm^{-1} band. The aromatic carbon-hydrogen group vibrates at 914 cm^{-1} [34].

The IR spectrum of the physical mixture of berberine and yeast cells was a combination of the IR spectra of empty yeast cells and berberine, separately. The IR spectra of the microcapsules was relatively the same as the spectrum of the empty yeast cells. These spectra could prove the fact that berberine was placed inside the yeast cells. This observation confirmed Shi et al. [5,7] studies. However we had some peak disappearances at 914 cm^{-1} and variation in the absorption bands of 1654 and 1545 cm^{-1} as a result of berberine-protein interactions in microcapsules spectra.

Conclusions

In this study, S. cerevisiae were introduced as a novel carrier for berberine as a model. It has shown that yeast microcapsules were loaded with berberine up to $40.2 \pm 0.2\%$ w/w. Three analytic methods indicated that berberine located inside the cells mainly by hydrophobic interactions with the yeast cell membrane and cell wall.

Competing interests
The authors declare that they have no competing interests.

Authors' contributions
RS participated in project design, carried out analytic experiments and participated in drafting the manuscript. BS FB supervised the whole project, supported the culture of microorganism, and participated in drafting the manuscript. OR participated in project design and drafting the manuscript. ZK contribution in analytical methods, commented the analytical results and participated in drafting the manuscript. All authors read and approved the final manuscript.

Acknowledgement
This work was supported by a grant from Mashhad University of Medical Sciences Research Council, Mashhad, Iran. The authors wish to thank the authorities in Mashhad University of Medical Sciences, Biotechnology Research center and School of Pharmacy for their support. This project was part of Ph.D student thesis in School of Pharmacy. The authors have no conflicts of interest that are directly relevant to the content of this manuscript.

Author details
[1]Department of Drug and Food Control, School of Pharmacy, Mashhad University of Medical Sciences, Mashhad, Iran. [2]Biotechnology Research Centre, School of Pharmacy, Mashhad University of Medical Sciences, Mashhad, Iran. [3]Targetted Drug Delivery Research Centre, School of Pharmacy, Mashhad University of Medical Sciences, Mashhad, Iran.

References
1. Madene A, Jacquot M, Scher J, Desobry S: Flavour encapsulation and controlled release: a review. Int J Food Sci Tech 2006, 41:1–21.
2. Gibbs BF, Kermasha S, Alli I, Mulligan N: Encapsulation in the food industry: a review. Int J Food Sci Nutr 1999, 50:213–224.
3. Khodaverdi E, Khalili N, Zangiabadi F, Homayouni A: Preparation, characterization and stability studies of glassy solid dispersions of indomethacin using PVP and isomalt as carriers. Iran J Basic Med Sci 2012, 15(3):820–32.
4. Gouin S: Microencapsulation: industrial appraisal of existing technologies and trends. Trends Food Sci Tech 2004, 15:330–347.
5. Shi G, Rao L, Yu H, Xiang H, Yang H, Ji R: Stabilization of photosensitive resveratrol within yeast cell. Int J Pharmaceut 2008, 349:83–93.
6. Bishop JRP, Nelson G, Lamb J: Microencapsulation in yeast cells. J Microencapsul 1998, 15(6):761–773.
7. Shi G, Rao L, Yu H, Xiang H, Pen G, Long S, et al: Yeast-cell based microencapsulation of chlorogenic acid as a water-soluble antioxidant. J Food Eng 2007, 80:1060–1067.
8. Chow C, Palecet P: Enzyme encapsulation in permeabilized Saccharomyces cerevisiae cells. Biotechnol Progr 2004, 20:449–456.
9. De Nobel JG, Klis FM, Munnik T, Priem J, Van Den Ende H: An assay of the relative cell wall porosity of Saccharomyces cerevisiae, Kluveromyces lactis and Schizosaccharomyces pombe. Yeast 1990, 6:483–490.
10. Shamsa F, Ahmadiani A, Khosrokhavar R: Antihistaminic and anticholinergic activity of barberry fruit (Berberis vulgaris) in the guinea-pig ileum. J Ethnopharmacol 1999, 64:161–166.
11. Mazzini S, Bellucci MC, Mondelli R: Mode of binding of the cytotoxic alkaloid berberine with the double helix oligonucleotide D (AAGAATTCTT). Bioorg Med Chem 2003, 11:505–514.
12. Imanshahid M, Hosseinzadeh H: Pharmacological and therapeutic effects of berberis vulgaris and its active constituent, berberine. Phytother Res 2008, 22:999–1012.
13. Fatehi-Hassanabad Z, Jafarzadeh M, Tarhini A, Fatehi M: The antihypertensive and vasodilator effects of aqueous extract from Berberis vulgaris fruit on hypertensive rats. Phytother Res 2005, 19:222–225.
14. DerMaderosian A: The Review of Natural Products. St. Louis, Missouri: Facts and Comparisons; 2001.
15. Chiou WF, Chen J, Chen CF: Relaxation of corpus cavernosum and raised intracavernous pressure by berberine in rabbit. Br J Pharmacol 1998, 125:1671–1684.
16. Zeng XH, Zeng XJ, Li YY: Efficacy and safety of berberine for congestive heart failure secondary to ischemic or idiopathic dilated cardiomyopathy. Am J Cardiol 2003, 92:173–176.
17. Yesilada E, Küpeli E, Berberis crataegina DC: Root exhibits potent anti-inflammatory, analgesic and febri-fuge effects in mice and rats. J Ethnopharmacol 2002, 79:237–248.
18. Lee CJ, Lee JH, Seok JH, et al: Effects of baicalein, berberine, curcumin and hesperidin on mucin release from airway goblet cells. Planta Med 2003, 69:523–526.
19. Lin SS, Chung JG, Lin JP, et al: Berberine inhibits arylamine N-acetyltransferase activity and gene expression in mouse leukemia L 1210 cells. Phytomedicine 2005, 12:351–358.

20. Rabbani GH, Butler T, Knight J, Sanyal SC, Alam K: Randomized controlled trial of berberine sulfate therapy for diarrhea due to enterotoxigenic *Escherichia coli* and *Vibrio cholerae*. *J Infect Dis* 1987, **155**:979–984.

21. Rabbani GH: Mechanism and treatment of diarrhoea due to *Vibrio cholerae* and *Escherichia coli*: roles of drugs and prostaglandins. *Dan Med Bull* 1996, **43**:173–185.

22. Birdsall TC, Kelly GS: Berberine: therapeutic potential of an alkaloid found in several medicinal plants. *Altern Med Rev* 1997, **2**:94–103.

23. Khosla PK, Neeraj VI, Gupta SK, Satpathy G: Berberine, a potential drug for trachoma. *Rev Int Trach Pathol Ocul Trop* 1992, **69**:147–165.

24. Freile ML, Giannini F, Pucci G, et al: Antimicrobial activity of aqueous extracts and of berberine isolated from Berberis heterophylla. *Fitoterapia* 2003, **74**:702–705.

25. Kaneda Y, Torii M, Tanaka T, Aikawa M: In vitro effects of berberine sulphate on the growth and structure of *Entamoeba histolytica*, *Giardia lamblia* and *Trichomonas vaginalis*. *Ann Trop Med Parasitol* 1991, **85**:417–425.

26. Mahady GB, Pendland SL, Stoia A, Chadwick LR: In vitro susceptibility of *Helicobacter pylori* to isoquinoline alkaloids from sanguinaria canadensis and Hydrastis Canadensis. *Phytother Res* 2003, **17**:217–221.

27. Ghosh AK, Bhattacharya FK, Ghosh DK: *Leishmania donovani*: Amastigote inhibition and mode of action of berberine. *Exp Parasitol* 1985, **60**:404–413.

28. Seki T, Morohashi M: Effect of some alkaloids, flavonoids and triterpenoids, contents of Japanese-Chinese traditional herbal medicines, on the lipogenesis of sebaceous glands. *Skin Pharmacol* 1993, **6**:56–60.

29. Lord PG, Wheals AE: Variability in individual cell cycles of *Saccharomyces cerevisiae*. *J. Cell Sci* 1981, **50**:361–376.

30. Paramera EI, Konteles SJ, Karathanos VT: Microencapsulation of curcumin in cells of *Saccharomyces cerevisiae*. *Food Chem* 2010, **125**:892–902.

31. Laroche C, Gervais P: Achievement of rapid dehydration at specific temperatures could maintain high *Sacharomyces cerevisiae* viability. *Appl Microbiol Biot* 2003, **60**:743–747.

32. Burattini E, Cavanga M, Dell Anna R, Malvezzi Campeggi F, Monti F, Rossi F, et al: An FT-IR microspectroscopy study of autolysis in cells of the wine yeast *Saccharomyces cerevisiae*. *Vib Spectrosc* 2008, **47**:139–147.

33. Korber DR, Choi A, Wolfaardt GM, Caldwell DE: Bacterial plasmolysis as a physical indicator of viability. *Appl Environ Microb* 1996, **62**(11):3939–3947.

34. Barik A, Mishra B, Shen L, Mohan H, Kadam RM, Dutta S, et al: Evaluation of a new copper (II)–curcumin complex as superoxide dismutase mimic and its free radical reactions. *Free Radical Bio Med* 2005, **39**:811–822.

High dose insulin therapy, an evidence based approach to beta blocker/calcium channel blocker toxicity

Christina Woodward, Ali Pourmand* and Maryann Mazer-Amirshahi

Abstract

Poison-induced cardiogenic shock (PICS) as a result of beta-blocker (β-blocker) or calcium channel blocker (CCB) overdose is a common and potentially life-threatening condition. Conventional therapies, including fluid resuscitation, atropine, cardiac pacing, calcium, glucagon, and vasopressors often fail to improve hemodynamic status. High-dose insulin (HDI) is an emerging therapeutic modality for PICS. In this article, we discuss the existing literature and highlight the therapeutic success and potential of HDI. Based on the current literature, which is limited primarily to case series and animal models, the authors conclude that HDI can be effective in restoring hemodynamic stability, and recommend considering its use in patients with PICS that is not responsive to traditional therapies. Future studies should be undertaken to determine the optimal dose and duration of therapy for HDI in PICS.

Keywords: High dose insulin, Beta-blocker, Calcium channel blocker, Overdose

Introduction

Poison-induced cardiogenic shock (PICS) due to beta-blocker (β-blocker) or calcium channel blocker (CCB) overdose is a frequent and potentially lethal occurrence [1]. β-blockers are used widely for conditions such as hypertension, dysrhythmias, and coronary artery disease; in the United States there were 128 million prescriptions for β-blockers filled in 2009 according to IMS Health, making them the fifth most commonly prescribed medication class in the country [2]. CCBs are also frequently utilized for patients with cardiovascular disease and other conditions, with an estimated 98 million prescriptions filled in 2010 alone [3]. The most common cause of PICS is β-blocker toxicity, with 24,465 exposures to β-blockers reported by the American Association of Poison Control Centers' National Poison Data System in 2012 [4]. While less frequent, CCB overdose has been associated with the highest mortality rates amongst cardiovascular agents in the United States [5].

Importance

Conventional therapies, including fluid resuscitation, atropine, cardiac pacing, calcium, glucagon, and vasopressors often fail to improve hemodynamic status in PICS secondary to β-blocker and CCB overdose. Even if there is a response to such traditional therapies, the response is often transient in nature [6-8]. High-dose insulin (HDI) (using doses 10-fold greater than traditional therapy for hyperglycemia) is an emerging therapeutic modality for PICS. Although there is a paucity of clinical trials and existing data are currently limited to case series or animal models, HDI has shown great promise as an effective treatment for β-blocker and CCB toxicity [7,9-13].

Unlike other countries such as Iran, where there is a growing trend to treat acutely poisoned patients in specialized tertiary hospitals where the clinical staff is trained specifically in toxicology, many poisoned patients in the U.S. are not seen at the bedside by a medical toxicologist [14]. As such, it is of critical importance that emergency medicine physicians, intensivists, and support staff (nursing, pharmacy) be equipped with the knowledge and comfort to utilize HDI. HDI is a potentially life-saving therapeutic option; however, its popularity is not yet widespread and has been mainly restricted to use

* Correspondence: Pourmand@gwu.edu
Department of Emergency Medicine, George Washington University,
Washington, DC 20037, USA

as a rescue therapy after conventional methods fail [15]; this limitation is likely due to a lack of randomized, controlled trials and practitioner unfamiliarity. In this paper, we will review the existing literature and highlight the therapeutic success and potential of HDI.

Mechanism of toxicity

β-blockers act on beta-receptors through competitive inhibition, indirectly decreasing the production of cAMP and thereby limiting calcium influx through L-type calcium channels with a resulting negative effect on heart rate and cardiac contractility [1,16,17]. CCBs exert their therapeutic and toxic effects by the direct blockade of L-type calcium channels causing relaxation of the vascular smooth muscle with subsequent vasodilation, and in the case of verapamil and diltiazem, inhibition of the sinoatrial and atrioventricular nodes. Calcium channel blockade concurrently triggers the heart to switch to preferential carbohydrate metabolism as opposed to the free fatty acid oxidation that occurs in the myocardium in the non-stressed state [8,17-19]. The effects of calcium channel antagonism are also seen in other parts of the body [1,6,17]. For example, in the beta-islet cells of the pancreas, calcium channel antagonism inhibits insulin secretion, producing insulin resistance and hyperglycemia [8,17,18].

Calcium flux is crucial to many aspects of normal myocardial activity, including contractility, pacemaker function, and signal propagation. Both CCBs and β-blockers ultimately result in decreased myocardial cytosolic calcium [1,17]. Life- threatening cardiovascular effects such as profound vasodilation with decreased systemic vascular resistance, bradycardia, conduction delay, hypotension, and resulting cardiogenic shock have been well established in BB and CCB overdose [17,20,21]. Other adverse effects include hyperglycemia (more common in CCB overdose) and lactic acid accumulation leading to metabolic acidosis [6,9,22,23]. In addition, altered mental status, dysrhythmias, seizures and other adverse effects may occur depending upon the specific agent ingested [17].

Management of PCIS

The primary goal in the management of PCIS is to restore hemodynamic stability [9]. Treatment tends to be physician dependent, given the lack of clinical trials and established guidelines. Once the patients' airway, breathing, and circulation have been stabilized, initial therapy for CCB and β-blocker overdose generally includes aggressive gastrointestinal decontamination. Activated charcoal, gastric lavage, and whole-bowel irrigation are potential options for decontamination in hemodynamically stable patients; however, these therapies are relatively contraindicated in the setting of shock. In patients with evidence of cardiovascular compromise, intravenous crystalloids such as normal saline, are initially administered as a bolus. Patients with symptomatic bradycardia can be treated with atropine and cardiac pacing; however, patients with β-blocker and CCB overdose often do not respond to these interventions [17]. Calcium and glucagon administration are often attempted as part of initial resuscitation efforts. Catecholamines, such as norepinephrine, can be administered as hemodynamic status warrants. For patients who remain hemodynamically unstable after these initial therapies, second line treatment options include HDI, lipid emulsion therapy [24,25] and mechanical life support (including intra-aortic balloon pump, cardiopulmonary bypass, or extracorporeal membrane oxygenation) [1].

Mechanism of action

HDI has been postulated to improve hemodynamics in CCB and β-blocker overdose by several different mechanisms. Most notably, a number of studies have demonstrated that insulin administered in higher doses has strong positive inotropic properties [9,11,17,18,20,21,26]. HDI also assists myocardial uptake of carbohydrates, which is the preferred fuel substrate of the heart under stressed conditions [1,8,21,27] HDI also inhibits free fatty acid metabolism [27,28]. Additionally, exogenous insulin administration can help to overcome the insulin resistance and insulin deficiency that occurs in CCB toxicity [1]. HDI produces vasodilation, which improves local microcirculation [11,21] and aids systemic perfusion [9,11,20]. Studies have demonstrated accelerated oxidation of myocardial lactate and reversal of metabolic acidosis with HDI [9,26]. Response to catecholamines is also improved with addition of HDI [9]. While conventional therapy sometimes offers temporary improvement in hemodynamics, the hemodynamic stability achieved with HDI does not appear to be as transient in nature [21].

Dosing and administration

There are no official guidelines regarding insulin dosing in PICS and wide practice variation exists. However, one of the most common recommendations consists of a 1 unit/kg bolus dose followed by a continuous infusion at 0.5-1 unit/kg per hour, which can be titrated to response. Insulin doses up to 10 units/kg per hour have been successfully used to treat PICS [29]. A dextrose bolus of 0.5 g/kg can be administered with the initial insulin bolus in patients whose blood glucose is less than 400 mg/dL. A continuous dextrose infusion (0.5 g/kg per hour) should be initiated. It is preferable to administered concentrated dextrose solutions through a central venous catheter [17]. Supplemental intravenous dextrose (110–150 mg/dL or 6–8 mmol/L) can be administered as needed to maintain euglycemia; however, patients with CCB overdose may be hyperglycemic despite HDI

[9,15,21]. Blood glucose should be checked every twenty minutes during the first hour, and can then be checked hourly [9], with the goal of maintaining blood glucose levels in the upper range of normal [15]. The onset of action of HDI is thought to be 15–45 minutes, but may be delayed several hours [15,21]. Once initiated, HDI therapy is continued until hemodynamic stability is achieved. There are no established recommendations regarding the proper duration of therapy and treatment with HDI should be guided by the patient's hemodynamic status [21], with the goal of maintaining a heart rate of at least 50 beats/min and a systolic blood pressure of at least 100 mm Hg [9]. Case reports have documented variable duration of HDI, ranging from 9 hours to 49 hours [7,10,30].

Adverse effects

HDI is relatively well tolerated; the most common adverse effects include hypoglycemia and hypokalemia; however, these are rare and reversible when proper serum monitoring and replacement is undertaken [21,31]. Supplemental glucose is often required throughout the administration of HDI and for as long as 24 hours after cessation of therapy [21]. Some adult patients may need up to 30 g of supplemental glucose per hour to maintain normokalemia, in addition to potassium supplements [15]. Serum potassium should be checked hourly during insulin titration and may be extended to every 6 h following titration and electrolyte stability [21]. Intravenous potassium repletion is required when concentrations drop below 2.8 mEq/L [21], with a target goal of maintaining concentrations at 2.8-3.2 mEq/L [9]. In some case reports, patients have not required potassium supplementation at all [7], while other authors have described the need for potassium supplementation averaging 2.7 mmol/h (or 4.1 mmol per 100 units of insulin) [31]. Hypokalemia during HDI is representative of intracellular shifting of potassium as opposed to total body depletion [21]. Practitioners can observe hypokalemia through electrocardiogram changes, beginning with decreased T-wave amplitude and progressing to ST segment depression, T-wave inversion, prolongation of the PR interval, increased P wave amplitude, and U wave appearance [32]. Despite the known risk of adverse arrhythmias with hypokalemia, there have been few such events recorded in the literature when HDI is used in cases of PICS [21]. It is important to note that the adverse effects associated with HDI are also present with the use of insulin at regular doses, which physicians, pharmacists, and nurses are accustomed to addressing in conditions such as diabetic ketoacidosis.

Experimental and clinical data

Although prospective clinical studies in human subjects comparing the efficacy of HDI to conventional treatments are lacking, several experimental animal studies have demonstrated the utility of HDI in achieving hemodynamic stability. A series of studies in canines by Kline et al. consistently demonstrated improved inotropy when HDI was given after verapamil overdose [8,18,20,26]. In other studies, HDI successfully normalized heart rate [13] and reversed negative inotropy caused by propranolol overdose in canines [11,13]. Superior survival rates have been witnessed in various animal studies when HDI is administered in PICS [8,12,20,26,33]. In humans, several case reports have documented successful hemodynamic stabilization with insulin after initial failed treatment attempts with conventional therapy [6,7,25,34,35].

To date, there are no studies on the most appropriate way to wean HDI once hemodynamic stability has been achieved [21]. While some physicians opt for a slow taper, others advocate for abrupt cessation of HDI infusion as this method has been postulated to allow insulin concentrations to self-taper as lipid stores slowly release insulin [7,21]. Several case reports have documented worsening hypotension in patients with CCB overdose with early insulin withdrawal that was alleviated when the insulin infusion was subsequently increased [7,30]. In one reported case of verapamil overdose resulting in hypotension and a junctional rhythm, HDI was initiated 3.5 hours after presentation (0.5 IU/kg bolus and infusion at 0.5 IU/kg/h) following failure of blood pressure stabilization with intravenous fluids and metaraminol boluses, with subsequent improvement in blood pressure and conversion to normal sinus rhythm within 30 minutes [30]. Following abrupt termination of HDI 5.5 hours after presentation the patient again became hypotensive, therefore HDI was restarted at 8.5 hours as well as an adrenaline infusion which again achieved hemodynamic stability. HDI was continued until 30.5 hours and the patient remained stable throughout this time. In another case report of verapamil overdose resulting in initial hypotension and third degree heart block, HDI up to 70 units per hour was initiated after 45 minutes of refractory hypotension despite calcium chloride and glucagon, with subsequent improvement in blood pressure [7]. Eight hours after presentation, HDI was gradually weaned while maintaining glucagon and dopamine infusions, resulting in recurrent hypotension, which was improved when the dose of HDI was increased. HDI was continued for a total of 27.5 hours.

Treatment difficulty could be due to delayed initiation of insulin therapy, as rare case reports have documented treatment failure with HDI when initiated late, for example at the end of cardiopulmonary resuscitation or following multiple hours of alternative therapies [36,37]. Although many sources recommend a 1 unit/kg bolus dose followed by a continuous infusion at 0.5-1 unit/kg per hour [9,15,21], no ceiling effect has ever been established and higher doses have been postulated to be more effective [38], with good outcomes documented in patients receiving insulin boluses as high as 10 U/kg [39] and infusions as high as 22 U/kg/h [25].

Conclusions

Although clinical trial data in humans are lacking, available published reports suggest that HDI is effective at restoring hemodynamic stability in CCB and β-blocker overdose. As such, HDI should be considered in patients with PCIS who do not respond to traditional therapies and providers who care for poisoned patients should be familiar with this potentially life-saving therapy. Future studies should be undertaken to determine the optimal dosing regimen and duration of therapy for HDI in PICS.

Competing interests

The authors have no commercial associations or sources of support that might pose a conflict of interest.

Authors' contribution

All authors have made substantive contributions to the study, and all authors endorse the data and conclusions. All authors read and approved the final manuscript.

References

1. DeWitt CR, Waksman JC: Pharmacology, pathophysiology, and management of calcium channel blocker and beta blocker toxicity. *Toxicol Rev* 2004, 23:223–238.
2. *Consumer Reports health best buy drugs: treating high blood pressure and heart disease: the beta-blockers;* 2011. http://www.consumerreports.org/health/resources/pdf/best-buy-drugs/CU-Betablockers-FIN060109.pdf.
3. *The Huffington Post: calcium-channel blockers, blood pressure medication, might raise breast cancer risk;* 2014. http://www.huffingtonpost.com/2013/08/06/calcium-channel-blockers-breast-cancer-bloodpressure_n_3712936.html?
4. Mowry JB, Spyker DA, Cantilena LR Jr, Bailey JE, Ford M: 2012 Annual Report of the American Association of Poison Control Centers' National Poison Data System (NPDS): 30th Annual Report. *Clin Toxicol (Phila)* 2013, 51:949–1229.
5. Watson WA, Litovitz TL, Klein-Schwartz W, Rodgers GC Jr, Youniss J, Reid N, Rouse WG, Rembert RS, Borys D: 2003 annual report of the American Association of Poison Control Centers Toxic Exposure Surveillance System. *Am J Emerg Med* 2004, 22:335–404.
6. Boyer EW, Duic PA, Evans A: Hyperinsulinemia/euglycemia therapy for calcium channel blocker poisoning. *Pedatr Emerg Care* 2002, 18:36–37.
7. Yuan TH, Kerns WP, Tomaszewski CA, Ford MD, Kline JA: Insulin-glucose as adjunctive therapy of severe calcium channel antagonist poisoning. *J Toxicol Clin Toxicol* 1999, 37:463–474.
8. Kline JA, Leonova E, Raymond RM: Beneficial myocardial metabolic effects of insulin during verapamil toxicity in the anesthetized canine. *Crit Care Med* 1995, 23:1251–1263.
9. Mégarbane B, Karyo S, Baud FJ: The role of insulin and glucose (hyperinsulinaemia/euglycaemia) therapy in acute calcium channel antagonist and beta-blocker poisoning. *Toxicol Rev* 2004, 23:215–222.
10. Marques I, Gomes E, de Oliveria J: Treatment of calcium channel blocker intoxication with insulin infusion: case report and literature review. *Resuscitation* 2003, 57:211–213.
11. Reikerås O, Gunnes P, Sørlie D, Ekroth R, Jorde R, Mjøs OD: Haemodynamic effects of low and high doses of insulin during beta-receptor blockade in dogs. *Clin Physiol* 1985, 5:455–467.
12. Kerns W, Schroeder JD, Williams C, Tomaszewski CA, Raymond RM: Insulin improves survival in a canine model of acute beta-blocker toxicity. *Ann Emerg Med* 1997, 29:748–757.
13. Krukenkamp I, Sorlie D, Silverman N, Pridjian A, Levitsky S: Direct effect of high-dose insulin on the depressed heart after beta-blockade or ischemia. *Thorac Cardiovasc Surg* 1986, 34:305–309.
14. Zamani N, Mehrpour O: Outpatient treatment of the poisoned patients in Iran; may it be a feasible plan? *DARU J Pharm Sci* 2013, 21(1):45.
15. Lheureux PE, Zahir S, Gris M, Derrey AS, Penaloza A: Bench-to-bedside review: hyperinsulinaemia/euglycaemia therapy in the management of overdose of calcium-channel blockers. *Crit Care* 2006, 10:212.
16. Love JN, Howell JM, Litovitz TL, Klein-Schwartz W: Acute beta blocker overdose: factors associated with the development of cardiovascular morbidity. *J Toxicol Clin Toxicol* 2000, 38:275–281.
17. Nelson L, Hoffman R, Flomenbaum N, Goldfrank L, Howland MA: *Goldfrank's Toxicologic Emergencies.* 9th edition. New York, NY: McGraw-Hill; 2010.
18. Kline JA, Leonova E, Williams TC, Schroeder JD, Watts JA: Myocardial metabolism during graded intraportal verapamil infusion in awake dogs. *J Cardiovasc Pharmacol* 1996, 27:719–726.
19. Downing SE: The heart in shock. In *Handbook of Shock and Trauma.* Edited by Altura BM, Lefer AM, Schumer W. New York: Raven Press; 1983:5–28.
20. Kline JA, Tomaszewsi CA, Schroeder JD, Raymond RM: Insulin is a superior antidote for cardiovascular toxicity induced by verapamil in the anesthetized canine. *J Pharm Exp Ther* 1993, 267:744–750.
21. Engebretsen KM, Kaczmarek KM, Morgan J, Holger JS: High-dose insulin therapy in beta-blocker and calcium channel-blocker poisoning. *Clin Toxicol (Phila)* 2011, 49:277–283.
22. Buss WC, Savage DD, Stepanek J, Little SA, McGuffee LJ: Effect of calcium channel antagonists on calcium uptake and release by isolated rat cardiac mitochondria. *Eur J Pharmacol* 1988, 152:247–253.
23. Rafael J, Patzelt J: Binding of diltiazem and verapamil to isolated rat heart mitochondria. *Basic Res Cardiol* 1987, 82:246–251.
24. Stellpflug SJ, Fritzlar SJ, Cole JB, Engebretsen KM, Holger JS: Cardiotoxic overdose treated with intravenous fat emulsion and high-dose insulin in the setting of hypertrophic cardiomyopathy. *J Med Toxicol* 2011, 7:151–153.
25. Stellpflug SJ, Harris CR, Engebretsen KM, Cole JB, Holger JS: Intentional overdose with cardiac arrest treated with intravenous fat emulsion and high-dose insulin. *Clin Toxicol* 2010, 48:227–229.
26. Kline JA, Raymond RM, Leonova ED, Williams TC, Watts JA: Insulin improves heart function and metabolism during non-ischemic cardiogenic shock in awake canines. *Cardiovasc Res* 1997, 34:289–298.
27. Farah AE, Alousi AA: The actions of insulin on cardiac contractility. *Life Sci* 1981, 29:975–1000.
28. Tune JD, Mallett RT, Downey HF: Insulin improves contractile function during moderate ischemia in canine left ventricle. *Am J Physiol* 1998, 274(5 Pt 2):H1574–H1581.
29. Holger JS, Stellpflug SJ, Cole JB, Harris CR, Engebretsen KM: High-dose insulin: a consecutive case series in toxin-induced cardiogenic shock. *Clin Toxicol* 2011, 49:653–658.
30. Boyer EW: *2000 Poisoning Data.* Boston: Massachusetts Poison Control Center; 2000.
31. Greene SL, Gawarammana I, Wood DM, Jones AL, Dargan PI: Relative safety of hyperinsulinaemia/euglycaemia therapy in the management of calcium channel blocker overdose: a prospective observational study. *Intensive Care Med* 2007, 33:2019–2024.
32. Levis JT: ECG diagnosis: hypokalemia. *Perm J* 2012, 16(2):57.
33. Holger JS, Engebretsen KM, Fritzlar SJ, Patten LC, Harris CR, Flottemesch TJ: Insulin versus vasopressin and epinephrine to treat beat-blocker toxicity. *Clin Toxicol* 2007, 45:396–401.
34. Vergugge LB, van Wezel HB: Pathophysiology of verapamil overdose; new insights into the role of insulin. *J Cardiothoracic Vasc Anesth* 2007, 21:406–409.
35. Boyer EW, Shannon M: Treatment of calcium channel blocker intoxication with insulin infusion. *N Eng J Med* 2001, 344:1721–1722.
36. Levine MD, Boyer E: Hyperinsulinemia-euglycemia therapy a useful tool in treating calcium channel blocker poisoning. *Crit care* 2006, 10:149.
37. Herbert J, O'Malley C, Tracey J, Dwyer R, Power M: Verapamil overdosage unresponsive to dextrose/insulin therapy. *J Toxicol Clin Toxicol* 2001, 39:293–294.

38. Cole JB, Stellpflug SJ, Ellsworth H, Anderson CP, Adams AB, Engebretsen KM, Holger JS: **A blinded, randomized, controlled trial of three doses of high-dose insulin in poison-induced cardiogenic shock.** *Clin Toxicol (Phila).* 2013, **51**:201–207.
39. Place R, Carlson A, Leikin J, Hanashiro P: **Hyperinsulin therapy in the treatment of verapamil overdose.** *J Toxicol Clin Toxicol* 2000, **38**:576–577.

The cytotoxic activities of 7-isopentenyloxycoumarin on 5637 cells via induction of apoptosis and cell cycle arrest in G2/M stage

Fereshteh Haghighi[1], Maryam M Matin[1,2*], Ahmad Reza Bahrami[1,2], Mehrdad Iranshahi[3], Fatemeh B Rassouli[1] and Azadeh Haghighitalab[1]

Abstract

Background: Bladder cancer is the second common malignancy of genitourinary tract, and transitional cell carcinomas (TCCs) account for 90% of all bladder cancers. Due to acquired resistance of TCC cells to a wide range of chemotherapeutic agents, there is always a need for search on new compounds for treatment of these cancers. Coumarins represent a group of natural compounds, which some of them have exerted valuable anti-tumor activities. The current study was designed to evaluate anti-tumor properties and mechanism of action of 7-isopentenyloxycoumarin, a prenyloxycoumarin, on 5637 cells (a TCC cell line).

Results: MTT results revealed that the cytotoxic effects of 7-isopentenyloxycoumarin on 5637 cancerous cells were more prominent in comparison to HDF-1 normal cells. This coumarin increased the amount of chromatin condensation and DNA damage in 5637 cells by 58 and 33%, respectively. The results also indicated that it can induce apoptosis most probably via activation of caspase-3 in these cells. Moreover, propidium iodide staining revealed that 7-isopentenyloxycoumarin induced cell cycle arrest at G2/M stage, after 24 h of treatment.

Conclusion: Our results indicated that 7-isopentenyloxycoumarin had selective toxic effects on this bladder cancer cell line and promoted its effects by apoptosis induction and cell cycle arrest. This coumarin can be considered for further studies to reveal its exact mechanism of action and also its anti-cancer effects *in vivo*.

Keywords: Bladder cancer, Cytotoxicity, 7-isopentenyloxycoumarin, Apoptosis, Cell cycle

Background

About 7 million people die from different types of cancer, which makes it the second cause of death worldwide every year [1]. Bladder cancer is the second most common genitourinary malignancy with a higher incidence in men. More than 90% of all bladder cancers are transitional cell carcinomas (TCCs). Although cisplatin-based combination chemotherapies like MVAC (methotrexate-vinblastine-adriamycin-cisplatin) are the standard treatments in patients with TCC, harnessing metastatic bladder cancer still remains one of the main challenges in urologic oncology [2,3]. The resistance of TCC cells to a wide range of

chemotherapeutic agents is the main reason for the failure of such treatments [4].

Apoptosis, also known as programmed cell death, is a naturally occurring process that plays a central role in the normal development and homeostasis of all multi-cellular organisms [5]. Apoptosis is accompanied by cell shrinkage, reduction of cellular volume, nuclear fragmentation, chromatin condensation, plasma membrane blebbing and engulfment by phagocytes *in vivo* [6]. There are two main apoptotic pathways in mammals: the extrinsic or death receptor pathway and the intrinsic or mitochondrial pathway. Both mechanisms end at the point of execution phase, which is initiated by the cleavage of executioner caspases and results in the apoptotic morphology. Caspase-3 is one of the most important executioner caspases, which is activated in both extrinsic and intrinsic pathways [7].

* Correspondence: Matin@um.ac.ir
[1]Department of Biology, Faculty of Science, Ferdowsi University of Mashhad, Mashhad, Iran
[2]Cell and Molecular Biotechnology Research Group, Institute of Biotechnology, Ferdowsi University of Mashhad, Mashhad, Iran
Full list of author information is available at the end of the article

Coumarins are a large group of natural compounds that are mainly found in the plant families of Rutaceae, Apiaceae and Umbelliferae as well as some bacteria and fungi [8]. Biological properties of coumarins include anti-coagulant, anti-viral, anti-microbial, anti-inflammatory, anti-oxidant and anti-tumor activities [9-12]. Induction of cell cycle arrest by coumarins is also reported frequently [9-11]. Prenyloxycoumarins represent a class of secondary metabolites that based on the length of their carbon chains, are categorized in three groups; C5 (isopentenyl), C10 (geranyl) and C15 (linear, mono- or bicyclic ses-quiterpenyl) [8]. One of these studied coumarins is 7-isopentenyloxycoumarin (7-IP) [13].

7-IP, a secondary metabolite with an isopentenyl chain fixed at C7 of the 1, 2-benzopyrone ring, exerts valuable and promising anti-microbial, anti-inflammatory and anti-cancer effects [14]. The chemopreventive [15], neuropro-tective [16] and anti-genotoxic [17] properties of 7-IP have been shown previously. This coumarin was first isolated by Prokopenko from the fruit of *Libanotis intermedia* in 1966. In nature, 7-IP is biosynthesized from 7-hydroxycoumarin and dimethylallyl diphosphate [14] and is widespread in edible vegetables and fruits such as grapefruit, lemon, orange, mandarin and many other plants [18].

In this study, 7-IP was synthesized by a reaction between 7-hydroxycoumarin and its relevant prenyl bromide. Here, we evaluated its toxic effects on 5637 and HDF-1 cell lines by MTT assay. Since, there is no report on the mechanism of action of 7-IP, we report the effects of this coumarin in more details by DAPI staining, comet assay, caspase-3 activity and cell cycle analysis.

Methods
Chemical synthesis
7-IP (Figure 1A) was synthesized as described by Askari *et al.* [13]. Briefly, it was synthesized by a reaction be-tween 7-hydroxycoumarin (Figure 1B) and isopentenyl

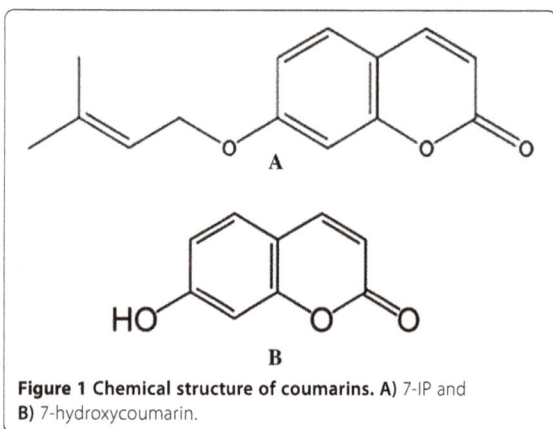

Figure 1 Chemical structure of coumarins. A) 7-IP and **B)** 7-hydroxycoumarin.

bromide in the presence of DBU (1, 8-diazabicyclo [5.4.0]undec-7-ene), in acetone at room temperature. The purity and chemical structure of 7-IP was then assessed by ^{1}H- and ^{13}C-NMR spectroscopy (Additional file 1: Table S1 and Additional file 2: Table S2).

Preparation of different 7-IP concentrations
To prepare different concentrations of 7-IP (10 to 100 µg/ml), 2 mg of the powder was dissolved in 500 µl dimethyl sulfoxide (DMSO, Merck, Germany), and diluted with complete culture medium before experiments. Since the solvent has cytotoxic effects, the control treatments were run at the same time with equivalent solutions of DMSO.

Cell lines and cell culture
Human 5637 cells (a TCC subline) were obtained from Pasteur Institute (Tehran, Iran). These epithelial like cells were first derived in 1974 of a primary bladder carcinoma from a 68- year old Caucasian man. HDF-1 (human der-mal fibroblast) cells, derived from human skin fibroblasts, were a generous gift from Royan Institute (Tehran, Iran). All cells were maintained in Dulbecco's modified Eagle's medium (DMEM, Gibco, Scotland) supplemented with 10% heat-inactivated fetal bovine serum (FBS, Gibco, Scotland) for 5367 cells, and 15% FBS for HDF-1 cells. 5637 and HDF-1 cells were grown at 37°C in a humidsified atmosphere of 10% and 5% CO_2 in air, respectively. To subculture the cells, they were washed with phosphate buffered saline (PBS) and incubated with 0.25% trypsin/ 1 mM ethylenediaminetetraacetic acid (EDTA) (Gibco, Scotland) for 5 min. Detached cells were resuspended in fresh serum-containing medium to inactivate the trypsin and transferred to new labeled flasks.

Cell viability assay
Cell viability was determined by MTT assay [19]. In this method, tetrazolium dye, 3-(4,5-Dimethyl-2-thiazolyl)-2,5-diphenyl-2*H*-tetrazolium bromide, is reduced by mito-chondrial enzymes to insoluble purple formazan in living cells. The absorbance of the colored product (after dissolv-ing in DMSO) can be determined by a spectrophotometer. Briefly, 5637 and HDF-1 cells were seeded at a density of 1.3×10^4 and 1.0×10^4 cells/well in 96-well tissue culture plates (Orange Scientific, France), respectively. The cells were allowed to attach and grow for 24 h. In order to identify the half maximal inhibitory concentration (IC_{50}) values of 7-IP, cells were treated with increasing concen-trations (10 to 100 µg/ml) of the compound for 24, 48 and 72 h. To perform MTT assay, 5 mg MTT dye (Sigma Aldrich, Germany) was dissolved in 1 ml PBS, filtered through a 0.22 µm filter (Orange Scientific, France) and used freshly before each experiment. Then 20 µl MTT solution (500 µg/ml final concentration) was added to

each well and plates were incubated at 37°C for 4 h. After this period, the remaining MTT solution was removed and 150 µl DMSO was added to each well to dissolve the formazan crystals. The absorbance of each well was then measured at 545 nm using an enzyme linked immuno-sorbent assay (ELISA) plate reader (Awareness, USA). The percentage of cell viability was calculated by dividing the mean absorbance of each treatment (7-IP) to the mean absorbance of its controls (DMSO) multiply by 100.

Morphological alterations

Cells treated with various concentrations of 7-IP were observed under a light inverted microscope (Olympus, Japan) for morphological changes after 24, 48 and 72 h of the treatments.

Apoptosis assay with DAPI staining

In order to evaluate the apoptotic effects of 7-IP semi-quantitatively, DAPI (4′, 6-diamidino-2-phenylindole dichloride) staining was performed. To do so, 5637 cells were grown to 80% confluency in 6-well tissue culture plates (Orange Scientific, France). Then the cells were treated with 65 µg/ml 7-IP and its equivalent amount of DMSO (1.625%) for 72 h. Cells were then washed gently with PBS and fixed with 4% paraformaldehyde (Sigma, Germany) for 10 min at room temperature. After that cells were washed with PBS, permeabilized with 0.1% Triton X-100 (Merck, Germany) and stained with 2 µg/ml DAPI (Merck, Germany) at 37°C for 10 min. Approximately, 700 cells from each treatment were visualized and counted under a fluorescent microscope (Olympus, Japan). Chromatin condensation was considered as a specific criterion for apoptotic morphology.

Alkaline comet assay

To investigate the DNA-damaging effects of 7-IP, the alkaline version of comet assay, which is a rapid, reliable and quantitative technique for detection of possible DNA lesions at the individual eukaryotic cells, was performed [20]. Briefly, untreated 5637 and HDF-1 cells, and cells treated for 72 h with 65 µg/ml 7-IP and its DMSO control were trypsinized and centrifuged at 1100 g for 10 min. The cell pellets were resuspended in 50 µl PBS and then mixed with 50 µl of 1.5% (w/v) low melting point agarose (LMA, Fermentas, Germany) and spread on glass slides precoated with 1% (w/v) normal melting point agarose (NMA, Helicon, Russia). Four slides were prepared for each treatment. The slides were kept for 20 min at 4°C to allow the agarose to solidify. After 20 min 100 µl of 0.75% (w/v) LMA was added to each slide, and kept for another 20 min at 4°C. When the gel was solidified, slides were submerged in freshly prepared lysing buffer (2.5 M NaCl, 100 mM Na$_2$EDTA, 10 mM Tris, 2% (v/v) Triton X-100, pH 10) for at least 4 h at 4°C. Then the slides were placed in an electrophoresis chamber filled with freshly prepared cold alkaline electrophoresis buffer (1 mM EDTA, 0.3 N NaOH, pH 13) and incubated for 30 min at 4°C. Electro-phoresis was conducted at 300 mA and 25 V for 20 min at 4°C. Slides were then washed with ice-cold neutralizing buffer (0.4 M Tris–HCl, pH 7.5) for three times, dried with 96% ethanol and stained with ethidium bromide (20 µg/ml). The slides were viewed and analyzed with a fluorescent microscope (Olympus, Japan). One hundred cells per slide were evaluated and the mean of comet tail (a product of fraction of DNA in tail and tail length) was determined using TriTek Cometscore version 1.5 software. The DNA damage was expressed as % DNA in tail.

Caspase-3 activity assay

Caspase-3 activity was assessed using caspase-3 colorimet-ric assay kit (Abcam, USA) according to manufacturer's protocol. Briefly, 5637 cells were treated with 65 µg/ml of 7-IP and its equivalent amount of DMSO for 12 h. Cells treated with 15 µg/ml of cisplatin for 24 h were used as a positive control. After the period of treatments, cells were trypsinized and centrifuged at 1100 g for 10 min. Cell pel-lets were suspended in 1 ml cold PBS and centrifuged at 4000 g for 5 min at 4°C. In order to extract total protein, cell pellets were resuspended and lysed with 100 µl of chilled lysis buffer and incubated on ice for 10 min. Cell lysates were then centrifuged at 10000 g for 1 min at 4°C. The concentration of proteins was measured by Bradford assay. Then 50 µl of 2× reaction buffer containing 10 mM DTT and 5 µl of 4 mM caspase-3 substrate (DEVD-pNA) were added to 200 µg protein from each sample and incubated at 37°C for 4 h. The p-NA light emission was quantified using ELISA plate reader at 405 nm. Compari-son of the absorbance of p-NA from an apoptotic sample with an uninduced control allowed determination of the fold increase in caspase-3 activity.

Cell cycle analysis

The cell cycle distribution was assayed by flow cytome-try after DNA staining with propidium iodide (PI). 5637 cells were treated with 65 µg/ml 7-IP and its equivalent amount of DMSO. After 24 h of treatments, floated cells were harvested and attached cells were trypsinized, washed with a protein-containing buffer (PBS + 5% FBS) and centrifuged at 1100 g for 10 min. The cell pellets were resuspended in 500 µl PBS containing 5% FBS and centrifuged at 200 g for 7 min at 4°C. After that cells were stained with a solution containing 100 µg/ml PI (Sigma Aldrich, Germany), 0.1% Triton X-100, 0.1% so-dium citrate (Merck, Germany) and RNase (100 µg/ml) (Merck, Germany) in ice cold PBS. The samples were then incubated at 4°C in dark for 1 h and flow cytomet-ric analyses were performed using a FACSCalibur (BD

Biosciences, USA) instrument and WinMDI version 2.9 software.

Statistical analyses

Data generated from experiments were collected in a completely randomized design. All assays were carried out at least three times. Statistical procedures were performed using Microsoft Office Excel (2007) SPSS, version 16.0 (SPSS software Inc., Chicago, IL, USA) and SAS, version 9.1 (SAS Institute, Inc., Cary, N.C., USA) softwares. A one-way analysis of variance (ANOVA) according to general linear model procedure of SAS software was performed to evaluate possible differences among the treatments. The statistical significant differences among means between each group were determined by using Tukey's single-step multiple comparison test. Differences among treatment means were compared at P-value of < 0.001. Values are expressed as mean $\pm$ SD.

Results

IC_{50} value determination of 7-IP in 5637 and HDF-1 cell lines

The cytotoxic effects of 7-IP were assessed by MTT assay in 5637 and HDF-1 cells exposed to 10–100 µg/ml of this coumarin for three consecutive days. Cell survival analyses showed that 7-IP had a concentration and time-dependent inhibitory effect on the growth of 5637 cells (Figure 2A). By increasing the concentrations, cell via-bilities were significantly different ($P < 0.001$) especially after 48 and 72 h of treatments. The IC_{50} values of this coumarin were calculated as 76, 76 and 65 µg/ml after 24, 48 and 72 h of treatments, respectively.

To assess the cytotoxic effects of 7-IP on normal cells, HDF-1 cells were used. As shown in Figure 2B, although this coumarin induced cell death in these non-cancerous cells, but its cytotoxic effects were not significant in com-parison to 5637 cells. Statistical analysis revealed that the slight cytotoxic effects of 7-IP on HDF-1 cells were not dose-dependent except at higher concentrations.

Morphological alterations

The cytotoxic effects of 7-IP were confirmed by mor-phological observations. As shown in Figure 3 (A-C), 5637 cells treated with 65 µg/ml 7-IP for 72 h, revealed prominent cytoplasmic granulation and cell number was significantly decreased as compared with control and untreated cultures. In the case of HDF-1 cells, there were no significant changes between cells treated with 100 µg/ml of 7-IP with control and untreated groups (Figure 3 D-F).

7-IP induces apoptosis in 5637 cells

To determine what kind of cell death has been induced by 7-IP, the chromatin condensation and DNA damage

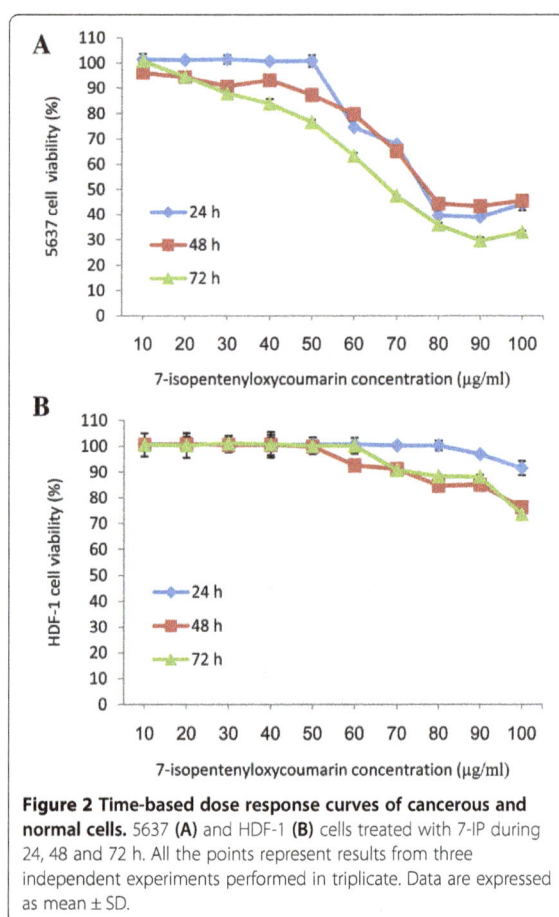

Figure 2 Time-based dose response curves of cancerous and normal cells. 5637 (**A**) and HDF-1 (**B**) cells treated with 7-IP during 24, 48 and 72 h. All the points represent results from three independent experiments performed in triplicate. Data are expressed as mean ± SD.

were assessed using DAPI staining and alkaline comet assay, respectively. Based on MTT results, 5637 cells were treated with 65 µg/ml 7-IP and equivalent amount of DMSO for 72 h. As shown in Figure 4 (A-C) cells treated with this compound, showed highly condensed chromatin and nuclear fragmentation in comparison to control and untreated cells. Quantitative results revealed that 89% of cells treated with 65 µg/ml 7-IP presented condensed chromatin, which was significantly ($P < 0.001$) higher than control (31%) and untreated (7.5%) cultures (Figure 4D).

Furthermore, detecting DNA damage inducing effects of 7-IP in 5637 cells by comet assay, showed comet tail in a high percentage of individual cells treated with this coumarin (Figure 5 A-C). Data analysis showed that 7-IP induced approximately 43% DNA damage, significantly ($P < 0.001$) higher than that induced by its DMSO control (11%, Figure 5G). In order to investigate the genotoxic effects of 7-IP in non-cancerous cells, comet assay was also performed in HDF-1 cells treated with the same amount of the compound. As shown in Figure 5 (D-F) the difference between comet tail in HDF-1 and 5637 cells

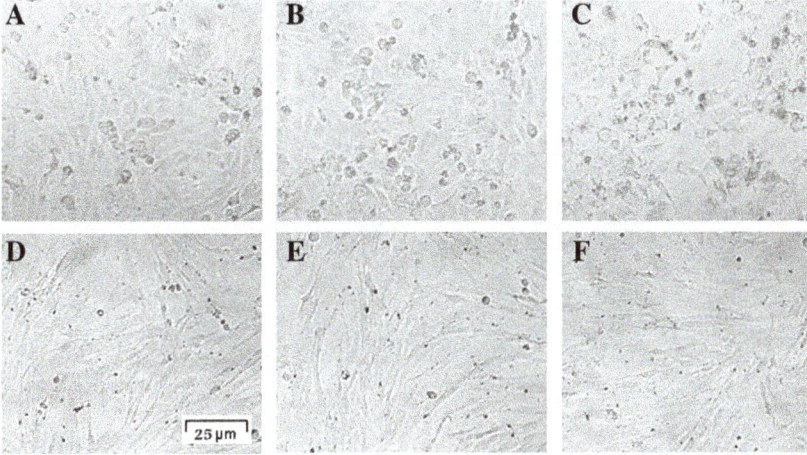

Figure 3 Light microscopic images of 5637 and HDF-1 cells. Untreated 5637 cells **(A)**. 5637 cells treated with 1.625% DMSO **(B)** represent little morphological changes as compared with untreated cells. 5637 cells treated with 65 µg/ml 7-IP **(C)** revealed prominent cytoplasmic granulation and cell death. Untreated HDF-1 cells **(D)**. HDF-1 cells treated with 2.5% DMSO **(E)**. HDF-1 cells treated with 100 µg/ml 7-IP after 72 h with little changes in their morphology **(F)**.

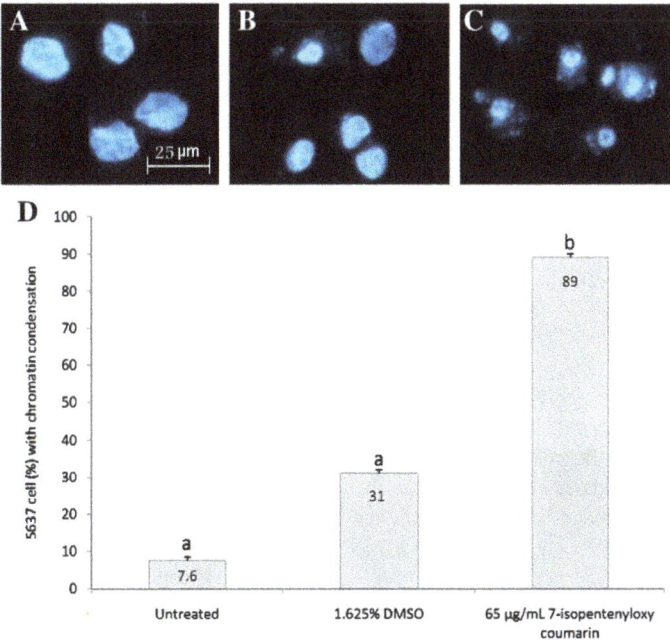

Figure 4 Investigating the apoptotic morphology of cells by DAPI staining. Chromatin condensation of 5637 cells without any treatment **(A)**, treated with 1.625% DMSO **(B)** and treated with 65 µg/ml 7-IP **(C)** for 72 h. The percentages of condensed chromatin, 72 h after treatments are compared with untreated and control groups **(D)**. Data are expressed as mean ± SD. The assay was done three times. Distinct letters indicate significant differences ($P < 0.001$) between cells treated with 65 µg/ml 7-IP and other cultures.

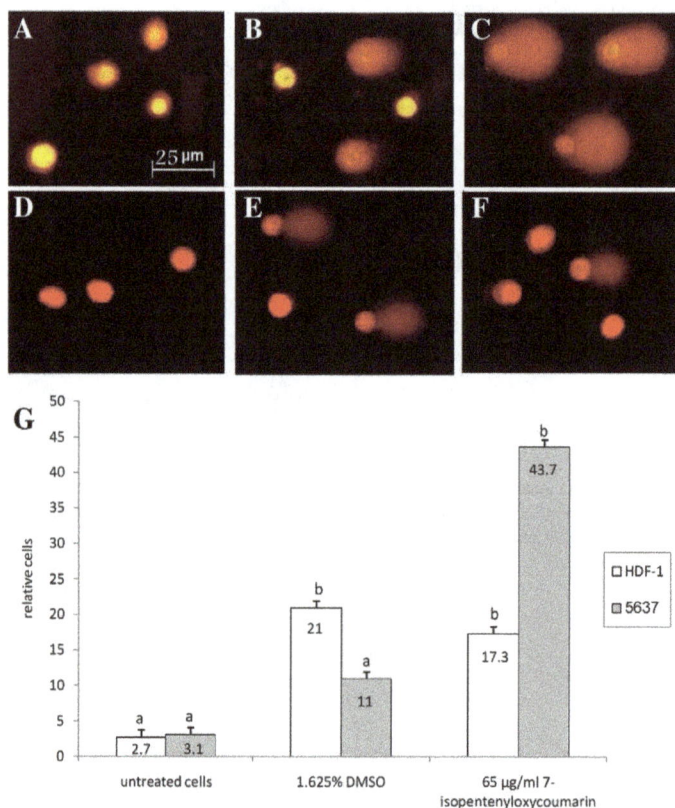

Figure 5 Evaluating the DNA damaging effects of 7-IP by comet assay. DNA damage of 5637 and HDF-1 cells without any treatment **(A and D)**, treated with 1.625% DMSO **(B and E)** and treated with 65 μg/ml 7-IP **(C and F)** for 72 h, respectively. The percentages of damaged DNA, 72 h after treatments are compared with untreated and control groups in both 5637 and HDF-1 cells **(G)**. Data are expressed as mean ± SD. The assay was repeated three times. Distinct letters show significant differences ($P < 0.001$) between different groups.

was obvious, treated HDF-1 cells represented a very small comet tail (Figure 5F). Statistical analysis revealed that the effect of 7-IP to induce DNA damage in HDF-1 cells (17%) is probably due to the presence of DMSO as a solvent since the DMSO control group induced the DNA damage by 21% (Figure 5G).

7-IP activates caspase-3

To confirm the apoptotic effects of 7-IP, the activity of caspase-3 enzyme was also analyzed. After 12 h of incubation, the caspase activity in 7-IP-treated 5637 cells was increased approximately 2.5 folds as compared with untreated culture (Figure 6), significantly ($P < 0.001$) higher than DMSO-treated group.

7-IP arrests 5637 cells at G2/M stage

To further study the anti-proliferative properties of 7-IP, its effects on cell cycle progression were evaluated by flow cytometry after PI staining. 5637 cells were treated with 65 μg/ml 7-IP and its equivalent amount of DMSO for 24 h. As shown in Figure 7, treatment with this

compound caused an increase in the percentage of cells in G2/M correlating with decreased number of cells in G1 as compared with DMSO and untreated cultures. Thus, exposure to 7-IP led to cell cycle arrest at G2/M stage (Figure 7C). Percentages of cells at different stages of cell cycle are presented in Table 1.

Discussion

Cancer is a consequence of unregulated cell growth with high morbidity and mortality worldwide. Despite major advances in cancer therapy, its treatment is far from being satisfactory and more research on new compounds and strategies to fight this disease is urgently needed.

As mentioned before, coumarins represent a large class of natural compounds with various biological activities, among which prenyloxycoumarins exert valuable anti-tumor properties both *in vitro* and *in vivo* [8,12,21].

In search for anti-cancer agents to treat bladder cancer, 7-IP was tested for its cytotoxicity on 5637 and HDF-1 cells (as control) *in vitro*. This compound belongs to prenyloxycoumarins with various biological properties, which

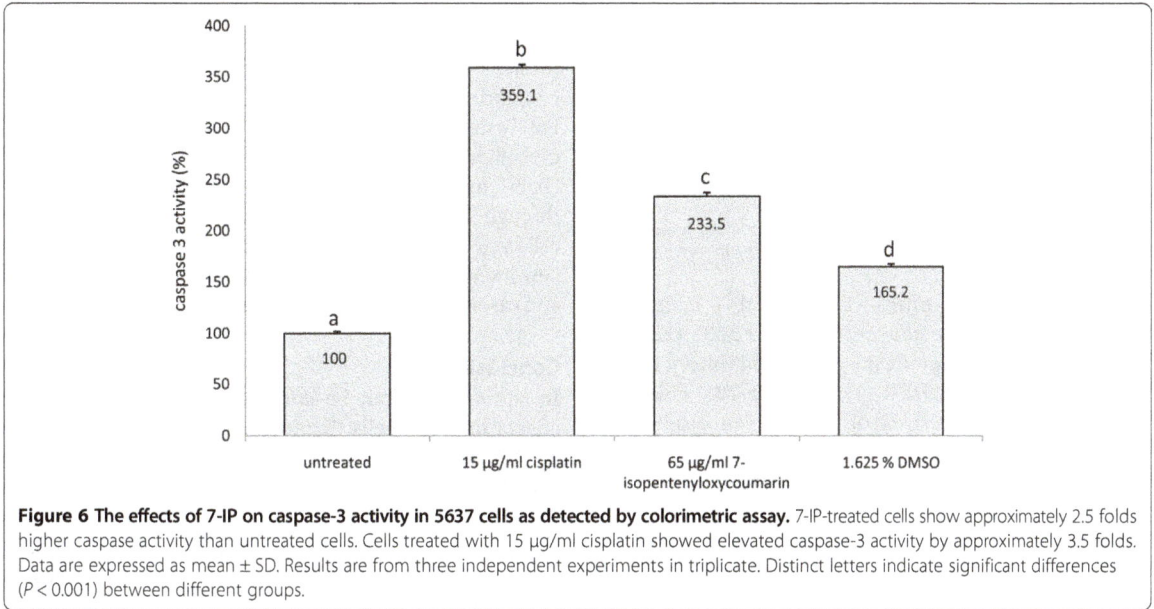

Figure 6 The effects of 7-IP on caspase-3 activity in 5637 cells as detected by colorimetric assay. 7-IP-treated cells show approximately 2.5 folds higher caspase activity than untreated cells. Cells treated with 15 μg/ml cisplatin showed elevated caspase-3 activity by approximately 3.5 folds. Data are expressed as mean ± SD. Results are from three independent experiments in triplicate. Distinct letters indicate significant differences (*P* < 0.001) between different groups.

can be synthesized both naturally and chemically [13]. Although this coumarin derivative exerts various biological properties, there is no report on its toxic effects and mechanism of action on bladder cancer cells in the literature. Our results revealed that the IC_{50} value of 7-IP in 5637 cells was 65 μg/ml (>100 μM) after 72 h of treatment, which is less than vinblastine but higher than vincristine and cisplatin [22]. Similar results were reported by Bruyere and coworkers who showed that 7-IP had IC_{50} values more than 100 μM in various human cancer cell lines [23]. Furthermore, Kawaii and colleagues determined low cytotoxicity of 7-IP on other cancers including lung, melanoma and leukemia [24]. On the other hand, Kofians and colleagues reported the ID_{50} values of 7-IP on KB and NSCLC-N6 cell lines, as 10.6 and 9.9 μg/ml, respectively

[25]. Considering different reports on toxic effects of 7-IP, it can be concluded that depending on the cell line, the cytotoxicity of this coumarin would be different. High IC_{50} value of 7-IP in 5637 cells can be explained by the multi-drug resistance (MDR) of these cells [26,27]. Several ATP-binding cassette (ABC) transporters have been discovered, including multidrug resistance-associated proteins (MRPs) and P-glycoproteins, which play critical roles in MDR [28]. For instance, it has been reported that TCC cells over express MDR1 and MRP2 proteins, two members of MRP family [29]. Therefore, it is possible that 7-IP is exported from 5637 cells by these efflux pumps, so high amounts of this compound are required to be accumulated inside the cell, in order to induce cytotoxicity. To investigate the anti-cancer

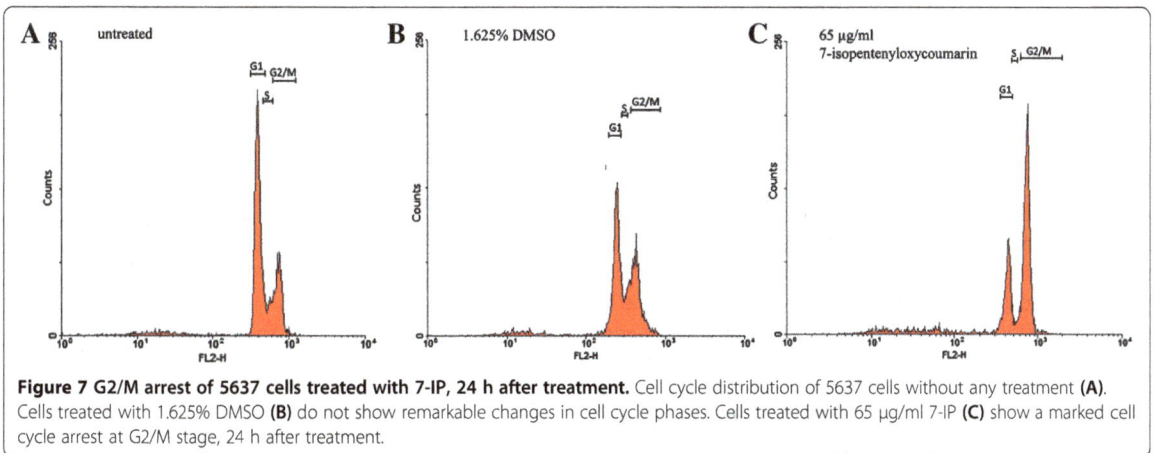

Figure 7 G2/M arrest of 5637 cells treated with 7-IP, 24 h after treatment. Cell cycle distribution of 5637 cells without any treatment (**A**). Cells treated with 1.625% DMSO (**B**) do not show remarkable changes in cell cycle phases. Cells treated with 65 μg/ml 7-IP (**C**) show a marked cell cycle arrest at G2/M stage, 24 h after treatment.

Table 1 Effects of 7-IP on 5637 cell cycle distribution

Treatment	Percentage of cells		
	G1 (Mean ± SD)	S (Mean ± SD)	G2/M (Mean ± SD)
untreated	55.7 ± 6.16[a]	13.3 ± 1.20[a]	32.5 ± 0.88[a]
1.625% DMSO	43 ± 0.87[b]	12 ± 0.41[a]	36 ± 1.53[a]
65 µg/ml 7-IP	22.4 ± 1.63[c]	5.2 ± 1.47[b]	53.5 ± 2.54[b]

Percentages of cells in each stage of cell cycle is represented as mean ± SD. Results are from three independent experiments. Distinct letters in each column indicate statistical significant differences (P < 0.001) between groups.

properties of 7-IP, non-cancerous HDF-1 cells were treated with the same concentrations as 5637 cells and results revealed no significant growth-inhibitory effects of this coumarin in HDF-1 cells (Figure 2B). This confirms the selective activity of 7-IP in cancerous 5637 cells.

Results of DAPI staining and comet assay also revealed that, in comparison with control cultures, 65 µg/ml 7-IP significantly (P < 0.001) increased both chromatin condensation and DNA damage in 5637 cells, which were in agreement with morphological observations and MTT results and indicate that cells are undergoing apoptotic cell death [30,31]. Moreover, to evaluate genotoxic effects of 7-IP in HDF-1 cells, comet assay was also performed in these cells. Comet results revealed that the DNA damaging effects of 7-IP were due to its solvent DMSO and there was no significant difference (P < 0.001) between these two groups. Thus, 7-IP does not have any significant toxic or genotoxic effects on normal HDF-1 cells.

To confirm the type of cell death, caspase-3 activity (the executioner upon which many apoptotic pathways converge) was evaluated using caspase-3 colorimetric assay kit. As shown in Figure 6, caspase activity in 7-IP-treated 5637 cells was elevated. The relative caspase-3 activity was increased about 2.5 folds in cells treated with this compound in comparison to untreated cells; which was also significantly increased compared to cells treated with equivalent amount of DMSO (P < 0.001).

Cell cycle analysis was performed by flow cytometry after PI staining to investigate the effects of 7-IP in more details. It was shown that this compound arrested 5637 cells in G2/M stage of the cell cycle (Figure 7C), which is similar to the effects of other anti-cancer drugs like taxol, doxorubicin and vincristine [32-34]. It is well established that progression of cell cycle is a tightly ordered and regulated process involving multiple checkpoints. Upregulation of cyclin B1/Cdc2 kinase activity, which regulates the entry and progression of the mitotic phase in eukaryotic cells, is known to be involved in the G2/M stage transition of the cell cycle. On the other hand, cells are arrested in M stage when microtubule network is disrupted [35]. Since 7-IP arrests 5637 cells in G2/M stage of the cell cycle, it is possible that this compound may act on cell cycle checkpoints or acts like a microtubule

inhibitor, preventing further cell division and subsequently initiates cell death by apoptosis. Our results are similar to other studies that determined the ability of different coumarins in caspase-3 activation and cell cycle arrest. For instance, Barthomeuf and colleagues showed that umbelliprenin (another prenyloxycoumarin with a farnesyl chain) markedly inhibited proliferation of M4Beu cells through induction of caspase-dependent apoptosis and cell-cycle arrest [9]. Another study by Chuang and his coworkers revealed that coumarin induced cell cycle arrest and caspase-3 dependent apoptosis in HeLa cells [10].

Conclusion

In summary, it can be concluded that 7-IP had toxic effects on 5637 cells. Exploring the anti-tumor activity of 7-IP showed that this coumarin has selective cytotoxic effects on 5637 cancerous cells in comparison to normal HDF-1 cells. Further studies in 5637 cells revealed that 7-IP induces chromatin condensation, DNA damage and apoptosis most probably via activation of caspase-3 and arrests the cell cycle at G2/M stage. Further studies are needed to determine its exact mechanism of action. For example, since antioxidants have different effects in cancer treatment [36], it is important to explore this property of 7-IP and its mechanism of action. Moreover, since *in vitro* conditions are very different from *in vivo* environments, in order to evaluate 7-IP effects on biological systems, an approved method on animal models is required [37].

Our study represents the first report describing 7-IP as an anti-tumor agent for bladder cancer cells *in vitro*. Although 7-IP was synthesized in this study, but considering the fact that it is widespread in edible vegetables and fruits, the present study could be regarded as a topic for future studies aiming to put in evidence dietary feeding chemopreventive effects on baldder cancer.

Additional files

Additional file 1: Table S1. 1H-NMR data for 7-isopentenyloxycoumarin (CDCl3, 500 MHz).

Additional file 2: Table S2. 13 C-NMR data for 7-isopentenyloxycoumarin (CDCl3, 125.7 MHz).

Abbreviations
DAPI: 4′, 6-diamidino-2-phenylindole dichloride; DMEM: Dulbecco's modified Eagle's medium; DMSO: Dimethyl sulfoxide; EDTA: Ethylenediaminetetraacetic acid; ELISA: Enzyme linked immunosorbent assay; FBS: Fetal bovine serum; HDF1: Human dermal fibroblast; IC$_{50}$: Half maximal inhibitory concentration; 7-IP: 7-isopentenyloxycoumarin; LMA: Low melting agarose; MTT: 3-(4,5-Dimethyl-2-thiazolyl)-2,5-diphenyl-2H-tetrazolium bromide; NMA: Normal melting agarose; NMR: Nuclear magnetic resonance; PBS: Phosphate buffered saline; PI: Propidium iodide; SD: Standard deviation; TCC: Transitional cell carcinoma.

Competing interests
The authors have no conflict of interests to declare.

Authors' contributions

MMM conceived the strategy of study and supervised the project. FH performed the experimental work and data interpretation. ARB gave consultation on designing the study, complemented the data. MI provided the compound and gave consultation. FBR and AH were involved in performing the experimental work and data interpretation. All authors read and approved the final manuscript.

Authors' information

Fereshteh Haghighi, M.Sc. in Cell and Molecular Biology; Maryam M. Matin, Ph.D. in Molecular Biotechnology and Associate Professor at Ferdowsi University of Mashhad; Ahmad Reza Bahrami, Ph.D. in Molecular Biotechnology, Head of Institute of Biotechnology and Professor at Ferdowsi University of Mashhad; Mehrdad Iranshahi, Ph.D. in Pharmacognosy and Associate Professor at Mashhad University of Medical Sciences, Fatemeh B. Rassouli, Ph.D. in Cell and Molecular Biology and Azadeh Haghighitalab, M.Sc. in Cell and Molecular Biology.

Acknowledgments

This work was supported by a grant from Ferdowsi University of Mashhad. The authors would like to thank Dr. Parsaee, Dr. Tayarani-Najjaran, Mrs. Saeinasab, Mr. Malaekeh-Nikouei and Mr. Nakhaei for their excellent support and technical help. We are also grateful to Dr. Sadeghi for his great support and statistical advice.

Author details

[1]Department of Biology, Faculty of Science, Ferdowsi University of Mashhad, Mashhad, Iran. [2]Cell and Molecular Biotechnology Research Group, Institute of Biotechnology, Ferdowsi University of Mashhad, Mashhad, Iran. [3]Biotechnology Research Center and School of Pharmacy, Mashhad University of Medical Sciences, Mashhad, Iran.

References

1. Coseri S: Natural products and their analogues as efficient anticancer drugs. Mini Rev Med Chem 2009, 9:560–571.
2. Bolenz C, Becker A, Trojan L, Schaaf A, Cao Y, Weiss C, Alken P, Michel MS: Optimizing chemotherapy for transitional cell carcinoma by application of bcl-2 and bcl-xL antisense oligodeoxynucleotides. Urol Oncol 2007, 25:476–482.
3. Nicholson BE, Frierson HF, Conaway MR, Seraj JM, Harding MA, Hampton GM, Theodorescu D: Profiling the evolution of human metastatic bladder cancer. Cancer Res 2004, 64:7813–7821.
4. Behnam Rassouli F, Matin MM, Iranshahi M, Bahrami AR, Neshati V, Mollazadeh S, Neshati Z: Mogoltacin enhances vincristine cytotoxicity in human transitional cell carcinoma (TCC) cell line. Phytomedicine 2009, 16:181–187.
5. Kannan K, Jain SK: Oxidative stress and apoptosis. Pathophysiology 2000, 7:153–163.
6. Kroemer G, Galluzzi L, Vandenabeele P, Abrams J, Alnemri ES, Baehrecke EH, Blagosklonny MV, El-Deiry WS, Golstein P, Green DR, Hengartner M, Knight RA, Kumar S, Lipton SA, Malorni W, Nunez G, Peter ME, Tschopp J, Yuan J, Piacentini M, Zhivotovsky B, Melino G: Classification of cell death: recommendations of the Nomenclature Committee on Cell Death 2009. Cell Death Differ 2009, 16:3–11.
7. Elmore S: Apoptosis: a review of programmed cell death. Toxicol Pathol 2007, 35:495–516.
8. Curini M, Cravotto G, Epifano F, Giannone G: Chemistry and biological activity of natural and synthetic prenyloxycoumarins. Curr Med Chem 2006, 13:199–222.
9. Barthomeuf C, Lim S, Iranshahi M, Chollet P: Umbelliprenin from Ferula szowitsiana inhibits the growth of human M4Beu metastatic pigmented malignant melanoma cells through cell-cycle arrest in G1 and induction of caspase-dependent apoptosis. Phytomedicine 2008, 15:103–111.
10. Chuang JY, Huang YF, Lu HF, Ho HC, Yang JS, Li TM, Chang NW, Chung JG: Coumarin induces cell cycle arrest and apoptosis in human cervical cancer HeLa cells through a mitochondria- and caspase-3 dependent

mechanism and NF-kappaB down-regulation. In Vivo 2007, 21:1003–1009.
11. Lopez-Gonzalez JS, Prado-Garcia H, Aguilar-Cazares D, Molina-Guarneros JA, Morales-Fuentes J, Mandoki JJ: Apoptosis and cell cycle disturbances induced by coumarin and 7-hydroxycoumarin on human lung carcinoma cell lines. Lung Cancer 2004, 43:275–283.
12. Riveiro ME, De Kimpe N, Moglioni A, Vazquez R, Monczor F, Shayo C, Davio C: Coumarins: old compounds with novel promising therapeutic perspectives. Curr Med Chem 2010, 17:1325–1338.
13. Askari M, Sahebkar A, Iranshahi M: Synthesis and purification of 7-prenyloxycoumarins and herniarin as bioactive natural coumarins. Iranian J Basic Med Sci 2009, 12:63–69.
14. Epifano F, Pelucchini C, Curini M, Genovese S: Insights on novel biologically active natural products: 7-isopentenyloxycoumarin. Nat Prod Commun 2009, 4:1755–1760.
15. Baba M, Jin Y, Mizuno A, Suzuki H, Okada Y, Takasuka N, Tokuda H, Nishino H, Okuyama T: Studies on cancer chemoprevention by traditional folk medicines XXIV. Inhibitory effect of a coumarin derivative, 7-isopentenyloxycoumarin, against tumor-promotion. Biol Pharm Bull 2002, 25:244–246.
16. Epifano F, Molinaro G, Genovese S, Ngomba RT, Nicoletti F, Curini M: Neuroprotective effect of prenyloxycoumarins from edible vegetables. Neurosci Lett 2008, 443:57–60.
17. Rezaee R, Hashemzaie M, Iranshahi M, Behravan E, Behravan J, Soltani F: Evaluation of antigenotoxic effect of 7-hydroxy coumarin and 7-isopentenyloxy coumarin on human peripheral lymphocytes exposed to oxidative stress. Toxicol Lett 2011, 205:108.
18. Epifano F, Curini M, Menghini L, Genovese S: Natural coumarins as a novel class of neuroprotective agents. Mini Rev Med Chem 2009, 9:1262–1271.
19. van Meerloo J, Kaspers GJ, Cloos J: Cell sensitivity assays: the MTT assay. Methods Mol Biol 2011, 731:237–245.
20. Collins AR: The comet assay for DNA damage and repair: principles, applications, and limitations. Mol Biotechnol 2004, 26:249–261.
21. Epifano F, Genovese S, Menghini L, Curini M: Chemistry and pharmacology of oxyprenylated secondary plant metabolites. Phytochemistry 2007, 68:939–953.
22. Rassouli FB, Matin MM, Iranshahi M, Bahrami AR: Investigating the cytotoxic and apoptosis inducing effects of monoterpenoid stylosin in vitro. Fitoterapia 2011, 82:742–749.
23. Bruyere C, Genovese S, Lallemand B, Ionescu-Motatu A, Curini M, Kiss R, Epifano F: Growth inhibitory activities of oxyprenylated and non-prenylated naturally occurring phenylpropanoids in cancer cell lines. Bioorg Med Chem Lett 2011, 21:4174–4179.
24. Kawaii S, Tomono Y, Ogawa K, Sugiura M, Yano M, Yoshizawa Y, Ito C, Furukawa H: Antiproliferative effect of isopentenylated coumarins on several cancer cell lines. Anticancer Res 2001, 21:1905–1911.
25. Kofinas C, Chinou I, Loukis A, Harvala C, Roussakis C, Maillard M, Hostettmann K: Cytotoxic coumarins from the aerial parts of Tordylium apulum and their effects on a non-small-cell bronchial carcinoma line. Planta Med 1998, 64:174–176.
26. Gottesman MM: How cancer cells evade chemotherapy: sixteenth Richard and Hinda Rosenthal Foundation Award Lecture. Cancer Res 1993, 53:747–754.
27. Shoemaker RH, Curt GA, Carney DN: Evidence for multidrug-resistant cells in human tumor cell populations. Cancer Treat Rep 1983, 67:883–888.
28. Choi CH: ABC transporters as multidrug resistance mechanisms and the development of chemosensitizers for their reversal. Cancer Cell Int 2005, 5:30–35.
29. Wu C, Zhang W, Chang J, Zhao Z, Sun G, Han R: MDR1/P-glycoprotein overexpression in bladder transitional cell carcinoma and its correlation with expression of survivin and Fas. Chin J Onco 2006, 3:191–195.
30. Hasegawa M, Yagi K, Iwakawa S, Hirai M: Chitosan induces apoptosis via caspase-3 activation in bladder tumor cells. Jpn J Cancer Res 2001, 92:459–466.
31. Nguyen SM, Lieven CJ, Levin LA: Simultaneous labeling of projecting neurons and apoptotic state. J Neurosci Methods 2007, 161:281–284.
32. Das GC, Holiday D, Gallardo R, Haas C: Taxol-induced cell cycle arrest and apoptosis: dose–response relationship in lung cancer cells of different wild-type p53 status and under isogenic condition. Cancer Lett 2001, 165:147–153.

33. Ling YH, el-Naggar AK, Priebe W, Perez-Soler R: **Cell cycle-dependent cytotoxicity, G2/M phase arrest, and distruption of p34cdc2/cyclin B1 activity induced by doxorubicin in synchronized p388 cells.** *Mol Pharmacol* 2012, **81**:832–841.
34. Blajeski AL, Phan VA, Kottke TJ, Kaufmann SH: **G1 and G2 cell-cycle arrest following microtubule depolymerization in human breast cancer cells.** *J Clin Invest* 2002, **110**:91–99.
35. Dash BC, El-Deiry WS: **Phosphorylation of p21 in G/M promotes cyclin B -Cdc2 kinase activity.** *Mol Cell Biol* 2005, **25**:3364–3387.
36. Abdollahi M, Shetab-Boushehri SV: **Is it right to look for anti-cancer drugs amongst compounds having antioxidant effect?** *DARU* 2012, **20**:61.
37. Shetab-Boushehri SV, Abdollahi M: **Current concerns on the validity of *in vitro* models that use transformed neoplastic cells in pharmacology and toxicology.** *Int J Pharmacol* 2012, **8**:594–595.

Non-addictive opium alkaloids selectively induce apoptosis in cancer cells compared to normal cells

Monireh Afzali[1], Padideh Ghaeli[2], Mahnaz Khanavi[3], Maliheh Parsa[1], Hamed Montazeri[1], Mohammad Hossein Ghahremani[1] and Seyed Nasser Ostad[1*]

Abstract

Background: Cytotoxic effects of some of the members of papaveraceae family have been reported in Iranian folk medicine. Recent reports has indicated that alkaloids fraction of opium may be responsible for its cytotoxic effect; however, the mechanism of this effect is not fully understood. This study has been designed to investigate the selective cytotoxic, genotoxic and also apoptosis induction effects of noscapine, papaverine and narceine, three non-addictable opium alkaloids, on HT29, T47D and HT1080 cancer cell lines. Mouse NIH3T3 cell line was chosen to present non-cancerous cells and Doxorubicin was selected as the positive control.

Methods: Cells were treated by different concentrations of Noscapine, Papaverine, Narceine and doxorubicin; viability was assessed by MTT assay. The genotoxicity and apoptosis induction were tested with comet assay and Annexin-V affinity when the concentration of each these drugs is less than its IC50. In addition, the DNA damage and caspase activity of the T47D cells were examined and the results were compared.

Results: This study noted the cytotoxicity and genotoxicity of noscapine and papaverine, specifically on cancerous cell lines. Furthermore, papaverine induces apoptosis in all studied cancer cell lines and noscapine showed this effect in T47D and HT29 cells but not in NIH-3 T3 cells as noncancerous cell line. narceine also showed genototoxicity in the studied cell lines at its IC50 concentration.

Conclusions: This experiment suggests that noscapine and papaverine may be of use in cancer treatment due to their specific cytotoxicity and genotoxicity. However, further in vivo studies are needed to confirm its usefulness in cancer treatment.

Keywords: Cancer cell, Cytotoxicity, Genotoxicity, Narceine, Noscapine, Papverine

Background

The agents which have the potential for induction of apoptosis may be considered as good candidates for cancer therapy due to their effect on the uncontrolled proliferation of malignant cells. In spite of excellent anti-tumor activities of common chemotherapy drugs, treatment will be restricted in some cases due to drug-resistance, low therapeutic index, severe side effects and different routes of administration [1]. Recently, in search for new treatments for cancer, there has been an emphasis on herbal and natural compounds. Cytotoxic effects of some members of Papaveraceae family have been considered in Iranian and Indian medicine [2]. *Papaverine somniferum L.* (opium poppy) has been traditionally used in Chinese and Indian herbal medicine to cure some disorders including chronic cough, dysentery, diarrhea, rectum prolapse and gastrointestinal problems [3]. The contents of opium alkaloids include morphine, codeine, tebaine, noscapine, papaverine, narceine as well as little percentage of some other compounds [4]. Many studies revealed a remarkable anti-tumor activity of the alkaloid noscapine, a naturally-occurring benzylisoquinoline alkaloid that constitutes about 2-10% of the alkaloid content of opium [5,6]. Furthermore, the anti-tumor activities of noscapine and its tubulin-binding property have been mentioned in many studies [7-12]. Noscapine inhibits the progression of melanoma, lymphoma, leukemia, breast cancer, colon cancer, ovarian carcinoma, glioblastoma, non-small cell lung

* Correspondence: ostadnas@tums.ac.ir
[1]Department Toxicology & Pharmacology, Faculty of Pharmacy, Toxicology & Poisoning Research Center, Tehran University of Medical Sciences, 14155/6451 Tehran, Iran
Full list of author information is available at the end of the article

cancer and prostate cancer while it has a little or no significant toxicity to the kidney, heart, liver, bone marrow, spleen and small intestine [8,12-16]. Papverine and narceine are two other benzylisoquinoline alkaloids constituting 0.5-3% and <0.5% of the alkaloid contents of opium, respectively. Papaverine has been used clinically as smooth muscle relaxant, anti-spasmodic for gastro-intestinal disorders, cough suppressant and for treatment of erectile dysfunction (an unlabeled use). Although cytotoxic effect of papaverine and some of its derivatives has been observed in breast cancer, melanoma and prostate cancer [17-20], their mechanism of action has not been fully understood. Based on our knowledge, no previous study has examined the anti-cancer activities of narceine.

In this study three different human cancer cell lines have been chosen. HT29 colorectal carcinoma and T47D breast cancer cells as two of the most common types of human tumors and HT1080 fibrosarcoma cells as one of the most resistant cell lines to anti-cancer therapy. In addition, non-cancerous NIH-3 T3 cell line has been chosen to compare the effect of the agents between cancerous and non-cancerous cells and doxorubicin has been chosen as positive control. The purpose of this study is to show whether papaverine and narcein have selective cytotoxicity, genotoxicity and induction of apoptosis in cancerous cell lines as has been demonstrated in noscapine and was claimed in the traditional medicine.

Methods
Cell lines and chemicals
T47D (Breast, ductal-carcinoma, Human), HT-29 (Colon, epithelial-like carcinoma, Human), HT-1080 (connective tissue, fibro sarcoma, Human) and NIH-3 T3 (Swiss mouse embryo fibroblast) cell lines were all obtain from National Cell Bank (Pasture institute of Iran, Tehran). The cells were cultured in RPMI 1640 medium (Biosera, England) that was supplemented with 10% heat-inactivated fetal bovine serum (FBS; Biosera, England) as well as antibiotic vials containing 100 U/ml penicillin and 100 μg/ml streptomycin (Gibco, USA); then were incubated in a humidified atmosphere with 5% CO_2 at 37°C.

The materials used in the present study and the manufacturers provided them are as following: noscapine hydrochloride, agarose and low melting point agarose (LMP) from Sigma-Aldrich (USA), papaverine hydrochloride and ethanol from TEMAD Co. (Tehran, Iran), narceine trihydrate from Seqchem (UK), doxorubicin from Sobhan-daru (Tehran, Iran), MTT (3-[4,5-dimethylthiazol-2yl] -2,5-diphenyl tetrazolium bromide) powder and Caspase Assay fluorometric kit from Roche (Germany) and annexine V-PE apoptosis detection kit from Abcam (UK).

In vitro cytotoxicity assay
The cells in logarithmic phase of growth were seeded into 96-well plates at a density of 10^4 cells per well and allowed to incubate overnight at 37°C. Cells were treated with different concentrations of noscapine, papaverine, narceine and doxorubicin and were incubated for 48 hours and then cell viability was determined by MTT assay. Briefly, 25 μl of 5 mg/ml MTT solution in phosphate-buffered saline was added and incubated for four hours at 37°C. The medium was removed and 100 μl dimethylsulf-oxide (DMSO) was added to each well. The formazan salts were quantified by reading the absorbance at a test wave-length of 570 nm and a reference wavelength of 690 nm [21-23]. The IC50 values were calculated from their cyto-toxity dose–response curves.

Single cell gel electrophoresis (SCGE)/comet
The treated cells were diluted with RPMI 1640 + 10% FBS to final concentration of 175000 cells/ml. Cells were treated with 0.4% methanol in the CO_2 incubator for 3 hours. Each sample of 50 ul was harvested; then, immediately suspended in 450 μl of solution composed of 10 μl PBS and 75 μl 0.5% LMP agarose. The samples were then immediately coated on a uniform background of each rough microscope slide that had been previously prepared by 1% agarose. The agarose on the microscope slides was allowed to harden at 4°C for 10 minutes. After coating with supportive layer (LMP), slides were then placed in a chilled (4°C) lysis buffer (2.5 M sodium chloride, 100 mM EDTA, pH = 10, 10 mM Trise base, 1% sodium lauryl sarcosinate, 0.01% triton x-100) for 30 minutes to unwind the nuclear DNA at 4°C and drip dried. Slides were then immersed in the same buffer for 30 minutes at 24 V and 250 mA at room temperature. DNA damage was recognized by ethidium bromide and florescence microscope after neutralizing the gel with Tris buffer [24-26]. Pictures were captured electronically with an image analysis system and analyzed for fluorescence intensity. DNA damage was evaluated using the tail length and compared with the control group.

Examination of PS exposure
Surface exposure of phosphatidyl serine (PS) by apoptotic cells was examined according to manufacturer's protocol. Briefly, cells were seeded in 6-well plates (3 × 10^5 Cells/well) and treated with the agents for 24 hours. Cells were collected and resuspended in binding buffer (10 mM HEPES/NaOH, pH 7.4, 140 mM NaCl, 2.5 mM $CaCl_2$) then were incubated with Annexin V-FITC and PI for 15 minutes at room temperature and darkness. The fluorescent intensity of the cells was measured in FL1 (for FITC) and FL2 (for PI) using flow cytometry technique.

DNA fragmentation

Following drug treatments, 2×106 cells were collected and incubated in lysis buffer in ice for 20 minutes. The cells were centrifuged at 4°C at 12000 g for 30 minutes and then the supernatant was extracted after being centrifuged using 1:1 mixture of phenol: chloroform. Two equivalences of cold ethanol with one-tenth equivalence of sodium acetate were added; nucleic acid contaminant was decanted and exposed to water-RNase solution for 30 minutes at 37°C. The samples were electrophoresed through 1.5% agarose gel that contained ethidium bromide at 5 V for 5 minutes and then the voltage increased to 100 V for an hour [27].

Caspase activity assay

The caspase activity was investigated based on the Homogeneous Caspases Assay fluorimetric kit. According to the protocol, the cells were cultured in a "black microplate with clear bottom" and were treated. Caspase Substrate in lysis buffer was added and was then incubated at 37°C for 2 hours. The free substrate was determined fluorimetrically at 521 nm and the activity of caspases was quantified by a calibration curve.

Statistical analysis

The results were analyzed using one way ANOVA followed by Tukey-Kramer Posttest. The p-value less than 0.05 ($p < 0.05$) was considered significant.

Any experimental research that is reported in this manuscript have been approved by ethics committee of pharmaceutical sciences research center of Tehran University of Medical Sciences.

Results

Cytotoxicity of noscapine, papaverine, narceine and doxorubicin on breast cancer, colorectal carcinoma and connective tissue fibro sarcoma cell lines and non-cancerous cell line

The MTT curve showed that noscapine and papaverine had a dose-dependent cytotoxic effect on T47D, HT-29 and HT-1080 cell lines, with no cytotoxic effect on non-cancerous NIH-3 T3 cells. Narceine did not show any toxic effect on the studied cell lines and doxorubicin-induced cytotoxicity was demonstrated on both cancerous and noncancerous cells. The results are presented in Figure 1.

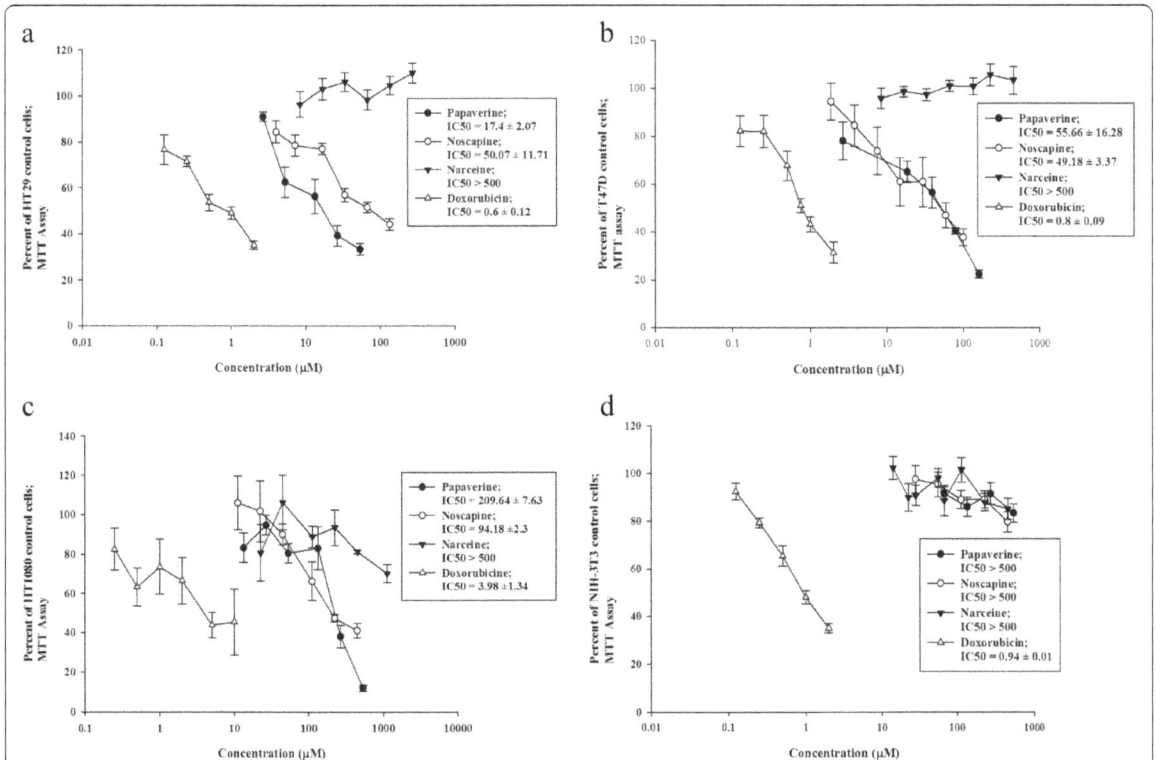

Figure 1 Cytotoxic effects of opium alkaloids and doxorubicin on cell lines. Cell viability in each treatment group was determined by MTT assay at 570 nm in reference standard at 690 nm. The IC50 values were calculated based on their cytotoxicity dose–response curve using Sigmaplot software and the results are expressed as Mean ± SD. **a**: HT29, **b**: T47D, **c**: HT1080 and **d**: NIH-3 T3.

Effect of noscapine, papaverine and narceine on DNA damage

The cells were evaluated with an image analysis system (CASP Comet assay Software Project) and the results are expressed in terms of L tail (length of tail) and are presented in Figure 2. Noscapine and papaverine selectively enhanced DNA damage on cancerous cells when compared with noncancerous cells ($p < 0.001$). On the other hand, DNA damage was observed on all the cell lines after administration of doxorubicin ($p < 0.001$). However, narceine induced DNA damage only on HT-1080 cells.

Effect of noscapine, papaverine, narceine on induction of apoptosis

Cell membrane asymmetry was investigated by translocation of phosphatidylserine to the cell surface in order to determine whether or not apoptosis was the major mechanism of cell death [28,29]. Based on this method, the apoptosis percentage has been reported and was compared with that in the control group (Figure 3). Results showed that doxorubicin has induced apoptosis in all the cell lines. However, noscapine and papaverine have induced apoptosis on HT-29 and T47D without any significant effect on NIH-3 T3 cell lines. However, the effects of narceine were different from the other two alkaloids. Narceine showed no apoptotic effect on the cell lines.

DNA fragmentation in T47D cells treated by noscapine, papaverine, narceine and compared to doxorubicin

To further determine if apoptosis was the major mechanism of the drug-induced cell death, DNA fragmentation was investigated in T47D cells. Figure 4 shows clear

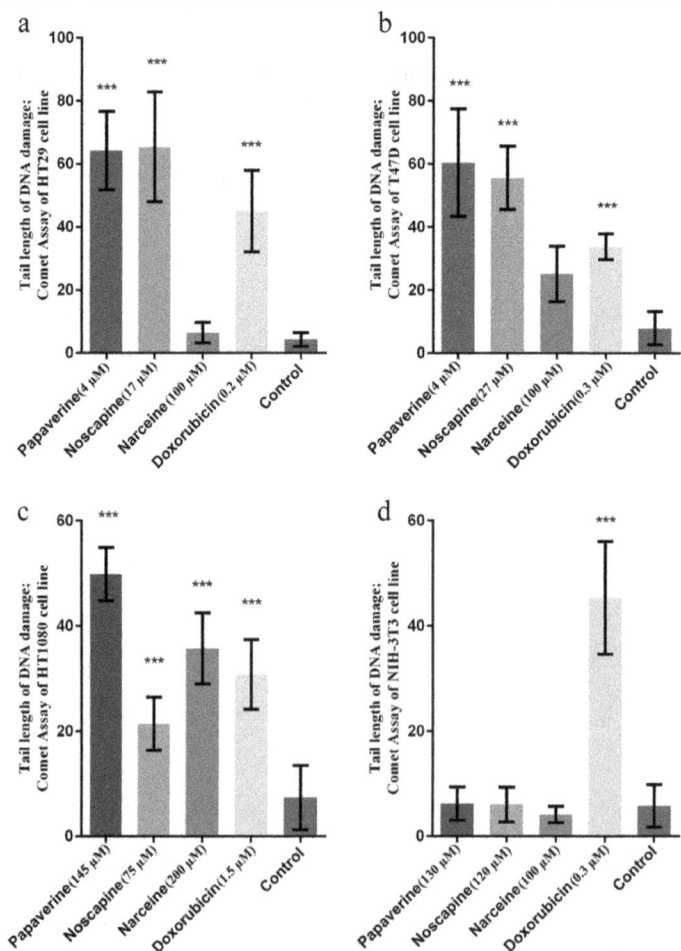

Figure 2 The DNA damage detected in treated cells compared to control group. The concentrations less than IC50 were used for treatment. The tail length of comet assay has been shown (Mean ± SD) and p-value has been reported. **a**: HT29, **b**: T47D, **c**: HT1080 and **d**: NIH-3 T3.

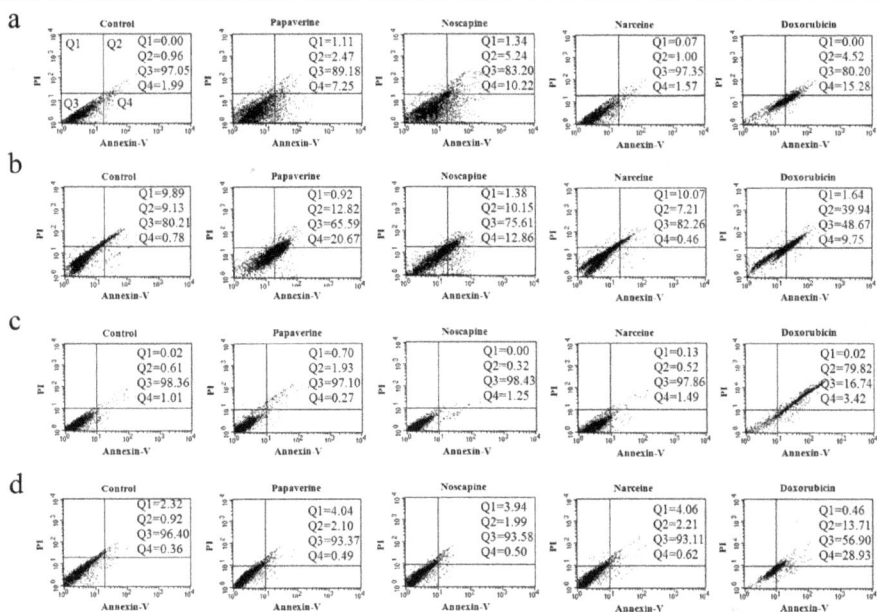

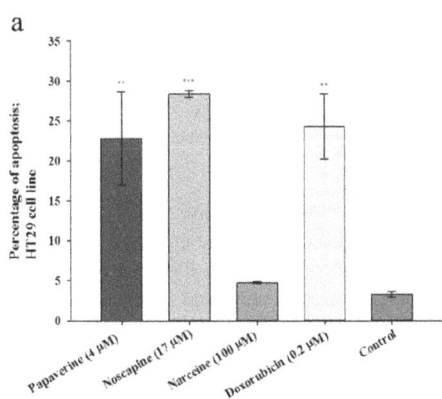

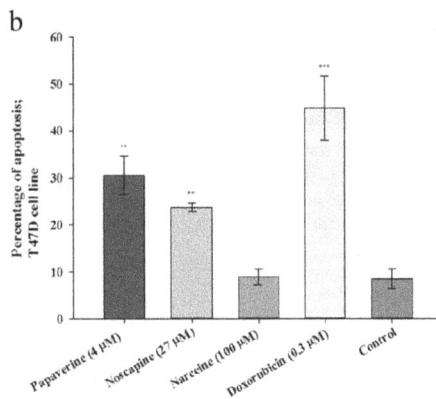

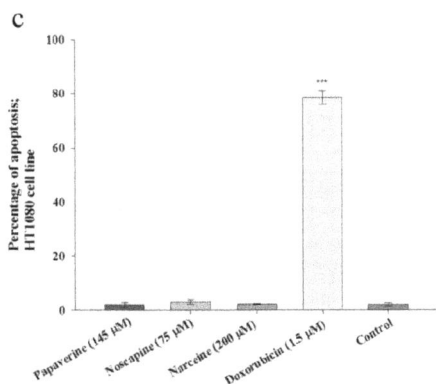

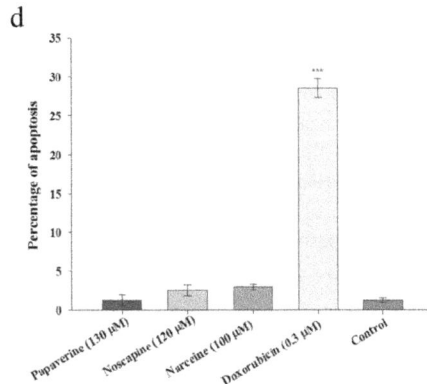

Figure 3 The membrane asymmetry comparison between treated cells compared to control group. The concentrations less than IC50 were used for treatment. The percentage of cell population of each quadrant has been shown and the quantitative average of percentage of apoptotic cells of repeated examinations (Mean ± SD) and p-value has been reported. **a**: HT29, **b**: T47D, **c**: HT1080 and **d**: NIH-3 T3.

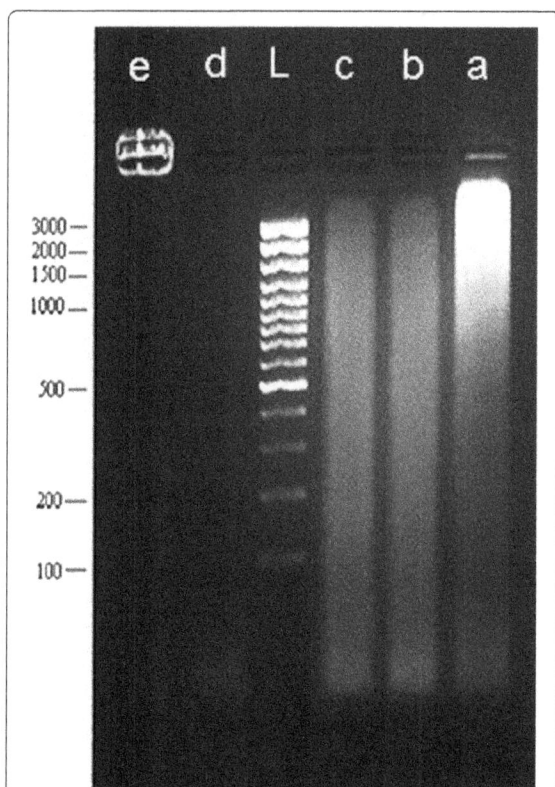

Figure 4 Internucleosomal fragmentation of T47D cells. The cells were treated with a: doxorubicin, b: noscapine, c: papaverine and d: narceine then DNA laddering was measured after 48 hours. e: negative control and L: Laddering marker are presented in figure as well.

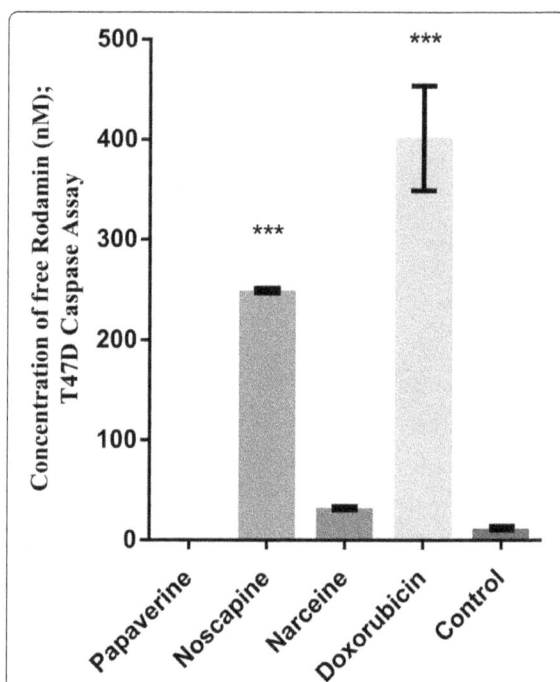

Figure 5 The activity of caspase-3 after 48 hours incubation of post-treatment T47D cells. Data are reported as mean ± SD. It is shown significant increase in caspase 3 activities after treatment by doxorubicin and noscapine ($p < 0.001$).

DNA fragmentation in cells treated by doxorubicin as positive control. Noscapine and papaverine induced DNA fragmentation in smaller sizes which were distinguishable from negative control group.

Caspase activity in T47D cells treated by noscapine, papaverine, narceine and compared to doxorubicin

Caspase-3 activity was measured by the cleavage of the substrate -Rodamin110- fluorimerically and was quantified by calibration curve (Figure 5). According to Figure 5 and in opposite to doxorubicin and noscapine, papaverine did not increase caspase activity.

Discussion

The present study noted that noscapine and papaverine had dose-dependent cytotoxic effects on cancer cell lines, without any cytotoxic effect on noncancerous NIH-3 T3 cells. Minor, non-significant increases are visible in cytotoxicity curves that maybe related to the non-specific toxicity caused by high concentrations of all

three alkaloids used in this study. Therefore the selective toxicity observed in the present project as well as the unselective doxorubicin-induced toxicity could have affected both cancerous and noncancerous cells. To determine whether or not apoptosis was considered as the major cell death pathway, the cell lines were examined by using annexin -V affinity, Comet assay, DNA laddering and Caspase assay. The annexin V assay has been widely accepted as a marker of apoptosis. Annexin V, a calcium-dependent phospholipid-binding protein, binds to PS residues on the cell membrane that are translocated to the outside of the cell due to apoptosis [28,29]. DNA damage is a hallmark of cell death [30] and alkaline single cell gel electrophoresis (SCGE) or comet assay is a very sensitive assay for detection of some kinds of DNA damage including single strand DNA breakage, alkaline-labile sites and other damage that generates DNA breaks [25,30]. Based on the results of this study, noscapine and papaverine induced DNA damage followed by apoptosis on HT-29 and T47D cell lines without significant effect on NIH-3 T3 as a noncancerous cell line. Apoptotic effect of noscapine was confirmed by the results of DNA fragmentation and caspase assay. It should be mentioned that even though many other studies have previously noted apoptosis induced by noscapine on cancer cells, a limited number of research has focused on noncancerous cell lines [12,31]. Recently, noscapine has been recognized as a kinetic stabilizer compound. Interestingly, noscapine binds to different site of tubulin when compared to other known tubulin-binding agents. Additionally, even though noscapine's binding to tubulin site is not very strong, it is adequate enough to arrest the cell cycle [31]. Therefore, this feature might explain the selective cytotoxicity of noscapine. Based on the results of the present study and in contrast to noscapine and what was expected, papaverine did not increase caspase activity. Several studies have shown the apoptotic effect of papaverine [17,19,20,32]. However, a study on human promyelocytic leukemia HL60 cells declined cytotoxic and apoptotic effects of this alkaloid [33]. According to the results of DNA damage and apoptotic annexin-V assays, papaverine produced genotoxicity through induction of apoptosis in cancer cells. This lack of caspase activity has been also reported previously by Rubis et al. [20]. The results of the later study as well as our study may indicate that caspase-independent apoptosis pathways are involved in the programmed cell death related to papaverine. Further studies seem to be necessary to better clarify the exact mechanisms of papaverine-dependent apoptosis. Furthermore, in spite of DNA damage in HT-1080 after alkaloids treatment (Figure 2), apoptosis was not confirmed as a cell death pathway in this cell line. This contradiction might be related to intracellular repair system. However, the effects of narceine were different from those seen with the other two alkaloids on the cells in our study. Among the cells tested in this study, only HT-1080 cells were affected by DNA damage induced by narceine. However this damage did not result in apoptosis. It should be mentioned that all the findings about narceine were obtained despite the fact that no cytotoxicity was present when MTT assay was performed. Part of these findings may be related to other pathways of cell toxicity or death. However, more studies are needed to determine anti-tumor activity of narceine.

Conclusion

In the present study, we demonstrated that noscapine and papaverine inserted selective cytotoxicity effects on cancer cell lines in comparison to doxorubicin which showed unselective cytotoxic effects on both malignant and non-malignant cell lines. This effect may present a new approach for using non-addictive opium alkaloids in the treatment of cancer. Further investigations are needed to clarify and confirm the selective cytotoxic effects of these alkaloids on other noncancerous cell lines.

Competing interests
The authors declare that they have no competing interests.

Authors' contributions
MA carried out the practical activities, participated in the design of the study and drafted the manuscript. PG helped to draft and edited the manuscript. MK participated in the sequence alignment. MP participated in practical activities, data analysis and helped to draft the manuscript. HM participated in practical activities and data analysis. MHG participated in design of the study, data analysis and helped to draft the manuscript. SNO participated in study design, coordination and data analysis and helped to draft the manuscript. All authors read and approved the final manuscript.

Acknowledgment
This project was supported by of deputy of research at Tehran University of medical sciences (TUMS) (grant number 8960) and was a part of Dr. Afzali's thesis toward graduation to receive Pharm.D degree.

Author details
[1]Department Toxicology & Pharmacology, Faculty of Pharmacy, Toxicology & Poisoning Research Center, Tehran University of Medical Sciences, 14155/6451 Tehran, Iran. [2]Department Clinical Pharmacy, Faculty of Pharmacy & Rational Drug Use Research Center, Tehran University of Medical Sciences, 14155/6451 Tehran, Iran. [3]Department Pharmacognosy, Faculty of Pharmacy, Tehran University of Medical Sciences, 14155/6451 Tehran, Iran.

References

1. Goodman LS, Gilman A, Brunton LL, Parker KL, Blumenthal DK, Buxton ILO. Goodman & Gilman's manual of pharmacology and therapeutics. New Delhi: McGraw-Hill; 2008.
2. Aruna K, Sivaramakrishnan V. Anticarcinogenic effects of some Indian plant products. Food Chem Toxicol. 1992;30:953–6.
3. Healthcare T. PDR for Herbal Medicines. 4, illustrated edn. Montvale: Thomson Healthcare; 2007.
4. Evans WC. Trease and Evans. WB Saunders Harcourt Publishers Ltd. 2002;292:357–75.
5. Aneja R, Miyagi T, Karna P, Ezell T, Shukla D, Vij Gupta M, et al. A novel microtubule-modulating agent induces mitochondrially driven caspase-dependent apoptosis via mitotic checkpoint activation in human prostate cancer cells. Eur J Cancer. 2010;46:1668–78.
6. Ye K, Ke Y, Keshava N, Shanks J, Kapp JA, Tekmal RR, et al. Opium alkaloid noscapine is an antitumor agent that arrests metaphase and induces apoptosis in dividing cells. P Natl Acad Sci. 1998;95:1601.
7. Zhou J, Gupta K, Aggarwal S, Aneja R, Chandra R, Panda D, et al. Brominated derivatives of noscapine are potent microtubule-interfering agents that perturb mitosis and inhibit cell proliferation. Mol Pharmacol. 2003;63:799–807.
8. Aneja R, Lopus M, Zhou J, Vangapandu SN, Ghaleb A, Yao J, et al. Rational design of the microtubule-targeting anti-breast cancer drug EM015. Cancer Res. 2006;66:3782–91.
9. Aneja R, Vangapandu SN, Lopus M, Chandra R, Panda D, Joshi HC. Development of a novel nitro-derivative of noscapine for the potential treatment of drug-resistant ovarian cancer and T-cell lymphoma. Mol Pharmacol. 2006;69:1801–9.
10. Heidari N, Goliaei B, Moghaddam PR, Rahbar-Roshandel N, Mahmoudian M. Apoptotic pathway induced by noscapine in human myelogenous leukemic cells. Anticancer Drugs. 2007;18:1139–48.
11. Jaiswal AS, Aneja R, Connors SK, Joshi HC, Multani AS, Pathak S, et al. 9-bromonoscapine-induced mitotic arrest of cigarette smoke condensate transformed breast epithelial cells. J Cell Biochem. 2009;106:1146–56.
12. Mahmoudian M, Rahimi-Moghaddam P. The anti-cancer activity of noscapine: a review. Recent Pat Anticancer Drug Discov. 2009;4:92–7.
13. Aneja R, Ghaleb AM, Zhou J, Yang VW, Joshi HC. p53 and p21 determine the sensitivity of noscapine-induced apoptosis in colon cancer cells. Cancer Res. 2007;67:3862–70.
14. Jackson T, Chougule MB, Ichite N, Patlolla RR, Singh M. Antitumor activity of noscapine in human non-small cell lung cancer xenograft model. Cancer Chemother Pharmacol. 2008;63:117–26.
15. Chougule M, Patel AR, Sachdeva P, Jackson T, Singh M. Anticancer activity of Noscapine, an opioid alkaloid in combination with Cisplatin in human non-small cell lung cancer. Lung Cancer. 2011;71:271–82.

16. Chougule MB, Patel AR, Jackson T, Singh M. Antitumor activity of noscapine in combination with doxorubicin in triple negative breast cancer. PloS one. 2011;6:e17733.

17. Helson L, Lai K, Young CW. Papaverine-induced changes in cultured human melanoma cells. Biochem Pharmacol. 1974;23:2917–20.

18. Goto T, Matsushima H, Kasuya Y, Hosaka Y, Kitamura T, Kawabe K, et al. The effect of papaverine on morphologic differentiation, proliferation and invasive potential of human prostatic cancer LNCaP cells. Int J Urol. 1999;6:314–9.

19. Nohl H, Rohr-Udilova N, Gille L, Bieberschulte W, Jurek D, Marian B, et al. Ubiquinol and the papaverine derivative caroverine prevent the expression of tumour-promoting factors in adenoma and carcinoma colon cancer cells induced by dietary fat. Biofactors. 2005;25:87–95.

20. Rubis B, Kaczmarek M, Szymanowska N, Galezowska E, Czyrski A, Juskowiak B, et al. The biological activity of G-quadruplex DNA binding papaverine-derived ligand in breast cancer cells. Invest New Drugs. 2009;27:289–96.

21. Morgan DML. Tetrazolium (MTT) assay for cellular viability and activity. Methods Mol Biol. 1997;79:179–83.

22. Plumb JA. Cell sensitivity assays: the MTT assay. Methods mol med. 2004;88:165–70.

23. Burton JD. The MTT assay to evaluate chemosensitivity. Methods Mol Med. 2005;110:69–78.

24. Lah B, Gorjanc G, Nekrep FV, Marinsek-Logar R. Comet assay assessment of wastewater genotoxicity using yeast cells. Bull Environ Contam Toxicol. 2004;72:607–16.

25. Kopjar N, Milas I, Garaj-Vrhovac V, Gamulin M. Alkaline comet assay study with breast cancer patients: evaluation of baseline and chemotherapy-induced DNA damage in non-target cells. Clin Exp Med. 2006;6:177–90.

26. Dhawan A, Bajpayee M, Parmar D. Comet assay: a reliable tool for the assessment of DNA damage in different models. Cell Biol Toxicol. 2009;25:5–32.

27. DNA Fragmantation Assays for Apoptosis Protocol. [hedricklab.ucsd.edu/Protocol/DNAFRAG.html]

28. Miller E. Apoptosis Measurement by Annexin V Staining. In: Langdon SP, editor. Cancer cell culture: methods and protocols, vol. Volume 88. Totowa: Springer; 2004. p. 191–202.

29. Jones S, Howl J. Applications of cell-penetrating peptides as signal transduction modulators for the selective induction of apoptosis. In: Langel U, editor. Methods in molecular biology, vol. Volume 683. Clifton: springer; 2011. p. 291–303.

30. Roos WP, Kaina B. DNA damage-induced cell death by apoptosis. Trends Mol Med. 2006;12:440–50.

31. Dhiman N, Sood A, Sharma A. Noscapine: An Anti-Mitotic Agent. 2013.

32. Gao YJ, Stead S, Lee RMKW. Papaverine induces apoptosis in vascular endothelial and smooth muscle cells. Life Sciences. 2002;70:2675–85.

33. Rosenkranz V, Wink M. Induction of apoptosis by alkaloids, non-protein amino acids and cardiac glycosides in human promyelotic HL-60 cells. Zeitschrift fur Naturforschung C-Journal of Biosciences. 2007;62:458.

A new formulation of cannabidiol in cream shows therapeutic effects in a mouse model of experimental autoimmune encephalomyelitis

Sabrina Giacoppo[1†], Maria Galuppo[1†], Federica Pollastro[2], Gianpaolo Grassi[3], Placido Bramanti[1] and Emanuela Mazzon[1*]

Abstract

Background: The present study was designed to investigate the efficacy of a new formulation of alone, purified cannabidiol (CBD) (>98 %), the main non-psychotropic cannabinoid of Cannabis sativa, as a topical treatment in an experimental model of autoimmune encephalomyelitis (EAE), the most commonly used model for multiple sclerosis (MS). Particularly, we evaluated whether administration of a topical 1 % CBD-cream, given at the time of symptomatic disease onset, could affect the EAE progression and if this treatment could also recover paralysis of hind limbs, qualifying topical-CBD for the symptomatic treatment of MS.

Methods: In order to have a preparation of 1 % of CBD-cream, pure CBD have been solubilized in propylene glycoland basic dense cream O/A. EAE was induced by immunization with myelin oligodendroglial glycoprotein peptide (MOG35–55) in C57BL/6 mice. After EAE onset, mice were allocated into several experimental groups (Naïve, EAE, EAE-1 % CBD-cream, EAE-vehicle cream, CTRL-1 % CBD-cream, CTRL-vehicle cream). Mice were observed daily for signs of EAE and weight loss. At the sacrifice of the animals, which occurred at the 28th day from EAE-induction, spinal cord and spleen tissues were collected in order to perform histological evaluation, immunohistochemistry and western blotting analysis.

Results: Achieved results surprisingly show that daily treatment with topical 1 % CBD-cream may exert neuroprotective effects against EAE, diminishing clinical disease score (mean of 5.0 in EAE mice vs 1.5 in EAE + CBD-cream), by recovering of paralysis of hind limbs and by ameliorating histological score typical of disease (lymphocytic infiltration and demyelination) in spinal cord tissues. Also, 1 % CBD-cream is able to counteract the EAE-induced damage reducing release of CD4 and CD8α T cells (spleen tissue localization was quantified about 10,69 % and 35,96 % of positive staining respectively in EAE mice) and expression of the main pro-inflammatory cytokines as well as several other direct or indirect markers of inflammation (p-selectin, IL-10, GFAP, Foxp3, TGF-β, IFN-γ), oxidative injury (Nitrotyrosine, iNOS, PARP) and apoptosis (Cleaved caspase 3).

Conclusion: All these data suggest an interesting new profile of CBD that could lead to its introduction in the clinical management of MS and its associated symptoms at least in association with current conventional therapy.

Keywords: Cannabis sativa L, Multiple sclerosis, CBD-cream, Inflammation, Oxidative stress

* Correspondence: emazzon.irccs@gmail.com
†Equal contributors
[1]IRCCS Centro Neurolesi "Bonino-Pulejo", Via Provinciale Palermo, contrada Casazza, 98124 Messina, Italy
Full list of author information is available at the end of the article

Background

Cannabidiol (CBD) is the major non psychotropic constituent naturally present in *Cannabis sativa* L. plant isolated across the 1930s and 1940s, but chemically identified only in the 1960s by Mechoulam et al. [1]. As well documented from *Cannabis sativa* L. it is also possible to extract over 100 different cannabinoids compounds considered as its most important bioactive constituents and mainly known for their psychoactive effects [2]. Among these the main studied is the Δ^9-tetrahydrocannabinol (Δ^9-THC). This class of compounds have their effect mainly by interacting with specific receptors: the cannabinoid receptor type 1 (CB1), found on neurons and glial cells in various parts of the brain, and the cannabinoid receptor type 2 (CB2), found mainly in the body's immune system [3, 4]. On the contrary, CBD has a very low affinity for these receptors (100 fold less than Δ^9-THC) and when it binds it produces little to no effect [5].

CBD is able to exert multiple pharmacological actions via no-CB1 and no-CB2 receptors involving intracellular pathways that play a key role in neuronal physiology [6, 7]. In particular, many actions of CBD seem to be mediated by binding transient receptor potential vanilloid type 1 (TRPV1) [8], G protein-coupled receptor 55 (GPR55) [6, 9] and 5-hydroxytryptamine receptor subtype 1A (5-HT1A) [10]. These additional and novel cannabinoid receptors (no-CB1 and no-CB2) have been identified in CB1 and CB2- knockout mice and are expressed in both central and peripheral nervous system [11, 12].

Moreover, CBD has proved to have several anti-inflammatory activities and regulates cell cycle and immune cells functions [13]. CBD is able to suppress the production of a wide range of pro-inflammatory cytokines, such as tumor necrosis factor (TNF)-α and interleukin-1 beta (IL-1β), chemokines, growth factors, as well as inhibition of immune cell proliferation, activation, maturation, migration and antigen presentation [14, 15]. CBD shows also a potent action in inhibiting oxidative and nitrosative stress, modulating the expression of inducible nitric oxide synthase (iNOS) and nitrotyrosine as well as reducing production of reactive oxygen species (ROS) [16].

Just about all these properties showed by CBD, have prompted researchers to test its effects in a number of conditions involving both inflammation and oxidative stress, like neurodegenerative diseases, demonstrating in cell cultures as well as in animal models evident neuroprotective effects [16, 17].

Among this kind of disorders, multiple sclerosis (MS) is one of those obviously induced and driven by an unusual response of the immune system cells (T and B-lymphocytes) against myelin sheats of neurons [18]. During MS myelin autoreactive peripheral T cells

migrate into the CNS and initiate cytotoxic, degenerative processes that include demyelination, oligodendrocyte cell death and axonal degeneration [15]. These effects lead to main clinical symptoms and neurological deficits [19].

According to the National MS Society, spasticity it is a common symptom in people suffering from MS. When MS damages the nerves that control muscles, it can result in spasticity that impairs movement and causes pain and stiffness. It usually occurs in the legs and can draw them up toward the body with painful cramping or cause spasms in the lower back, until losing the sensitivity of the limbs.

To date, current treatments for MS only offer palliative relief without providing a cure, and many are also associated with adverse effects that limit their long-term utility [20].

To overcome these limits, the interest of researchers was focused on finding alternative cure that could be less invasive and that may use for the treatment of MS and its correlated symptoms.

Numerous studies have been performed to evaluate the role of cannabinoids on treatment of EAE-associated spasticity as well as on modulation of the neurodegenerative process [21–25]. In this context, CBD has been proven to decrease peripheral inflammation and neuroinflammation in EAE mice when systemically given at the time of symptomatic disease [25]. In addition CBD is able to affect disease progression and ameliorated clinical symptoms. Moreover, CBD-Glatiramer Acetate (GA) combination administered in nasal delivery system (NDS) resulted in a statistically significant decrease of clinical scores and inflammatory cytokine expression in EAE mice [26].

Moreover, according to the two most relevant double-blind, randomized, placebo-controlled trials, benefits from use of cannabinoids seen in animal studies have also been shown in the treatment of MS patients suffering spasticity, with a significant associated disability and quality of life impairment [27, 28].

To date, the only commercially available preparation containing cannabinoids is Sativex® (GW Pharma, Ltd, Salisbury, Wiltshire, UK), an oral spray containing a mixture of two extracts in approximately a 1:1 ratio standardized to contain 2.7 mg of Δ^9-THC and 2.5 mg of CBD/ 0.1 mL in an aromatized water-ethanol solution. Sativex® is used to alleviate spasticity in adult MS patients who do not show appropriate response to other drugs during an initial trial period of therapy [29].

Compared to other routes of administration, its advantage is a faster plateau of plasma concentration. Also, it has been established that coadministration of CBD and Δ^9-THC can reduce unwanted effects of Δ^9-THC [30].

The aim of this work was to study for the first time the effects of a topical administration of alone, purified CBD, as a new treatment strategy for MS. In specific, we evaluated whether treatment with a topical 1 % CBD-cream given at the time of symptomatic disease onset, could ameliorate the progression of the disease, counteracting the overall cascade of events occurring after EAE induction in mice. In addition, we investigated whether 1 % CBD-cream treatment could enhance responsiveness to a mechanical stimulus and recover paralysis of the hind limbs, qualifying topical-CBD for the symptomatic treatment of MS.

By examining this profile of CBD, we strongly hope to provide new evidences about the efficacy of the new topical treatment and to contribute into delineating a clearer profile of the compound so that its use could be an alternative to oral and parenteral administration of drugs for treatment of autoimmune and neurodegenerative diseases, like MS.

Methods

Plant material

Cannabis sativa L, derived from greenhouse cultivation at CRA-CIN, Rovigo (Italy), where a voucher specimen is kept, was collected in November 2013. The isolation and manipulation of cannabinoids was done in accordance with their legal status (Authorization SP/106 23/05/2013 of the Ministry of Health, Rome, Italy).

Extraction and Isolation of CBD

Pure CBD (>98 %) was isolated from an Italian variety of industrial hemp (Carmagnola) according to the method of the cannabinoid purification reported in Taglialatela-Scafati O. et al. [31] with some modifications in order to avoid any trace of Δ^9-THC that could interfere in the trial or causes legal limitation.

Dried flowerheads of *Cannabis sativa* (500 g) were heated at 120 °C in a ventilated oven for 2.5 h to decarboxylate pre-cannabinoids. After cooling to room temperature, the plant material was extracted with acetone (210 L). Removal of the solvent left a gummy residue that was partitioned between 1:1 aqueous methanol (1 L) and petroleum ether (1 L). The defatted polar phase was concentrated and extracted with CH_2Cl_2. The organic phase was dried (Na_2SO_4) and evaporated to afford a black gum (10 g), which was purified by flash chromatography on RP-18 silica gel (Biotage equipment, 250 mL column, linear gradient, from methanol water 55:45 to 90:10). Overall, five fractions were collected. The more polar one was further fractionated by gravity column chromatography on silica gel, with use of acidified (0.5 % HOAc) petroleum ether/EtOAc mixtures. After four chromatographic steps, crude CBD (10 mg) was obtained from a fraction directly eluted. The crude fraction was further purified by HPLC (eluentn-hexane/EtOAc 7:3) to provide pure CBD (6, 7.0 mg, 14 ppm based on dried plant material).

Finally the purity of CBD of 98 % was estimated by HPLC analysis according to the method of American Herbal Pharmacopoeia as reported in Swift et al. [32].

Cream preparation

Pure CBD have been solubilized in propylene glycoland basic dense cream O/A to have a concentration of 1 % of CBD. Each application for both hind limbs regards a surface of about 1 cm².

Animals

Male C57BL/6 mice (Harlan Milan, Italy) 12 weeks of age and weighing 20–25 g were housed in individually ventilated cages with food and water *ad libitum*. The room was maintained at a constant temperature and humidity on a 12 h/12 h light/dark cycle.

Ethics statement

This study was carried out in strict accordance with the recommendations in the guide for the care and use of laboratory animals of the National Institutes of Health. The protocol was approved by the Ministry of Health "General Direction of animal health and veterinary drug" (Authorization 150/2014-B 28/03/2014). In particular, animal care was in compliance with Italian regulations on protection of animals used for experimental and other scientific purposes (D.M. 116/92) as well as with the EEC regulations (O.J. of E.C.L 358/1 12/18/1986). Also, it was minimized number of animals used for this experiment and their suffering.

Induction of Experimental Autoimmune Encephalomyelitis (EAE)

After anesthesia, induced with an anesthetic cocktail composed of tiletamine plus xylazine (10 ml/kg, ip), EAE was actively induced using Myelin Oligodendrocyte Glycoprotein peptide $(MOG)_{35-55}$ (MEVGWYRSPFSRVVH-LYRNGK; % peak area by HPLC ≥ 95, AnaSpec, EGT Corporate Headquarters, Fremont, CA, USA), according to Paschalidis et al. [33]. Mice were immunized subcutaneously with 300 μl/flank of the emulsion consisting of 300 μg of $(MOG)_{35-55}$ in phosphate-buffered saline (PBS) mixed with an equal volume of Complete Freund's Adjuvant (CFA) containing 300 μg heat-killed *M. Tubercolosis* H37Ra (Difco Laboratories Sparks, MD,USA). Immediately after $(MOG)_{35-55}$ injection, the animals received an ip injection of 100 μl of *B. Pertussis* toxin (Sigma-Aldrich, Milan, Italy) (500 ng/100 μl, i.p), repeated 48 h later. The disease follows a course of progressive degeneration, with visible signs of pathology consisting of flaccidity of the tail and loss of motion of the hind legs.

Experimental design

Mice were randomly allocated into the following groups (N = 40 total animals):

1. Naive group (N = 5): mice did not receive $(MOG)_{35-55}$ or other treatment;
2. EAE group (N = 10): mice subjected to EAE that did not receive pharmacological treatment;
3. EAE + 1 % CBD-cream treatment group (N = 10): EAE mice were subjected to one topical treatment of lower limbs with the 1 % CBD-cream every 24 h. In specific, before the beginning of treatment all animals were subjected to shaving of both hind limbs in outer thigh (area of 1 cm^2) to facilitate the absorption of cream. Indeed, at each treatment cream was spread in this area until fully absorbed, also to prevent that animals could eat or lick cream. Only after the animals were placed in their cages. The treatment was started after the onset of disease signs and then daily protracted until the sacrifice;
4. EAE + vehicle cream (no plus CBD) group (N = 5): mice subjected to the same condition of the above group, but treated every 24 h with one topical application of the basic cream without CBD until the sacrifice;
5. CTRL group + 1 % CBD-cream (N = 5): mice subjected to shaving of both hind limbs in outer thigh (area of 1 cm^2) and every 24 h subjected to one topical application with the 1 % CBD-cream that was spread until fully absorbed;
6. CTRL group + vehicle cream (no plus CBD) (N = 5): mice subjected to the same condition of the above group, but every 24 h treated with one topical application of the basic cream without CBD.

Of note, the last two groups were provided to verify if any beneficial effect was ascribed to the method of administration of the cream, such as spreading or whether treatment with 1 % CBD-cream or vehicle cream) could cause some allergic reaction in mice at cutaneous either at systemic level.

At the end of the experiment, which occurred at the 28th day from EAE-induction, animals were euthanized with ip of Tanax (5 ml/kg body weight). Also, spinal cord tissues and spleen were sampled and processed in order to evaluate parameters of disease.

Schematically, a plan of the experiment is shown in Fig. 1a.

Clinical disease score and body weight evaluation

14 days after EAE induction, mice show the first signs of MS disease, characterized by loss of tail tonus, hind limb paralysis and body weight loss. Clinical score was evaluated according to a standardized scoring system [34] as follows: 0 = no signs; 1 = partial flaccid tail; 2 = complete flaccid tail; 3 = hind limb hypotonia; 4 = partial hind limb paralysis; 5 = complete hind limb paralysis; 6 = moribund or dead animal. Animals with a score ≥ 5 were sacrificed to avoid animal suffering.

The first measurement of clinical disease score and body weight were taken on the day of EAE- induction (day zero), and all the subsequent measurements were recorded every 48 h until sacrifice. Also, the daily variation of these two parameters of disease has been expressed compared to day of EAE induction (day zero). The value day has been expressed as mean ± SEM of all animals for each experimental group.

Needle test

The test was aimed to assess mice's responsiveness to a mechanical stimulus. It starts with the filament of 0.02 g, applying force to the left paw three times for a total period of 30 s (about 2 s to the stimulus) and to evaluate the response of the mouse after each application. The same treatment is repeated on the right paw. Response to two on three stimuli is regarded as a positive reaction. Specifically, a positive response is a paw withdrawal from the stimulus. The maximum score for both paws has a value of 6. In specific, 7 tests were performed every 48 h in two weeks from the first administration of 1 % CBD-cream. Animals were subjected to these measurements every 48 h in order to avoid additional stress that could affect the results. The values are expressed as mean ± SEM of each group.

Blood sampling

At the time of sacrifice, following anesthesia blood samples were collected via cardiac injection in EDTA K2/gel tubes (BD Vacutainer® BD Diagnostic, Milan Italy) and centrifuged following at least 30 min from the collection at 10,000 g speed for 5 min. The achieved plasma was collected, aliquoted and stored at −20 °C to be used for detection of CBD.

Pharmacokinetic analysis

Pharmacokinetc analysis of CBD plasma concentration was performed by liquid chromatography followed by mass spectrometry detection according to a reported method [38] with some modifications.

May Grunwald Giemsa staining

At 28 days following EAE-induction, spinal cords were fully sampled from cervical to lumbar area and were fixed in 10 % (w/v) PBS-buffered formaldehyde. Spinal cord samples were first paraffin-embedded and cut into 7 μm-thick sections and then were deparaffinized with xylene, rehydrated, stained with May Grunwald Giemsa

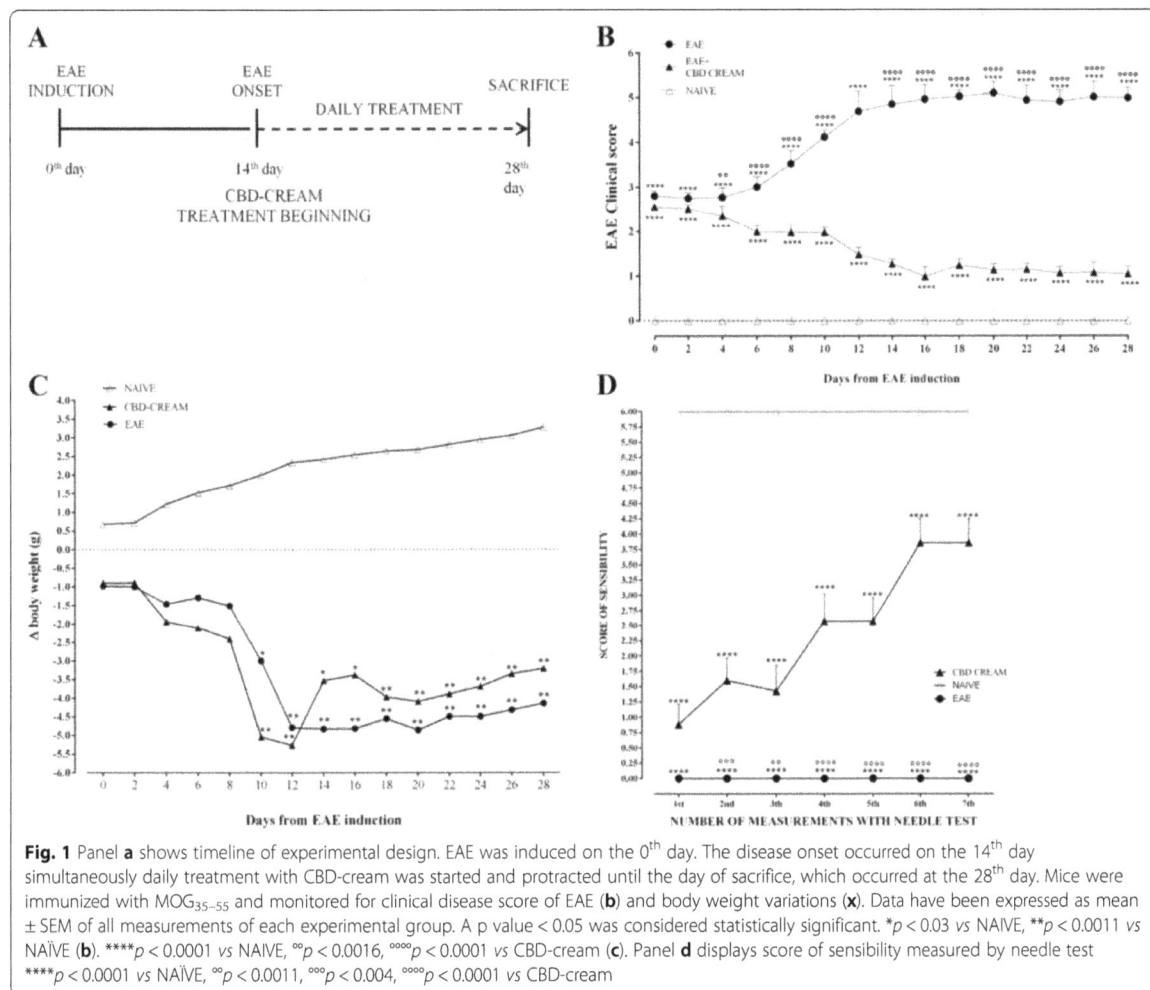

Fig. 1 Panel **a** shows timeline of experimental design. EAE was induced on the 0th day. The disease onset occurred on the 14th day simultaneously daily treatment with CBD-cream was started and protracted until the day of sacrifice, which occurred at the 28th day. Mice were immunized with MOG_{35-55} and monitored for clinical disease score of EAE (**b**) and body weight variations (**x**). Data have been expressed as mean $\pm$ SEM of all measurements of each experimental group. A p value < 0.05 was considered statistically significant. $*p < 0.03$ *vs* NAIVE, $**p < 0.0011$ *vs* NAÏVE (**b**). $****p < 0.0001$ *vs* NAIVE, $°°p < 0.0016$, $°°°°p < 0.0001$ *vs* CBD-cream (**c**). Panel **d** displays score of sensibility measured by needle test $****p < 0.0001$ *vs* NAÏVE, $°°p < 0.0011$, $°°°p < 0.004$, $°°°°p < 0.0001$ *vs* CBD-cream

and studied using light microscopy (Leica ICC50HD microscope).

May Grunwald Giemsa staining was performed according to the manufacturer's protocol (Bio-Optica, Milan, Italy) for the differentiation of cells present in lymphohemopoietic tissues. The staining solutions contain methylene blue (a basic dye), related azures (also basic dyes) and eosin (an acid dye). The first involves a blue/purple staining, the second involves a pink/red staining. The staining provides the nuclei of white blood cells and the granules of basophil granulocytes in blue, while red blood cells and eosinophil granules in red.

Luxol Fast Blue (LFB)
To show myelin and phospholipids in histological sections, LFB staining was performed according to the manufacturer's protocol (Bio-Optica, Milan, Italy). LFB affinity for central nervous system is usually ascribed to the bonds it forms with phospholipidic structures such

as lecithin and sphingomyelin. The staining provides: myelin in turquoise blue, neurons and glial nuclei in pink/violet and Nissl substance in pale pink.

Immunohistochemical evaluation
After deparaffinization with xylene, sections of spinal cord and spleen samples were hydrated. Detection of FOXP3, CD4, CD8α, GFAP, p-selectin, IL-1β, iNOS, nitrotyrosine and PARP-1 was carried out after boiling in citrate buffer 0.01 M pH 6 for 4 min. Endogenous peroxidase was quenched with 0.3 % (v/v) hydrogen peroxide in 60 % (v/v) methanol for 30 min. Nonspecific adsorption was minimized by incubating the section in 2 % (v/v) normal goat serum in PBS for 20 min.

Sections were incubated overnight with:

- anti-FOXP3 monoclonal antibody (1:100 in PBS v/v; Santa Cruz Biotechnology, Inc);

- anti-CD4 polyclonal antibody (1:100 in PBS v/v; Santa Cruz Biotechnology, Inc);
- anti-CD8α polyclonal antibody (1:100 in PBS v/v; Santa Cruz Biotechnology, Inc);
- anti-GFAP monoclonal antibody (1:50 in PBS v/v; Cell Signaling Technology);
- anti-p-selectin polyclonal antibody (1:100 in PBS v/v; Santa Cruz Biotechnology, Inc);
- anti-IL-1β polyclonal antibody (1:100 in PBS v/v; Santa Cruz Biotechnology, Inc);
- anti iNOS polyclonal antibody (1:100 in PBS v/v; Santa Cruz Biotechnology, Inc);
- anti-nitrotyrosine polyclonal antibody (1:100 in PBS v/v; Millipore);
- anti-PARP-1 polyclonal antibody (1:100 in PBS v/v; Santa Cruz Biotechnology, Inc).

Endogenous biotin or avidin binding sites were blocked by sequential incubation for 15 min with biotin and avidin (DBA, Milan, Italy), respectively. Sections were washed with PBS and incubated with secondary antibody. Specific labelling was detected with a biotin-conjugated goat anti-rabbit IgG and avidin–biotin peroxidase complex (Vectastain ABC kit, VECTOR). The immunostaining was developed with peroxidase substrate kit DAB (Vector Laboratories, Inc.) (brown color) and counterstaining with hematoxylin (blue background).

To verify the binding specificity, some sections were also incubated with only the primary antibody (no secondary) or with only the secondary antibody (no primary). In these cases no positive staining was found in the sections, indicating that the immunoreaction was positive in all the experiments carried out.

All sections were obtained using light microscopy (LEICA DM 2000 combined with LEICA ICC50 HD camera). Leica Application Suite V4.2.0 software was used as image computer program to acquire immunohistochemical pictures.

Western blot analysis

All the extraction procedures were performed on ice using ice-cold reagents. In brief, spinal cord tissues were suspended in extraction buffer containing 0.32 M sucrose, 10 mM Tris–HCl, pH 7.4, 1 mM EGTA, 2 mM EDTA, 5 mM NaN_3, 10 mM 2-mercaptoethanol, 50 mM NaF, protease inhibitor tablets (Roche Applied Science, Monza, Italy), and they were homogenized at the highest setting for 2 min. The homogenates were chilled on ice for 15 min and then centrifuged at 1000 g for 10 min at 4 °C, and the supernatant (cytosol + membrane extract from spinal cord tissue) was collected to evaluate content of cytoplasmic proteins.

The pellets were suspended in the supplied complete lysis buffer containing 1 % Triton X-100, 150 mM NaCl, 10 mM Tris–HCl, pH 7.4, 1 mM EGTA, 1 mM EDTA protease inhibitors (Roche), and then were centrifuged for 30 min at 15.000 g at 4 °C. Then, supernatant containing nuclear extract was collected to evaluate the content of nuclear proteins. Supernatants were stored at –80 °C until use. Protein concentration in homogenate was estimated by Bio-Rad Protein Assay (Bio-Rad, Segrate, Italy) using BSA as standard, and 20 μg of cytosol and nuclear extract from each sample were analyzed.

Proteins were separated on sodium dodecyl sulfate-polyacrylamide minigels and transferred onto PVDF membranes (Immobilon-P Transfer membrane, Millipore), blocked with PBS containing 5 % nonfat dried milk (PM) for 45 min at room temperature, and subsequently probed at 4 °C overnight with specific antibodies for TNF-α (1:500; Cell Signaling Technology), cleaved-caspase 3 (1:500; Cell Signaling Technology), GFAP (1:1000; Cell Signaling Technology), IL-6 (1:500; Abcam), IL-10 (1:250; Santa Cruz Biotechnology Inc), TGF-β (1:500; Abcam) and IFN-γ (1:250; Santa Cruz Biotechnology Inc) in 1x PBS, 5 % (w/v) non fat dried milk, 0.1 % Tween-20 (PMT). HRP-conjugated goat anti-mouse IgG, HRP-conjugated goat anti-rabbit IgG or HRP-conjugated chicken anti-rat were incubated as secondary antibody (1:2000; Santa Cruz Biotechnology Inc) for 1 h at room temperature.

To ascertain that blots were loaded with equal amounts of protein lysates, they were also incubated with antibody for GAPDH HRP Conjugated (1:1000; Cell Signaling Technology) and beta-actin (1:1000; Santa Cruz Biotechnology, Inc). The relative expression of protein bands, was visualized using an enhanced chemiluminescence system (Luminata Western HRP Substrates, Millipore) and protein bands were acquired and quantified with ChemiDoc™ MP System (Bio-Rad) and a computer program (ImageJ software) respectively.

Blots are representative of three separate and reproducible experiments. The statistical analysis was carried out on three repeated blots performed on separate experiments.

Statistical evaluation

GraphPad Prism version 6.0 program (GraphPad Software, La Jolla, CA) was used for statistical analysis of the data. The results were statistically analyzed using one-way ANOVA followed by a Bonferroni *post hoc* test for multiple comparisons. A p value less than or equal to 0.05 was considered significant. Results are expressed as the mean ± SEM of n experiments.

Results

Pharmacokinetic parameters of CBD after topical cream application

The summary of the pharmacokinetic parameters is showed in Table 1. The results of the *in vivo* experiment showed that the steady-state plasma concentration (C_{ss}) of CBD were 6.1 ± 1.9 ng/mL, which were attained at 14.9 ± 12.0 h (T_{lag}). Also, the maximum plasma concentration (C_{max}) was 8.3 ± 2.1 ng/mL and the temperature maximum (T_{max}) was 38.2 ± 18.9. Statistical analysis was performed by one-way analysis of variance followed by Bonferroni *post hoc* analysis. A *p* value less than or equal to 0.05 was considered significant. Data represent mean ± SD.

Clinical score and body weight

Clinical disease score (Fig. 1b) as well as body weight measurement (Fig. 1c) evaluation was assessed as parameters of disease. In both cases, CBD-treated EAE-affected mice show a trend of recovery over time compared to untreated EAE mice, in particular following the disease onset and until sacrifice. As displayed, mice belonging to the EAE group show a grading of disease with a clinical score as mean of 5.0 ± 0.329, while mice treated topically with 1 % CBD-cream revealed a lower grade of disability with a clinical score as mean of 1.5 ± 0.214. (Fig. 1b). In addition, in mice pharmacologically treated the recovery of the clinical score matches with an increase of body weight. Moreover, as expected, after EAE induction, a significant body weight loss was observed in EAE mice. Mice belonging to naive group have a normal increase in body weight as well as absence of motor deficit.

These data confirm both the disability in mice affected by EAE and the belief that chronic inflammation and autoimmune conditions in animals are associated with substantial feeding alterations.

Of note during the entire treatment period were not detected in mice treated with 1 % CBD-cream or vehicle cream (no plus CBD) allergic reactions in mice at cutaneous either at systemic level. Also, in order to confirm this, mice were subjected to every 48 h to little samples of blood from the tail to make a blood smear glass slide and calculate subsequent leukocyte formula, demonstrating any alteration in percentage of leukocytes.

Table 1 Pharmacokinetic parameters of CBD after topical treatment with 1 % CBD-cream

Pharmacokinetic parameter	CBD
C_{max} (ng/mL)	8.3 ± 2.1
T_{max} (hours)	38.2 ± 18.9
C_{ss} (ng/mL)	6.1 ± 1.9
T_{lag} (hours)	15.5 ± 12.0

CBD enhances responsiveness to a mechanical stimulus

Mice subjected to EAE show many clinical and pathological features of human MS, like paralysis of the hind limbs. In order to evaluate whether topical treatment with CBD can improve limbs sensitivity to a mechanical stimulus, we measured by needle test mechanical allodynia that may arise after peripheral nerve injury (Fig. 1d). To this purpose, a stimulus was applied on the paw plantar surface, evaluating the paw retraction response treshold.

In EAE mice treated topically with CBD a significantly increased response to mechanical stimulus was evident already from the first measurements. Moreover, EAE mice showed no response to mechanical stimulus applied to the paw plantar, while naive animals always responded by retracting the paw (Fig. 1d).

CBD improves histopathology of EAE

Since EAE is a demyelinating disease, CBD was evaluated for the protective effect on myelin sheath integrity by LFB staining at 28 days after EAE induction. Compared to naive animals and CTRL + CBD-cream (Additional files 1A and B, EAE mice exhibited markedly reduced myelin and axonal structures in the spinal cord (Fig. 2a). Also, treatment with 1 % CBD-cream, reduced demyelination and axonal loss in EAE mice with a high LFB positive staining (Fig. 2b).

The May-Grunwald Giemsa staining method was also used to evaluate inflammatory cells infiltration. The observed results clearly show considerable infiltration of lymphocytes cells in white matter of spinal cord samples taken from EAE mice (Fig. 2c, as shownn by square brackets) compared with naive mice and CTRL + CBD-cream (Additional files 1C and D). Remarkably, treatment with CBD-cream led to a complete resolution of inflammatory cells infiltration (Fig. 2d).

CBD modulates production of Treg cells and CD4 and CD8α Tcells

To assess whether CBD was able to modulate the production of Treg cells, we evaluated expression of the transcription factor Foxp3 by immunohistochemical analysis. Spinal cord sections from naive mice and CTRL + CBD-cream (Additional files 1E and F) did not show positive staining for Foxp3, which conversely, was positive in EAE mice (Fig. 2e). Sections obtained from 1 % CBD-cream treated group showed negative degree for Foxp3 (Fig. 2f).

In addition, to these observations, immunohistochemical analysis carried out in spleen sections, showed a positive staining for CD4 as well as for CD8α in EAE mice (Fig. 3a and b). Conversely, a negative staining for CD4 and CD8α was observed in EAE mice administered with 1 % CBD-cream (Fig. 3c and d) as well as in naïve mice and CTRL + CBD-cream (Additional files 2E, F, G and H).

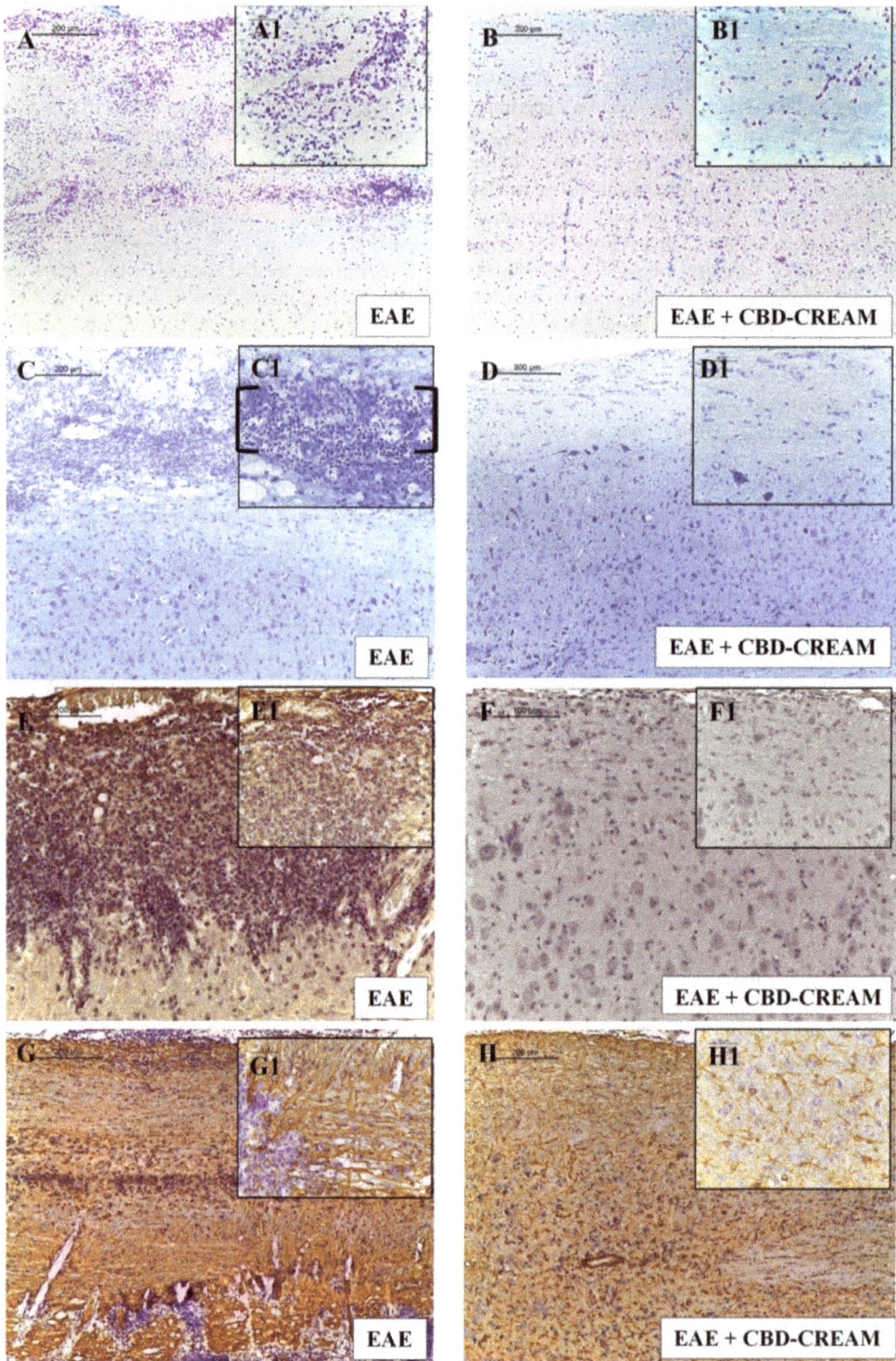

Fig. 2 (See legend on next page.)

(See figure on previous page.)
Fig. 2 LFB staining compared EAE group (**a**:10x, A1 magnification:40x) to EAE+ 1 % CBD-cream (**b**:10x, B1 magnification:40x). May-Grunwald Giemsa staining for EAE mice (**c**:10x, C1 magnification:40x) compared to mice treated with 1 % CBD-cream (**d**:10x, D1 magnification:40x). Immunohistochemical evaluation for Foxp3 in EAE (**e**:20x, E1 magnification:40x) and in EAE + 1 % CBD-cream mice (**f**:20x, F1 magnification:40x). Immunohistochemical evaluation for GFAP in EAE (**g**:10x, G1 magnification:40x) and in EAE + 1 % CBD-cream mice (**h**:10x, H1 magnification:40x)

Also, overall quantitative analysis of immunohistochemical images showed that tissue localization for CD8α was estimated about 35.96 % of positive staining in EAE mice, 3.63 % in EAE + 1 % CBD-cream mice and 0 in naïve group. Also, for CD4 tissue localization was estimated about 10.69 % of positive staining in EAE mice, 2.53 % in EAE + 1 % CBD-cream mice and 1.02 % in naïve ones. These images are representative of at least three experiments. Values shown are the mean of three different fields observed.

Effects CBD on GFAP expression

In order to investigate whether CBD can modulate astrocytic activation, we evaluated GFAP expression by immunohistochemical analysis. GFAP is considered a marker protein for astrogliosis, and a marked positive staining for GFAP was evident in the sections from EAE mice (Fig. 2g), compared to naive group and CTRL + CBD-cream (Additional files 1G and H). GFAP positive staining was significantly reduced in animals treated topically with CBD (Fig. 2h). Also, the same results were corroborated by western blot analysis on spinal cord tissues (Fig. 5e).

CBD modulates p-selectin expression

No positive staining for p-selectin was observed in longitudinal sections of spinal cord from naive mice and CTRL + CBD-cream (Additional files 1A and B), whereas

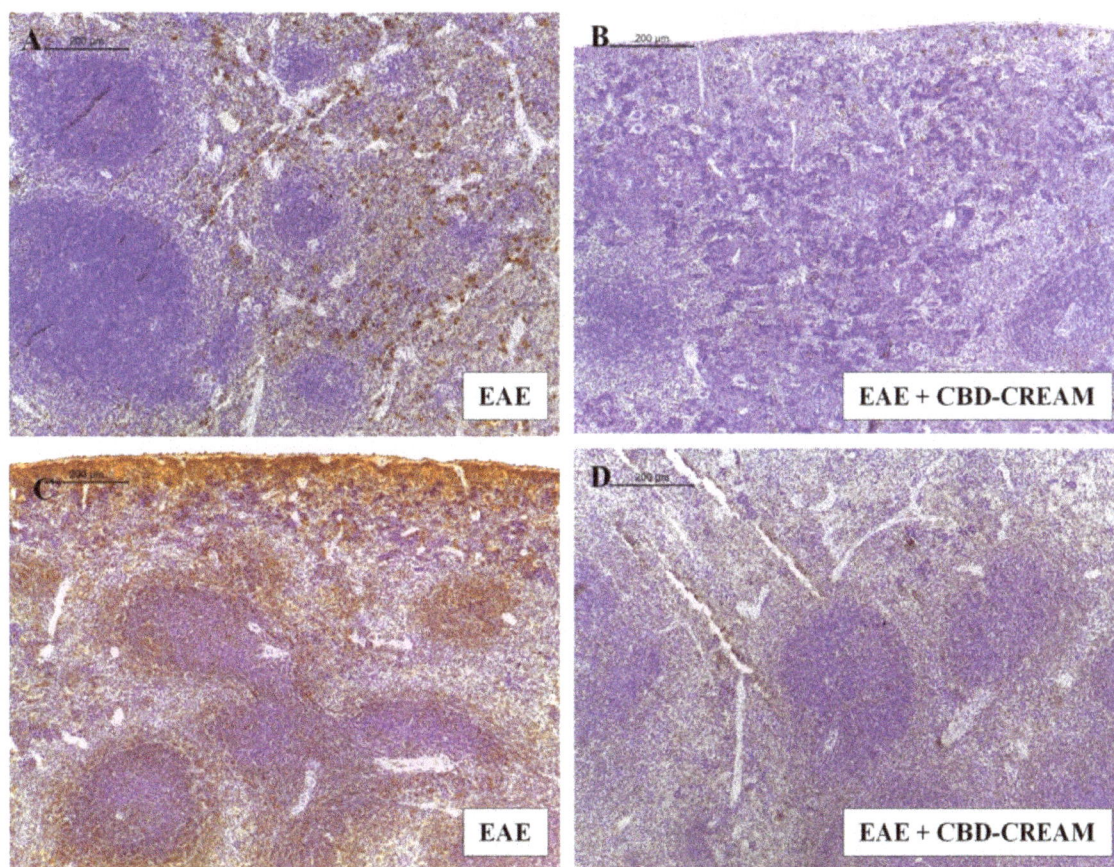

Fig. 3 Immunohistochemical analysis for CD4 in spleen tissues from EAE mice (**a**:10x, A1 magnification:40x) and mice treated with 1 % CBD-cream (**b**:10x, B1 magnification:40x). Immunohistochemical image for CD8α localization of EAE mice (**c**:10x, C1 magnification:40x) compared to CBD topical treated mice (**d**:10x, D1 magnification:40x) in spleen tissues

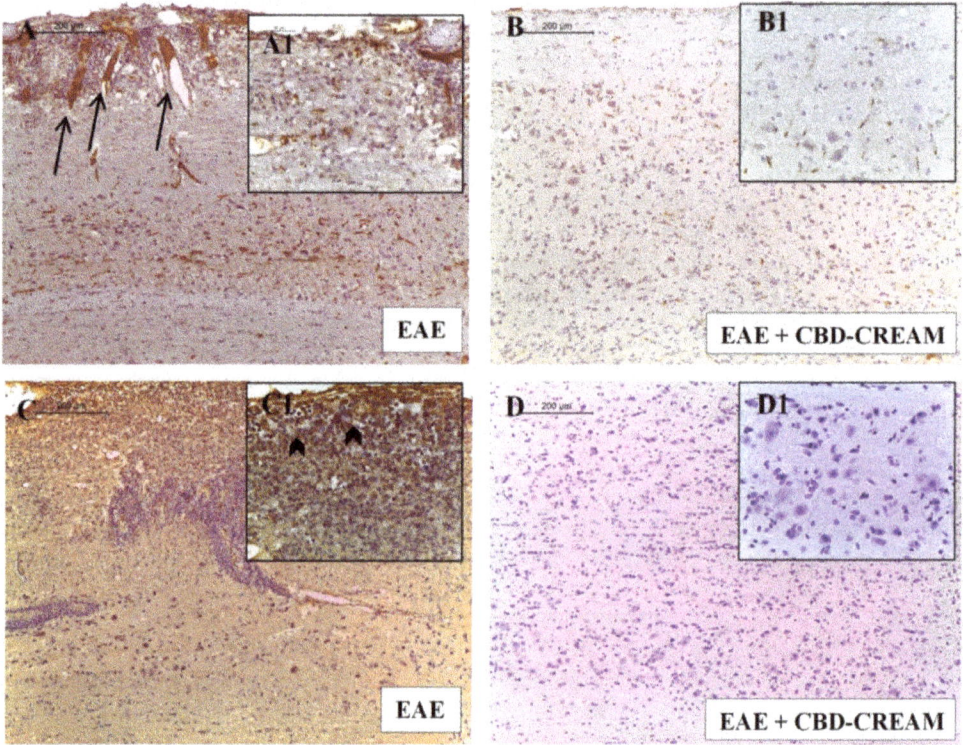

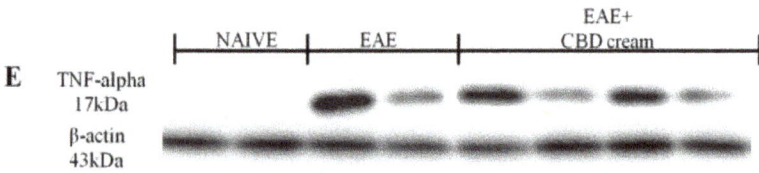

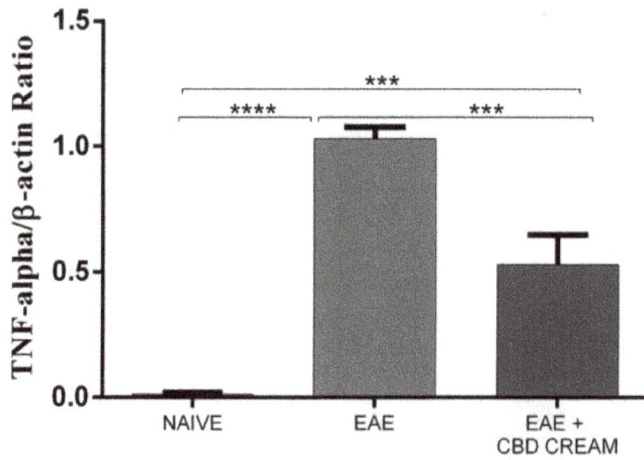

Fig. 4 (See legend on next page.)

(See figure on previous page.)
Fig. 4 Comparision of p-selectin immunohistochemical localization between EAE mice (**a**:10x, A1 magnification:40x) and EAE treated mice with 1 % CBD-cream (**b**:10x, B1 magnification:40x). Immunohistochemical analysis for IL-1β in spinal cord tissues from EAE mice (**c**:10x, C1 magnification:40x) and mice treated with 1 % CBD-cream (**d**:10x, D1 magnification:40x). Western blot analysis for TNF-α was showed in **e**. β-actin was used as internal control. ****$p < 0.0001$ *vs* EAE, ***$p < 0.0004$, ***$p < 0.0010$ *vs* EAE + 1 % CBD-cream

an intense positive staining in the vascular endothelium of EAE mice (Fig. 4a as shown by arrows) was observed. Conversely, negative staining for p-selectin was observed in spinal cord tissues from mice treated with 1 % CBD-cream (Fig. 4b).

CBD regulates inflammatory pathway

In order to investigate whether treatment with CBD can modulate the inflammatory processes triggered by EAE induction through regulating secretion of pro-inflammatory cytokines, the expression levels of IL-1β, IL-6, TNF-α, TGF-β and INF-γ in spinal cord samples were quantified by immunohistochemical and western blot analysis, respectively.

A positive staining for IL-1β was observed in spinal cord sections of EAE mice group (Fig. 4c arrowheads indicate positivity for inflammatory cells, including lymphocytes and neutrophils) when compared to naive mice (Additional files 1C and D), while no positive staining for cytokine expression was obtained in mice treated with CBD-cream (Fig. 4d). Additionally, by western blot analysis on homogenates of spinal cord tissues, a considerable increase in TNF-α release was established in EAE mice compared to naive animals. Conversely, levels of TNF-α were attenuated by 1 % CBD-cream administration. (Fig. 4e).

By Western blot, we found also appreciably increased expression of IL-6 in the spinal cord tissues from EAE

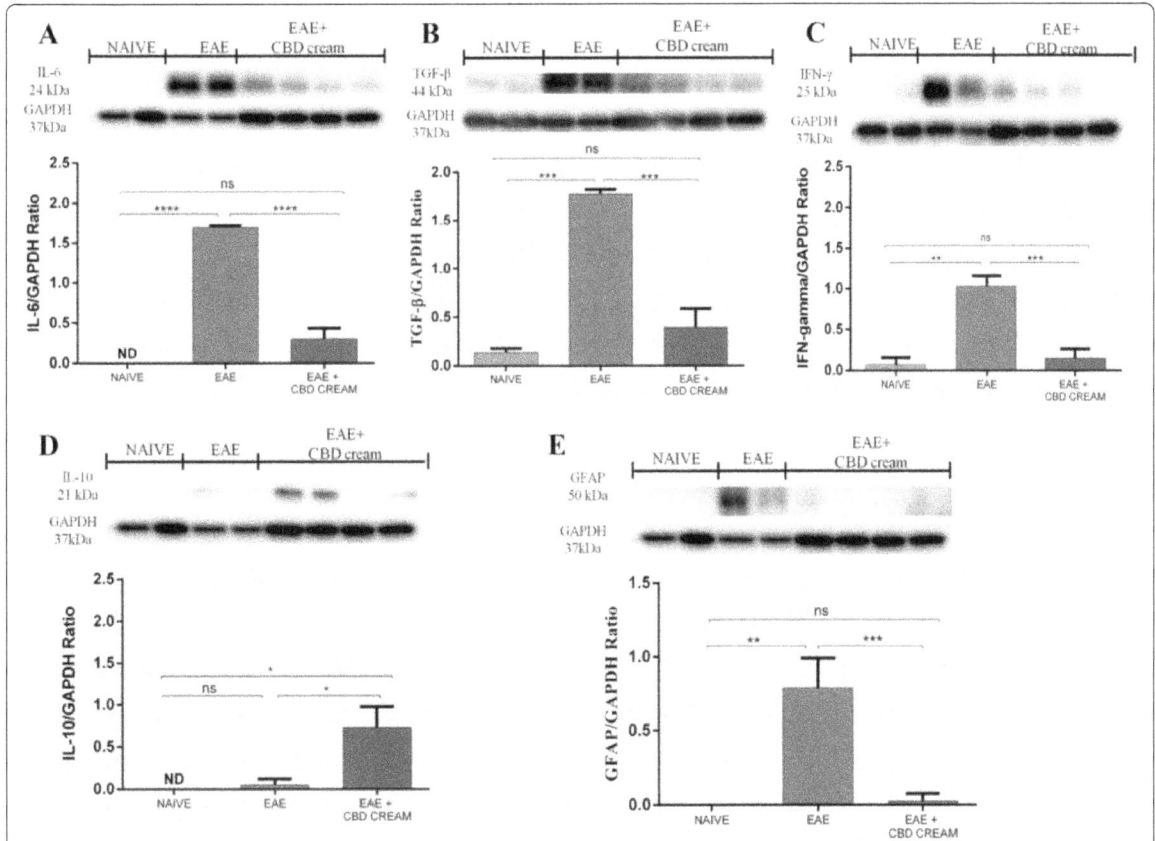

Fig. 5 Western blot analysis for IL-6 was showed in **a**. ****$p < 0.0001$ *vs* EAE, ****$p < 0.0001$ *vs* EAE + 1 % CBD-cream. Western blot analysis for TGF-β (**b**). ***$p < 0.0004$ *vs* EAE, ***$p < 0.0004$ *vs* EAE + 1 % CBD-cream. In **c** was displayed western blot analysis for IFN-γ. **$p < 0.0011$ *vs* EAE, ***$p < 0.0008$ *vs* EAE + 1 % CBD-cream. Western blot analysis for IL-10 (**d**). *$p < 0.0326$, *$p < 0.0415$ *vs* EAE + 1 % CBD-cream. In **e** was displayed western blot analysis for GFAP **$p < 0.0016$ *vs* EAE, ***$p < 0.0009$ *vs* EAE + 1 % CBD-cream. ND not detectable

mice On the contrary, topical treatment with 1 % CBD-cream diminished its levels (Fig. 5a).

Western blot analysis for TGF-β revealed that this signaling pathway is strongly activated following EAE-induction while 1 % CBD-cream treatment reduces the expression levels of this marker (Fig. 5b). Similarly, it was found an increased expression of INF-γ in EAE mice, decreased by 1 % CBD-cream treatment (Fig. 5c).

Also, by western blot analysis we investigated the role of IL-10 as antinflammatory cytokine, showing a basal level of IL-10 expression in samples obtained from EAE mice, whereas treatment of mice with 1 % CBD-cream significantly increased its expression. It was not observed an expression of IL-10 in naïve animals. (Fig. 5d).

CBD modulates production of nitrotyrosine, iNOS and PARP

CBD could also counteract the nitrosative stress resulting from the EAE-induction. Spinal cord sections obtained from EAE untreated mice exhibited positive staining for nitrotyrosine (Fig. 6a as shown by arrowheads), iNOS (Fig. 6c arrowheads shown positivity for

inflammatory cells) and PARP (Fig. 6e as shown by arrowheads) .Sections obtained from mice treated with 1 % CBD-cream showed negative staining for nitrotyrosine (Fig. 6b), iNOS (Fig. 6d) as well as PARP staining (Fig. 6f).

CBD reduces Cleaved-caspase 3 expression induced by EAE

By Western blot, we evaluated the activation of the caspase pathway, particularly, cleaved-caspase 3, which leads to programmed cell death by cleavage of cellular substrates. Cleaved-caspase 3 levels were appreciably increased in the spinal cord tissues from EAE mice. On the contrary, topical treatment with 1 % CBD-cream prevented EAE-induced cleaved-caspase 3 production (Fig. 6g).

Discussion

Cannabis sativa represents a great source of bioactive compounds whose potential for medicinal use is currently at the center of an intense research activity,

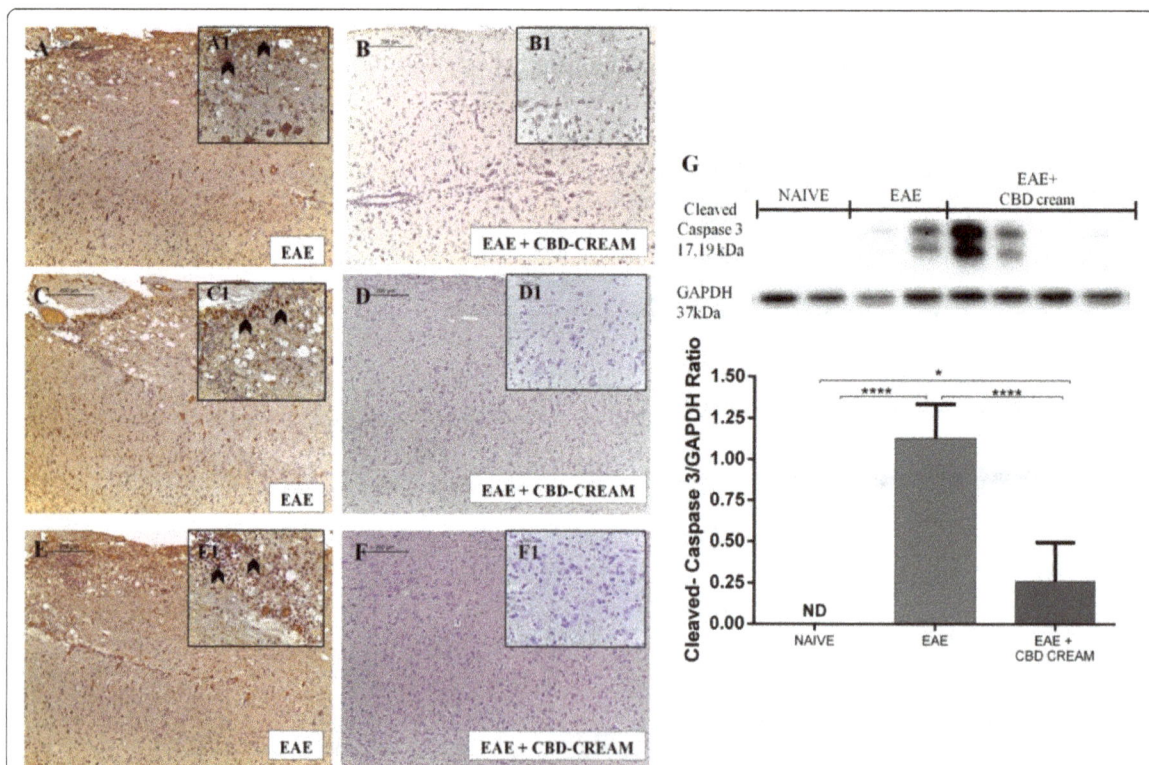

Fig. 6 Immunohistochemical image for nitrotyrosine localization of EAE mice (**a**:10x, A1 magnification:40x) compared to CBD topical treated mice (**b**:10x, B1 magnification:40x). Immunohistochemical evaluation for iNOS in EAE (**c**:10x, C1 magnification:40x) and in EAE + 1 % CBD-cream mice (**d**:10x, D1 magnification:40x). Immunohistochemical analysis for PARP in spinal cord tissues from EAE mice (**e**) and mice treated with 1 % CBD-cream (**f**). Panel **g** shows western blot analysis for Cleaved-caspase 3. GAPDH was used as internal control. ****$p < 0.0001$ vs EAE, *$p < 0.0244$, ****$p < 0.0001$ vs. EAE + CBD-cream. ND not detectable

especially for the management of neurodegenerative disorders, and MS in particular.

In this regard it is noteworthy to consider the recent introduction of Sativex®, a cannabinoid oromucosal spray containing a 1:1 ratio of THC and cannabidiol CBD, for the management of symptomatic treatment of chronic pain and spasticity in MS patients [29]. Despite this combination has been approved and in the current state introduced in several countries under this formulation, over the years the point of view of the scientific community regarding THC and CBD is changed. Although emerging evidence regarding putative therapeutic activities of cannabinoids, to date it remains to be overcome limits about unavoidable psychotropic effects, exhibited by many of them [30].

Several experimental studies have shown that CBD possesses many properties, often wrongly attributed by collective imagination just to THC alone and wide experimental evidences demonstrated that isolating non-psychotropic compounds by THC component provide beneficial effects for therapeutic use, mostly for CNS disorders [35, 36].

To date, although CBD pharmacodynamic remains still unclear, its pharmacokinetics appears better defined. It is known that when orally given, due to a marked first-pass effect, CBD bioavailability ranges between values of 13 and 19 % [37], hence the oral route is not ideal for the therapeutic delivery of CBD, but for this reason the intravenous administration is preferable. Even further intranasal administration could be more effective as results in the rapid attainment of the drug blood level, but it is more suitable for acute or breakthrough pain [38].

As CBD has low aqueous solubility and undergoes first-pass metabolism, alternative delivery routes would be necessary to achieve successful therapeutic effects.

An easy method of CBD administration would be through the topical route, thus maintaining a costant therapeutic drug level and reducing increased side effects because of the decreased peak plasma levels. It has been demonstrated, although only a few published studies, that cannabinoids are good candidates for topical delivery in the treatment of chronic conditions [39, 40].

For this reason, the present work was designed to define a new topical formulation of CBD, whose intrinsic potential as a molecule with a therapeutic effect has not yet completely understood.

Recent studies have already described beneficial effects of intraperitoneal administration of CBD alone or in mixture with other compounds in EAE mouse model with antinflammatory and antioxidant properties [23–25]. According to Rahimi et al. [41] intraperitoneally treatment with CBD in mixture with palmitoylethanolamide (PEA) during EAE onset reduced the severity of the neurobehavioral deficits of EAE. This effect of CBD and PEA was accompanied by decreased inflammatory cytokines expression, demyelination, axonal damage and inflammatory cytokine expression [41].

Also, in Kozela et al. study [25] it was found that systemic treatment with alone CBD during disease onset ameliorated the severity of the clinical signs of EAE. This effect of CBD was accompanied by diminished axonal damage and inflammation as well as microglial activation and T-cell recruitment in the spinal cord of EAE mice. Also, this effect seems not to be mediated via the known cannabinoid CB1 and CB2 receptors [25].

Similarly, our achieved results have demonstrated that topical formulation of CBD significantly modulates many intracellular pathways associated to EAE/MS etiopathology, by improving clinical features correlated with severity of the pathology.

One of the first hallmarks of disease in the MOG-induced EAE model is a reduction of body weight and onset of symptoms such as tail tonus and hind limb paralysis. As expected, mice belonging to EAE group showed the highest score of disease (about 5 points in the grading scale of disease) against 1,5 of EAE topical treated mice. The therapeutic effect in terms of wellness following the CBD administration as topical treatment was a reduced body weight loss associated with an improvement in the disease score. Therefore, 1 % CBD-cream has proven effective into reduce the main disease parameters.

Moreover, as known, EAE is associated with a complex series of processes triggered by neuroinflammation and the infiltration of immune cells into the CNS, followed by a dysfunction of neural activity and neuronal death [42]. Here, we confirmed findings of above cited studies, demonstrating that 1 % CBD-cream treatment acts counteracting leukocyte infiltration and microglial activation and improving neuroinflammation status. Hystopathology of spinal cord samples supported this view showing a marked remyelination following 1 % CBD-cream treatment. To better understand this aspect, we believe usefull to focus the attention on the above cited leukocyte infiltration key-event of EAE model and critical step into the establishment of inflammatory response and demyelinization [43].

In this context, adhesion molecules, as p-selectin, play a significant role in the induction of leukocyte-endothelial cell adhesion and extravasation of immune cells during pathological process [44]. Therefore, according to a supposed action on this pathway mediated by 1 % CBD-cream treatment, it was not surprising to find a modulated p-selectin immunolocalization.

Although as known that MS is a disease mediated by an autoimmune attack directed against components of the myelin sheath, the mechanisms that lead to loss of function associated with these immunologically events remain poorly understood. The activation of T cells and macrophages that secrete freely diffusable factors has an important role in the pathogenesis of MS. These factors are the proinflammatory cytokines and reactive oxygen and reactive nitrogen species [45, 46]. As expected we found increased levels of proinflammatory mediators including IL-1β, TNF-α, IL-6, IFN-γ and TGF-β in spinal cord from EAE mice. Remarkably, 1 % CBD-cream treatment significantly attenuates the expression of all these inflammatory markers and also regulates immune tolerance by increasing the production of antinflammatory cytokines, like IL-10. This confirms that CBD was able to decrease TNF-α, IL-2 and IFN-γ release from activated splenocytes and macrophages as reported in other studues [47–49].

Of note, this cytokine profile suggests it as an important factor in immunopathogenesis of MS, because the main feature of MS pathophysiology is the neuroinflammatory reaction.

As reported in literature it's probably that all these mediators are produced by Th17 cells, that play a key role in in autoimmune neuroinflammation and EAE development [50]. Also, it is generally considered that Th17-mediated inflammation is characterized by neutrophil recruitment into the CNS and neurons killing. In this context, mainly IFN-γ seems to have a pathological role in the development of this autoimmune disease [51]. Our results show that the MOG-induced EAE causes significant increases in IFN-γ expression. 1 % CBD-cream administration, significantly diminished the expression of this cytokine.

Moreover, several studies on MS evaluated immunosuppressive effect of cannabinoids demonstrated that they are able to exert their action modulating the induction of Tregulatory cells (Tregs) [13], normally involved in the maintenance of tolerance toward self-constituents, and limiting inflammatory responses against foreign antigens. Treg cell recruitment plays a key defensive role in suppression of Th1 effector cells, which are the main T cell subtype mediating disease pathogenesis.

To verify if treatment with CBD can modulate the production of Treg cells, we evaluated the expression of the transcription factor Foxp3, as an indirect marker of Treg. In accordance with a previous study [52], we confirmed a clear engagement of Treg cells during EAE, while treatment with CBD-cream is able to deplete Foxp3 positive cells. This leads to think that the immune system response is somehowe restrained by topic application of 1 % CBD-cream in EAE affected mice in correlation with a lower degree of autoimmune cells activity in these animals. Also, it is possible that 1 % CBD-cream stimulates Th0 cell to develop into a Treg phenotype.

This observation has special relevance if we consider that CD4 T cells expression is involved in cell-mediated immunity and in the pathogenesis of MS, with destruction of the axonal myelin sheath in several areas of CNS and spinal cord being mediated mainly by self-reactive CD4 T cells. As expected, we observed that both CD4 and also CD8α detections were apparent in untreated EAE mice, while topical treatment reveals the capability to counteract the release of cytotoxic T cells.

Corroborating these results, immunostaining for GFAP, a marker of astrocytic activation, involved in many processes of cellular function [53], was reduced in EAE mice treated with 1 % CBD-cream compared with untreated mice. This potentially can be correlated with the triggering of antioxidant mechanisms that, notoriously, interfere with GFAP upregulation occurring in astocytes.

Looking at this first report of achieved results we feel to state that CBD, acting as an antinflammatory agent, is capable to reduce the inflammatory signs of MS. Nevertheless, we have obtained deeper data characterizing the therapeutic properties of the 1 % CBD-cream preparation.

For this, we have to consider that CBD has a potent capability to attenuate oxidative and nitrosative stress in wide neurological disease models, although the underlying mechanism is still unclear.

As, it is known that several cellular mediators and proinflammatory cytokines can induce iNOS, enzyme present in actively demyelinating lesions, and that nitrates and nitrites are increased in the CSF and serum of patients with MS [54]. Therefore, several studies have suggested a role for NO and its oxidizing molecules (such as peroxynitrite) in the immunopathogenesis of MS as contributors of the inflammatory process [55] In accordance with these assumptions, we demonstrated that CBD reduces the expression of iNOS and nitrotyrosine in tissues from EAE treated mice, suggesting that this compound, at least in part, may be responsible for the reduction of cytokines production, that in turn counteract the rise of iNOS levels and the downstream cascade of events triggered by the inflammatory process, reducing thus oxidative stress.

The strong link between oxidative stress and apoptosis is well known, as is the concept that down-regulation of nitrosative stress and protection against apoptosis within the CNS represents an effective neuroprotective therapy for the MS treatment. In particular, PARP expression is correlated and in turn activated by cleaved-caspase 3. Positive staining for PARP, responsible of DNA breakdown in apoptosis, was found in EAE mice, while it was significantly reduced by topical treatment with CBD. In keeping with these observations, the expression of cleaved caspase 3, a major key regulator of apoptosis, was evaluated displaying an attenuated expression when CBD was topically administered.

All these results overall suggest and allow us to hypothesize that CBD has the capability to interfere with EAE-induced neuronal apoptotic death, attenuating, or even preventing the activation of cellular molecular mechanisms triggered by severe damage.

Moreover, in the current literature CBD has been shown to be a potent analgesic in animal models of hyperlgesia and mechanical allodynia, as possible candidate for the treatment of inflammatory pain and other common symptoms related to chronic pain [56]. These analgesic effects of CBD might be mediated by its modulation of TRPV1 receptor [57]. Furthermore, there are evidences that cannabinoids induce antinociception both via supraspinal mechanisms and the interaction with peripheral CB2 receptors and via activation of CB1 receptors at the spinal cord level [58]. However, CBD shows only marginal affinity for CB1 and CB2, and the potential involvement of the endocannabinoid system might be indirectly mediated by its effects on the enzymes of the endocannabinoid system.

We also confirmed that CBD has a beneficial effect on mechanical allodynia in EAE animals. Since mice subjected to EAE show paralysis of the hind limbs with a consequent loss of sensitivity, we evaluated the effects of a CBD topical treatment applied on the hind limbs of animals in recovering a response to a mechanical stimulus induced on the paw plantar surface. Amazingly, topical CBD significantly increased response to mechanical stimulus from the earliest measurements, recovering the responsiveness of the hind limbs.

We can also affirm that the protective effects of treatment are not due to the method of drug administration (shaving and/or spreading of the cream). Animals treated with cream that not containing the active ingredient did not show any improvement in recovering paralysis of the hind limbs. For us, this represent a data is of pivotal importance, and in the event that it will be clinically confirmed, this finding could open new opportunities for the treatment of MS.

Conclusions

Summarizing, we have shown that the topical administration of CBD can protect against the cascade of events (inflammation, oxidative injury and neuronal cell death) associated to the induction of EAE. Of note, topical CBD application was able to recover the hind limb lost sensitivity. This observation provides a rationale for evaluating its clinical translation that might represent a new concept in the management of MS.

Finally, we suggest that CBD, devoid of psychoactive activity, could be potentially, safe and effective non invasive alternatives for alleviating neuroinflammation and neurodegeneration.

Additional files

Additional file 1: Figure S1. LFB staining shows naive group (A:10x) and CTRL-CBD cream (B:10x). May-Grunwald Giemsa staining for naive mice (C:10x) and mice CTRL-CBD cream (D:10x). Immunohistochemical evaluation for Foxp3 in naive group (E:10x) and in CTRL-CBD cream (F:10x). Immunohistochemical evaluation for GFAP in naive mice (G:10x) and in mice CTRL-CBD cream (H:10x). (TIFF 18429 kb)

Additional file 2: Figure S2. Immunohistochemical localization for p-selectin in naive mice (A:10x) and CTRL-CBD cream (B:10x). Immunohistochemical analysis for IL-1β in spinal cord tissues from naive mice (C:10x) and for CTRL-CBD cream (D:10x). Immunohistochemical analysis for CD4 in spleen tissues from naive mice (E:10x) and for CTRL-CBD cream (F:10x). Immunohistochemical image for CD8α localization of naive mice (G:10x) and for CTRL-CBD cream (H:10x) in spleen tissues. (TIFF 19661 kb)

Abbreviations

CBD: Cannabidiol; EAE: Autoimmune encephalomyelitis; MS: Multiple sclerosis; MOG_{35-55}: Myelin oligodendrocyte glycoprotein peptide; Δ^9-THC: Δ^9-tetrahydrocannabinol; CB1: Cannabinoid receptor type 1; CB2: Cannabinoid receptor type 2; TRPV1: Transient receptor potential vanilloid type 1; GPR55: G protein-coupled receptor 55; 5-HT1A: 5-hydroxytryptamine receptor subtype 1A; TNF-α: Tumor necrosis factor-alpha; IL-1β: Interleukin-1beta; iNOS: Inducible nitric oxide synthase; ROS: Reactive oxygen species; GA: Glatiramer acetate; NDS: Nasal delivery system; CFA: Complete Freund's adjuvant; LFB: Luxol Fast Blue; C_{SS}: steady-state plasma concentration; Cmax: maximum plasma concentration; T_{max}: temperature maximum; PEA: palmitoylethanolamide; Tregs: regulatory T cells.

Competing interests

The authors declare that they have no competing interests

Authors' contributions

SG Drafting of the manuscript and molecular biology analysis, MG Experimental model and data analysis and interpretation, FP Extraction and isolation of CBD and manuscript supervision, GG Provided the Cannabis sativa L. plant, derived from greenhouse cultivation at CRA-CIN, Rovigo (Italy) and supervised the manuscript, PB Study concept and design: PB, EM Designed research, performed experimental procedures and produced all histological data. All authors read and approved the final manuscript.

Author details

¹IRCCS Centro Neurolesi "Bonino-Pulejo", Via Provinciale Palermo, contrada Casazza, 98124 Messina, Italy. ²Dipartimento di Scienze del Farmaco, Università del Piemonte Orientale, Largo Donegani 2, 28100 Novara, Italy. ³Consiglio per le Ricerca e la sperimentazione in Agricoltura – Centro di Ricerca per le Colture Industriali (CRA-CIN), Viale G. Amendola 82, 45100 Rovigo, Italy.

References

1. Mechoulam R, Shani A, Edery H, Grunfeld Y. Chemical basis of hashish activity. Science. 1970;169:611–2.
2. Elsohly MA, Slade D. Chemical constituents of marijuana: the complex mixture of natural cannabinoids. Life Sci. 2005;78:539–48.
3. Munro S, Thomas KL, Abu-Shaar M. Molecular characterization of a peripheral receptor for cannabinoids. Nature. 1993;365:61–5.
4. Van Sickle MD, Duncan M, Kingsley PJ, Mouihate A, Urbani P, Mackie K, et al. Identification and functional characterization of brainstem cannabinoid CB2 receptors. Science. 2005;310:329–32.
5. Thomas A, Baillie GL, Phillips AM, Razdan RK, Ross RA, Pertwee RG. Cannabidiol displays unexpectedly high potency as an antagonist of CB1 and CB2 receptor agonists in vitro. Br J Pharmacol. 2007;150:613–23.
6. Pertwee RG, Howlett AC, Abood ME, Alexander SP, Di Marzo V, Elphick MR, et al. International Union of Basic and Clinical Pharmacology. LXXIX.

Cannabinoid receptors and their ligands: beyond CB(1) and CB(2). Pharmacol Rev. 2010;62:588–631.

7. Zuardi AW. Cannabidiol: from an inactive cannabinoid to a drug with wide spectrum of action. Rev Bras Psiquiatr. 2008;30:271–80.

8. Costa B, Giagnoni G, Franke C, Trovato AE, Colleoni M. Vanilloid TRPV1 receptor mediates the antihyperalgesic effect of the nonpsychoactive cannabinoid, cannabidiol, in a rat model of acute inflammation. Br J Pharmacol. 2004;143:247–50.

9. Pertwee RG. GPR55: a new member of the cannabinoid receptor clan? Br J Pharmacol. 2007;152:984–6.

10. Russo EB, Burnett A, Hall B, Parker KK. Agonistic properties of cannabidiol at 5-HT1a receptors. Neurochem Res. 2005;30:1037–43.

11. Buckley NE. The peripheral cannabinoid receptor knockout mice: an update. Br J Pharmacol. 2008;153:309–18.

12. Valverde O, Karsak M, Zimmer A. Analysis of the endocannabinoid system by using CB1 cannabinoid receptor knockout mice. Handb Exp Pharmacol. 2005;117–45.

13. Rieder SA, Chauhan A, Singh U, Nagarkatti M, Nagarkatti P. Cannabinoid-induced apoptosis in immune cells as a pathway to immunosuppression. Immunobiology. 2010;215:598–605.

14. Jean-Gilles L, Gran B, Constantinescu CS. Interaction between cytokines, cannabinoids and the nervous system. Immunobiology. 2010;215:606–10.

15. Mechoulam R, Peters M, Murillo-Rodriguez E, Hanus LO. Cannabidiol–recent advances. Chem Biodivers. 2007;4:1678–92.

16. Iuvone T, Esposito G, De Filippis D, Scuderi C, Steardo L. Cannabidiol: a promising drug for neurodegenerative disorders? CNS Neurosci Ther. 2009;15:65–75.

17. Giacoppo S, Mandolino G, Galuppo M, Bramanti P, Mazzon E. Cannabinoids: new promising agents in the treatment of neurological diseases. Molecules. 2014;19:18781–816.

18. Siffrin V, Brandt AU, Herz J, Zipp F. New insights into adaptive immunity in chronic neuroinflammation. Adv Immunol. 2007;96:1–40.

19. Compston A, Coles A. Multiple sclerosis. Lancet. 2002;359:1221–31.

20. Weber MS, Menge T, Lehmann-Horn K, Kronsbein HC, Zettl U, Sellner J, et al. Current treatment strategies for multiple sclerosis - efficacy versus neurological adverse effects. Curr Pharm Des. 2012;18:209–19.

21. Malfitano AM, Proto MC, Bifulco M. Cannabinoids in the management of spasticity associated with multiple sclerosis. Neuropsychiatr Dis Treat. 2008;4:847–53.

22. Carrillo-Salinas FJ, Navarrete C, Mecha M, Feliu A, Collado JA, Cantarero I, et al. A cannabigerol derivative suppresses immune responses and protects mice from experimental autoimmune encephalomyelitis. PloS one. 2014;9:e94733.

23. Baker D, Jackson SJ, Pryce G. Cannabinoid control of neuroinflammation related to multiple sclerosis. Br J Pharmacol. 2007;152:649–54.

24. Kubajewska I, Constantinescu CS. Cannabinoids and experimental models of multiple sclerosis. Immunobiology. 2010;215:647–57.

25. Kozela E, Lev N, Kaushansky N, Eilam R, Rimmerman N, Levy R, et al. Cannabidiol inhibits pathogenic T cells, decreases spinal microglial activation and ameliorates multiple sclerosis-like disease in C57BL/6 mice. Br J Pharmacol. 2011;163:1507–19.

26. Duchi S, Ovadia H, Touitou E. Nasal administration of drugs as a new non-invasive strategy for efficient treatment of multiple sclerosis. J Neuroimmunol. 2013;258:32–40.

27. Zajicek JP, Sanders HP, Wright DE, Vickery PJ, Ingram WM, Reilly SM, et al. Cannabinoids in multiple sclerosis (CAMS) study: safety and efficacy data for 12 months follow up. J Neurol Neurosurg Psychiatry. 2005;76:1664–9.

28. Zajicek J, Ball S, Wright D, Vickery J, Nunn A, Miller D, et al. Effect of dronabinol on progression in progressive multiple sclerosis (CUPID): a randomised, placebo-controlled trial. Lancet Neurol. 2013;12:857–65.

29. Vaney C, Heinzel-Gutenbrunner M, Jobin P, Tschopp F, Gattlen B, Hagen U, et al. Efficacy, safety and tolerability of an orally administered cannabis extract in the treatment of spasticity in patients with multiple sclerosis: a randomized, double-blind, placebo-controlled, crossover study. Mult Scler. 2004;10:417–24.

30. Karniol IG, Shirakawa I, Kasinski N, Pfeferman A, Carlini EA. Cannabidiol interferes with the effects of delta 9 - tetrahydrocannabinol in man. Eur J Pharmacol. 1974;28:172–7.

31. Taglialatela-Scafati O, Pagani A, Scala F, De Petrocellis L, Di Marzo V, Grassi G, et al. Cannabimovone, a Cannabinoid with a Rearranged Terpenoid Skeleton from Hemp. Eur J Org Chem. 2010;11:2067–72.

32. Swift W, Wong A, Li KM, Arnold JC, McGregor IS. Analysis of cannabis seizures in NSW, Australia: cannabis potency and cannabinoid profile. PloS one. 2013;8:e70052.

33. Paschalidis N, Iqbal AJ, Maione F, Wood EG, Perretti M, Flower RJ, et al. Modulation of experimental autoimmune encephalomyelitis by endogenous annexin A1. J Neuroinflammation. 2009;6:33.

34. Rodrigues DH, Vilela MC, Barcelos LS, Pinho V, Teixeira MM, Teixeira AL. Absence of PI3Kgamma leads to increased leukocyte apoptosis and diminished severity of experimental autoimmune encephalomyelitis. J Neuroimmunol. 2010;222:90–4.

35. England TJ, Hind WH, Rasid NA, O'Sullivan SE. Cannabinoids in experimental stroke: a systematic review and meta-analysis. J Cereb Blood Flow Metab. 2015;35:348–58.

36. Hill AJ, Williams CM, Whalley BJ, Stephens GJ. Phytocannabinoids as novel therapeutic agents in CNS disorders. Pharmacol Ther. 2012;133:79–97.

37. Harvey DJ, Mechoulam R. Metabolites of cannabidiol identified in human urine. Xenobiotica. 1990;20:303–20.

38. Paudel KS, Hammell DC, Agu RU, Valiveti S, Stinchcomb AL. Cannabidiol bioavailability after nasal and transdermal application: effect of permeation enhancers. Drug Dev Ind Pharm. 2010;36:1088–97.

39. Lodzki M, Godin B, Rakou L, Mechoulam R, Gallily R, Touitou E. Cannabidiol-transdermal delivery and anti-inflammatory effect in a murine model. J Control Release. 2003;93:377–87.

40. Touitou E, Fabian B, Dany S, Almog S. Transdermal delivery of tetrahydrocannabinol. Int J Pharm. 1988;43:9–15.

41. Rahimi A, Faizi M, Talebi F, Noorbakhsh F, Kahrizi F, Naderi N. Interaction between the protective effects of cannabidiol and palmitoylethanolamide in experimental model of multiple sclerosis in C57BL/6 mice. Neuroscience. 2015;290:279–87.

42. Gold R, Linington C, Lassmann H. Understanding pathogenesis and therapy of multiple sclerosis via animal models: 70 years of merits and culprits in experimental autoimmune encephalomyelitis research. Brain. 2006;129:1953–71.

43. McFarland HF, Martin R. Multiple sclerosis: a complicated picture of autoimmunity. Nat Immunol. 2007;8:913–9.

44. Golias C, Tsoutsi E, Matziridis A, Makridis P, Batistatou A, Charalabopoulos K. Review. Leukocyte and endothelial cell adhesion molecules in inflammation focusing on inflammatory heart disease. In vivo. 2007;21:757–69.

45. Brosnan CF, Raine CS. Mechanisms of immune injury in multiple sclerosis. Brain Pathol. 1996;6:243–57.

46. Esposito G, De Filippis D, Maiuri MC, De Stefano D, Carnuccio R, Iuvone T. Cannabidiol inhibits inducible nitric oxide synthase protein expression and nitric oxide production in beta-amyloid stimulated PC12 neurons through p38 MAP kinase and NF-kappaB involvement. Neurosci Lett. 2006;399:91–5.

47. Malfait AM, Gallily R, Sumariwalla PF, Malik AS, Andreakos E, Mechoulam R, et al. The nonpsychoactive cannabis constituent cannabidiol is an oral anti-arthritic therapeutic in murine collagen-induced arthritis. Proc Natl Acad Sci U S A. 2000;97:9561–6.

48. Jan TR, Su ST, Wu HY, Liao MH. Suppressive effects of cannabidiol on antigen-specific antibody production and functional activity of splenocytes in ovalbumin-sensitized BALB/c mice. Int Immunopharmacol. 2007;7:773–80.

49. Kaplan BLF, Springs AEB, Kaminski NE. The profile of immune modulation by cannabidiol (CBD) involves deregulation of nuclear factor of activated T cells (NFAT). Biochem Pharmacol. 2008;76:726–37.

50. Lovett-Racke AE, Yang Y, Racke MK. Th1 versus Th17: are T cell cytokines relevant in multiple sclerosis? Biochim Biophys Acta. 1812;2011:246–51.

51. Hammarberg H, Lidman O, Lundberg C, Eltayeb SY, Gielen AW, Muhallab S, et al. Neuroprotection by encephalomyelitis: rescue of mechanically injured neurons and neurotrophin production by CNS-infiltrating T and natural killer cells. J Neurosci. 2000;20:5283–91.

52. Zorzella-Pezavento SF, Chiuso-Minicucci F, Franca TG, Ishikawa LL, da Rosa LC, Marques C, et al. Persistent inflammation in the CNS during chronic EAE despite local absence of IL-17 production. Mediators Inflamm. 2013;2013:519627.

53. Eng LF, Ghirnikar RS. GFAP and astrogliosis. Brain Pathol. 1994;4:229–37.

54. Lindquist S, Hassinger S, Lindquist JA, Sailer M. The balance of pro-inflammatory and trophic factors in multiple sclerosis patients: effects of acute relapse and immunomodulatory treatment. Mult Scler. 2011;17:851–66.

55. Cross AH, Manning PT, Stern MK, Misko TP. Evidence for the production of peroxynitrite in inflammatory CNS demyelination. J Neuroimmunol. 1997;80:121–30.

56.   Rahn EJ, Hohmann AG. Cannabinoids as pharmacotherapies for neuropathic pain: from the bench to the bedside. Neurotherapeutics. 2009;6:713–37.

57.   Costa B, Trovato AE, Comelli F, Giagnoni G, Colleoni M. The non-psychoactive cannabis constituent cannabidiol is an orally effective therapeutic agent in rat chronic inflammatory and neuropathic pain. Eur J Pharmacol. 2007;556:75–83.

58.   Calignano A, La Rana G, Giuffrida A, Piomelli D. Control of pain initiation by endogenous cannabinoids. Nature. 1998;394:277–81.

19

Artemia salina as a model organism in toxicity assessment of nanoparticles

Somayeh Rajabi[1], Ali Ramazani[1,2]*, Mehrdad Hamidi[3] and Tahereh Naji[1]

Abstract

Background: Because of expanding presence of nanomaterials, there has been an increase in the exposure of humans to nanoparticles that is why nanotoxicology studies are important. A number of studies on the effects of nanomatrials in *in vitro* and *in vivo* systems have been published. Currently cytotoxicity of different nanoparticles is assessed using the 3-(4,5-dimethylthiazol-2-yl)-2,5-diphenyltetrazolium bromide (MTT) assay on different cell lines to determine cell viability, a tedious and expensive method. The aim of this study was to evaluate the *Artemia salina* test in comparison with the MTT assay in the assessment of cytotoxicity of nanostructures because the former method is more rapid and convenient and less expensive.

Methods: At the first stage, toxicity of different nanoparticles with different concentrations (1.56–400 µg/mL) was measured by means of the brine shrimp lethality test. At the second stage, the effect of nanoparticles on the viability of the L929 cell line was assessed using the MTT assay. Experiments were conducted with each concentration in triplicate.

Results: The results obtained from both tests (*A. salina* test and MTT assay) did not have statistically significant differences ($P > 0.05$).

Conclusions: These findings suggest that the *A. salina* test may expedite toxicity experiments and decrease costs, and therefore, may be considered an alternative to the *in vitro* cell culture assay.

Keywords: *Artemia salina*, Toxicity, Nanoparticle, Cell culture

Background

Nanoscience is a novel science that is being developed to probe and manipulate matter on the scale of single atoms and molecules. Physicist Richard P. Feynman was the first to mention molecular machines built with atomic precision at a meeting of the American Physical Society in 1959 [1], and Noro Taniguchi, a professor at the University of Tokyo, coined the term nanotechnology in 1979 [2]. Nanotechnology is the use of nanoscience to design NMs (nanomaterials) and NPs (nanoparticles), with structural components between 1 and 100 nanometers; it is thought to be one of the key technologies of the 21st century [3,4]. In the above range, physicochemical characteristics of NPs in biological systems can vary. Some potential hazards have been identified in the life cycle

of NMs and NPs [5,6]. Growing research and development in nanotechnology have resulted in the identification of many unique properties of nanomaterials such as enhanced magnetic, catalytic, optical, electrical, and mechanical properties when compared to conventional formulations of the same materials [7]. While nanoparticles have a wide variety of functions, there has been increasing issues and debate amongst the regulatory and scientific community regarding the fate of nanoparticles in biological systems and associated side effects these agents might have on living organisms [8-12]. These materials are increasingly used for commercial purposes and leading to direct and indirect exposure of humans [13]. Any *in vivo* use of nanoparticles requires thorough understanding of the kinetics and toxicology of the particles, establishment of principles and test procedures to ensure safe manufacture and usage of nanomaterials, and comprehensive training of personnel in safety and potential hazards of nanotechnology [13]. Nanotoxicology research is applied

* Correspondence: ramazania@zums.ac.ir
[1]Cell and Molecular Biology Departments, Pharmaceutical Sciences Branch, Islamic Azad University, Tehran, Iran
[2]Biotechnology Departments, School of Pharmacy, Zanjan University of Medical Sciences, Zanjan, Iran
Full list of author information is available at the end of the article

to various fields including biology and pathology, but typically to pharmacology and to the use of NMs and nanodevices for diagnostic and therapeutic purposes. Therefore, a key goal for toxicologists is to identify *in vitro* and *in vivo* assays accurately reflecting the ability of NPs to induce toxic effects in the humans and in the environment. In addition, standardized tests for both *in vitro* and *in vivo* studies are needed to develop better and more rapid screening techniques and to predict toxicity [14,15]. The cytotoxicity effects of NPs were investigated in a multitude of animal models by means of *in vivo* tests employing the typical NP exposure routes, i.e., pulmonary, oral, dermal, and injection based [16]. The cost and labor intensiveness of the *in vivo* studies have led researchers to the use of *in vitro* methods for assessment of NPs cytotoxicity. In addition, animal rights advocates have criticized the use of animals in nanotechnology experiments. All *in vivo* studies must be conducted with the approval of regulatory bodies such as IACUC (an Institutional Animal Care and Use Committee) to ensure ethical treatment of animals [16]. For the above reasons, *in vitro* techniques are increasingly used for the analysis of cytotoxicity of NPs including cell culture, the WST-1 assay [17,18], XTT assay, MTT assay [19,20], LDH assay, BrdU assay, and fluorescence microscopy [21,22]. Currently, cytotoxicity testing of various NPs in cell culture involves the MTT assay, which determines cell viability based on mitochondrial function by measuring the activity of mitochondrial enzymes [23-27]. In this test, tetrazolium is reduced by mitochondrial succinate dehydrogenase of live cells to water-insoluble purple formazan crystals, which are subsequently solubilized using an organic solvent (e.g., dimethyl sulfoxide; DMSO) [28]. The cell viability is quantified based on absorbance of the solution at 570 nm. Therefore, the MTT assay requires solubilization steps with tetrazolium, which is toxic to cells and can interfere with some chemical reactions [28]. The cytotoxicity assays are often tedious and expensive, and there is a lack of a simple and rapid screening procedure. Nowadays, brine shrimp lethality assays are extensively used in research and applied toxicology [29]. There is a tendency to use an *Artemia salina* assay in toxicological tests that screen a large number of extracts for drug discovery in medicinal plants [30-33]. This is because in this case, aseptic techniques are not required, and thus *A. salina* assays could replace the more ethically challenging MTT assay that requires animal serum [34]. This assay was proposed by Michael and coworkers in 1959 and was later adopted by many laboratories as a method for preliminary estimation of toxicity [35]. *Artemia* is one of the most valuable test organisms available for ecotoxicity testing, and the available research suggests that several applications of *Artemia* to toxicology and ecotoxicology will continue to be used

widely [36]. Because of the rapidity, convenience, and low cost of *Artemia*-based assays, we decided to evaluate the *A. salina* test in comparison with the MTT assay in the assessment of cytotoxicity of different classes of NPs.

Materials and methods
Materials
Fetal bovine serum (FBS), phosphate-buffered saline (PBS), trypsin, penicillin, streptomycin, DMSO, 3-[4,5-dimethyl-thiazol-2-yl]-2,5-diphenyl tetrazolium bromide (MTT), Triton X-100, and the RPMI-1640 medium supplemented with 10% heat inactivated FBS were purchased from Sigma–Aldrich. The mouse fibroblast cell line (L929) was provided by Pasteur Institute of Iran.

Synthesis of NPs
Sixteen NPs from different classes (Table 1) were prepared by the Nanotechnology Laboratory of School of Pharmacy of Zanjan University of Medical Sciences. The zeta potential and particle size distribution of the prepared nanoparticles were determined by photon correlation spectroscopy (PCS) using a Nano/zetasizer (Malvern Instruments, Nano ZS, Worcestershire, UK) working on the dynamic light scattering (DLS) platform.

Cell culture and determination of cytotoxicity by MTT assay
The effect of NPs on the viability of L929 cells was assessed by means of the MTT assay. After thawing, the cells were cultured in the RPMI 1640 medium containing 10% FBS, penicillin (100 units/mL), and streptomycin (100 mg/mL) at 37°C in a humidified 5% CO_2 incubator. The cells were seeded in a 96-well plate at a density of 5,000 cells per well (the cells were stained with trypan blue and counted with haemocytometer). These cells were incubated overnight at 37°C before the cell viability test. A stock suspension of each NP at 50 mg/mL in distilled water was prepared. After that, fresh suspensions of different concentrations of NPs (two fold serial dilutions from 1.56–400 µg/mL) were made using serial dilution of the stock suspensions of NPs in the RPMI 1640 medium, immediately before use. We added 200 µL of a suspension (different concentrations of NPs) to each well of the microtiter plates. The cells were incubated for 24 h under the same conditions. Wells without any NPs served as a negative control. The experiments were performed in triplicate for each concentration. To assess cell survival, 100 µL of an MTT solution (2 mg/mL in PBS) was added to each well and incubated for 3 h at 37°C to produce insoluble formazan. Then, 100 µL of DMSO was added to dissolve formazan crystals, and the absorbance was measured on an Infinite M200 microplate reader (Tecan) at 570 nm, with 630 nm as a reference wavelength. The percentage of cell viability

Table 1 Names and characteristics of NPs used in this study

NPs class	NPs name	Size NPs (nm)	Zeta potential (mV)
Inorganic nanoparticles	Magnetic	55	- 31
	Nanosfer	97	+8.9
Lipid-base nanoparticles	Liposome	139.3	- 28
	Coated SLNs	464.6	+20
	Uncoated SLNs	176.3	- 45
	Nanogele + SLN	376.6	+4
Polymeric nanoparticles	Nanogele	270	+22
	Micellar	97.9	- 1.10
	PAMAM (G5)	6	+36.8
	PAMAM-FA	55	+36.4
	PAMAM-PEG-FA	70	9.12
Drug nanoparticles	Nanosuspansion Atorvastatin	269.8	ND
	Nanosuspansion Ibuprofen	160.9	ND
	Nanosuspansion Repaglinide	260.6	ND
	Nanosuspansion Cyclosporin	220.5	ND
	Nanosuspansion Azitromycin	270	ND

ND; not determined.

was calculated using the formula $(A_{test}/A_{control}) \times 100$, where A_{test} is the mean absorbance of treated cells and $A_{control}$ is the mean absorbance of a negative control.

Toxicity testing by *A. salina*

A. salina eggs were purchased from the Aquatic Animal Research Center, Urmia University, Urmia, Iran. Dried cysts were placed in a bottle containing artificial sea water which was prepared by dissolving 35 g of sodium chloride in 1 L of distilled water. After 36–48 h incubation at room temperature (28–30°C) under conditions of strong aeration and continuous illuminations [33], the larvae (nauplii) hatched within 48 h.

The evaluation of cytotoxicity of NPs in *A. salina* was performed according to the previous methods [30,33,37,38]. The assay was carried out on larvae of brine shrimp (*A. salina* Leach.). A stock solution of 50 mg of nanoparticles in 1 mL of distilled water was prepared. Then, fresh suspensions with different concentrations of NPs (two fold serial dilutions from 1.56–400 µg/mL) were made by means of serial dilution of the stock suspensions of NPs in artificial sea water (35 g/L) immediately before use. We added 200 µL of a suspension (different concentrations of NPs) to each well of the 96-well microtiter plates. After that, 10 nauplii per well were added in the 96-well plates and incubated at room temperature for 24 h. The numbers of surviving nauplii in each well were counted under a stereoscopic microscope after 24 h. The experiments were conducted in triplicate for each concentration. The negative control wells contained 10 nauplii and artificial sea water only.

The percentages of deaths were calculated by comparing the number of survivors in the test and control wells. The lethality was calculated using Abbott's formula as follows: % Lethality = [(Test – Control)/Control] × 100.

Statistical analysis

All experiments were done in triplicate and the results were calculated as a mean ± standard deviation (SD). The experimental data were processed using the paired sample *t*-test, Pearson correlation and linear regression analysis of the SPSS version 16.0 software for Windows. The toxicity of each nanoparticle was calculated from the 50% lethality dose (LD_{50}) by means of Finney's Probit analysis [39].

Results

Cytotoxicity of nanostructures by the MTT assay

The MTT assay is a viable method for assessing *in vitro* cytotoxicity of NPs. In this study, L929 cells were treated with different concentrations (0.78–200 µg/mL) of the 16 NPs (Table 1). Cell viability was determined 24 hours after the treatment. The results are presented in Table 2. Uncoated solid lipid nanoparticles (SLNs), Nanogel + SLN, Bare Nanogel, polyamidoamine (PAMAM; G5), and PAMAM-FA demonstrated moderate cytotoxicity. In contrast, the NPs with $IC_{50} > 200$ µg/mL were not toxic to the L929 cell line. The cytotoxicity was weak when the IC_{50} values were between 150 and 200 µg/mL.

Cytotoxicity of nanostructures in the brine shrimp assay

The brine shrimp lethality assay was also used to determine the cytotoxicity of NPs. According to the results

Table 2 NPs toxicity assay by *Artemia salina* and MTT assay

NPs name	*Artemia salina* assay, LC$_{50}$ (µg/m)	95% confidence limits for concentration		MTT assay, IC$_{50}$ (µg/ml)	95% confidence limits for concentration	
		Lower bound	Upper bound		Lower bound	Upper bound
Magnetic	698.710	431.764	2669.870	997.402	527.931	3340.601
Nanosfer	302.001	215.853	497.009	207.431	141.862	365.065
Liposome	751.249	432.851	6492.955	1002.666	543.931	4358.603
Coated SLNs	360.594	285.519	501.000	605.594	472.900	1248.021
Uncoated SLNs	239.040	192.979	310.917	149.018	90.886	328.486
Nanogele + SLN	19.656	15.141	24.908	113.903	58.153	380.573
Nanogele	40.440	8.221	95.196	130.171	77.672	285.277
Micellar	560.060	352.592	1801.667	686.002	263.396	1329.851
PAMAM (G5)	145.6	60.435	671.764	72.254	41.149	139.077
PAMAM-FA	213.316	185.467	839.316	99.783	61.360	130.925
PAMAM-PEG-FA	401.21	256.482	1002.310	270.585	129.042	496.556
Nanosuspansion Atorvastatin	417.349	272.658	1046.615	807.668	301.840	1080.114
Nanosuspansion Ibuprofen	373.526	285.877	559.357	156.433	117.536	244.043
Nanosuspansion Repaglinide	807.754	488.424	4335.993	297.756	221.995	527.574
Nanosuspansion Cyclosporin	531.961	368.036	1095.239	167.965	108.493	230.459
Nanosuspansion Azitromycin	110.316	57.555	231.560	162.512	168.114	249.652

(Table 2), of the 16 NPs that we screened for lethality in *A. salina*, only two NPs (Nanogel + SLN and Nanogel) showed strong toxicity (LC$_{50}$ < 100 µg/mL). In contrast, NPs of Uncoated SLN, PAMAM (G5), Nanosuspension Ibuprofen, and Nanosuspension Azithromycin exhibited moderate cytotoxicity (LC$_{50}$ ranged between 100 and 500 µg/mL), and the other NPs showed weak cytotoxicity in *A. salina* (LC$_{50}$ range 500–1000 µg/mL) [37,40]. Comparison between the results of two methods is indicated in Figure 1. As shown in Figure 1, the trend lines and the direction of the graphs are in same direction.

Discussion

Several assays for eco-toxicological testing of nanomaterials have been developed. Different model systems such as bacteria [41], fathead minnows [42], zebrafish embryos [43], copepod [44], Daphnia [45,46], and rainbow trout [47,48] have been reported [49]. In addition to standard tests, there is a need to establish better, rapid and convenient methods to predict the toxic effects of nanomaterials. Till now, A few studies have reported the toxicity effect of nanomaterials on *A. salina* [38,50-52]. These studies were investigated on metal nanoparticles

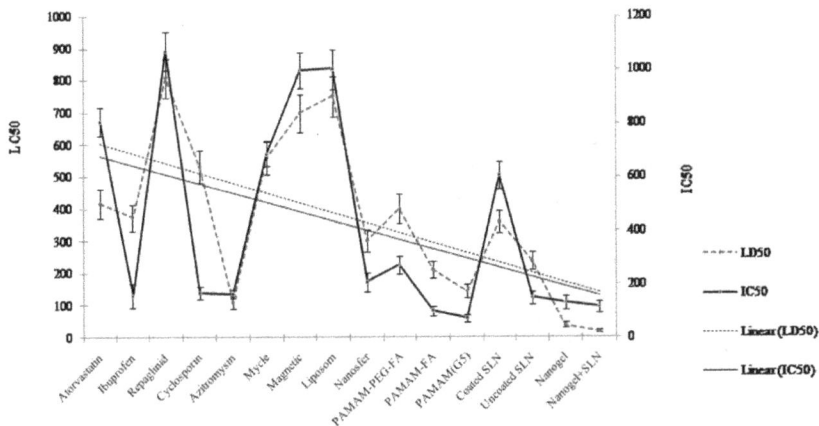

Figure 1 Comparison of *Artemia salina* and MTT assay results

and we want develop the *A. salina* assay for toxicity assessment of different class of nanomaterials especially those used for drug deliveries.

In this work, cytotoxicity of 16 NPs was assessed using two methods: the brine shrimp lethality assay and the MTT assay in L929 cells. According to the results (Figure 1) the correlation between the LC_{50} and IC_{50} values is significant ($R^2 = 0.72$, $P = 0.000$). This mean that 72% variability noted in MTT method could be accounted for by brine shrimp lethality assay and 28% is unaccounted for due to measurement error. There was not statistically significant difference between two assays when the results were compared with paired t test ($P = 0.402$). Also the comparison between LC_{50} and IC_{50} mean values statistically analyzed by chi square test and the result showed that there is no differences between two assay methods (P = 0.235). This mean that results obtained by brine shrimp lethality assay is comparable with MTT results. Both the ranking and the degree of cytotoxicity were similar between the brine shrimp lethality assay and the MTT assay. As it has been shown in Table 2, the ranges of 95% confidence limit are wide. The width of the confidence interval for an individual study depends to a large extent on the sample size. Larger studies tend to give more precise estimates of effects (and hence have narrower confidence intervals) than smaller studies. In order to obtain a more reliable estimate of the confidence interval it may be necessary to perform several independent assays and to combine these into one single confidence interval [53]. The results demonstrate the ability of the brine shrimp lethality assay to accurately quantify cytotoxicity of NPs and to replace the MTT assay, which is expensive and tedious. In this field, cytotoxicity assays and experimental procedures often lack a simple, convenient, and rapid screening method. On the other hand, the brine shrimp lethality assay has been used in toxicology research routinely for over thirty years [36]. The genus *Artemia* has a several advantages that make it ideal for general toxicity assays including wide geographical distribution, adaptability to extreme conditions, capability to use several nutrient resources, and availability of their cysts for collection [36]. The brine shrimp assay is convenient because it is rapid (24 h), economical, and simple. The eggs of *A. salina* are readily available at low cost and remain viable for years in dry storage. The assay easily accommodates a large number of nauplii for statistical validation and no special equipment is needed. Moreover, this assay does not require animal serum and thereby it prevents unnecessary use of animals in scientific experiments. In summary, it is possible to measure cytotoxicity of NPs using the brine shrimp lethality assay instead of the common *in vitro* cell culture assays.

Conclusion

This work shows that the brine shrimp lethality assay can be used to study toxicity of nanostructures. Self-sufficiency

and rapid results are important advantages of this method. *Artemia*-based toxicity assay of NPs are cheap, continuously available, simple and reliable and are thus an important answer to routine needs of toxicity screening, for industrial monitoring requirements or for regulatory purposes. Our data are expected to facilitate pharmacological and nanotoxicological research.

Competing interests
The authors declare that they have no competing interests.

Authors' contributions
SR carried out the experiments and drafted the manuscript. AR designed the study and participated in data analysis. MH participated in study design. TN helped in study design and manuscript preparation. All authors read and approved the final manuscript.

Acknowledgments
We thank the research deputy of Zanjan University of Medical Sciences (ZUMS) for financial support of this project.

Author details
[1]Cell and Molecular Biology Departments, Pharmaceutical Sciences Branch, Islamic Azad University, Tehran, Iran. [2]Biotechnology Departments, School of Pharmacy, Zanjan University of Medical Sciences, Zanjan, Iran. [3]Zanjan Pharmaceutical Nanotechnology Research Center, Zanjan University of Medical Sciences, Zanjan, Iran.

References
1.   Toumey CP. Reading Feynman into nanotechnology. Techné: Res Philos Technol. 2009;12:133–68.
2.   Singh M, Manikandan S, Kumaraguru A. Nanoparticles: a new technology with wide applications. Res J Nanosci Nanotechnol. 2011;1:1–11.
3.   Lloyd SM, Lave LB, Matthews HS. Life cycle benefits of using nanotechnology to stabilize platinum-group metal particles in automotive catalysts. Environ Sci Technol. 2005;39:1384–92.
4.   Yadav A, Ghune M, Jain DK. Nano-medicine based drug delivery system. J Advanced Pharm Educ Res. 2011;1:201–13.
5.   Drobne D. Nanotoxicology for safe and sustainable nanotechnology. Arh Hig Rada Toksikol. 2007;58:471–8.
6.   Ikramullah A, Salve D, Pai G, Rathore M, Joshi D. In vitro cytotoxicity testing of silver nano-particals in lymphocyte and sperm cells. Ind J Fund Appl Life Sci. 2013;3:44–7.
7.   Arora S, Rajwade JM, Paknikar KM. Nanotoxicology and in vitro studies: the need of the hour. Toxicol Appl Pharmacol. 2012;258:151–65.
8.   Sharma A, Madhunapantula SV, Robertson GP. Toxicological considerations when creating nanoparticle-based drugs and drug delivery systems. Expert Opin Drug Metab Toxicol. 2012;8:47–69.
9.   Hsieh SF, Bello D, Schmidt DF, Pal AK, Rogers EJ. Biological oxidative damage by carbon nanotubes: fingerprint or footprint? Nanotoxicology. 2012;6:61–76.
10. Wessels A, Van Berlo D, Boots AW, Gerloff K, Scherbart AM, Cassee FR, et al. Oxidative stress and DNA damage responses in rat and mouse lung to inhaled carbon nanoparticles. Nanotoxicology. 2011;5:66–78.
11. Mogharabi M, Abdollahi M, Faramarzi M. Toxicity of nanomaterials; an undermined issue. Daru. 2014;22:59.
12. Mostafalou S, Mohammadi H, Ramazani A, Abdollahi M. Different biokinetics of nanomedicines linking to their toxicity; an overview. Daru. 2013;21:14.
13. Nel A, Xia T, Madler L, Li N. Toxic potential of materials at the nanolevel. Science. 2006;311:622–7.
14. Dhawan A, Sharma V. Toxicity assessment of nanomaterials: methods and challenges. Anal Bioanal Chem. 2010;398:589–605.
15. Maccormack TJ, Clark RJ, Dang MK, Ma G, Kelly JA, Veinot JG, et al. Inhibition of enzyme activity by nanomaterials: potential mechanisms and implications for nanotoxicity testing. Nanotoxicology. 2012;6:514–25.

16. Suh WH, Suslick KS, Stucky GD, Suh YH. Nanotechnology, nanotoxicology, and neuroscience. Prog Neurobiol. 2009;87:133–70.

17. Dechsakulthorn F, Hayes A, Bakand S, Joeng L, Winder C. In vitro cytotoxicity assessment of selected nanoparticles using human skin fibroblasts. AATEX. 2007;14:397–400.

18. Gonzales M, Mitsumori LM, Kushleika JV, Rosenfeld ME, Krishnan KM. Cytotoxicity of iron oxide nanoparticles made from the thermal decomposition of organometallics and aqueous phase transfer with Pluronic F127. Contrast Media Mol Imaging. 2010;5:286–93.

19. Zanette C, Pelin M, Crosera M, Adami G, Bovenzi M, Larese FF, et al. Silver nanoparticles exert a long-lasting antiproliferative effect on human keratinocyte HaCaT cell line. Toxicol In Vitro. 2011;25:1053–60.

20. Sauer UG, Vogel S, Hess A, Kolle SN, Ma-Hock L, van Ravenzwaay B, et al. In vivo-in vitro comparison of acute respiratory tract toxicity using human 3D airway epithelial models and murine 3T3 monolayer cell systems. Toxicol In Vitro. 2013;27:174–90.

21. Decker T, Lohmann-Matthes ML. A quick and simple method for the quantitation of lactate dehydrogenase release in measurements of cellular cytotoxicity and tumor necrosis factor (TNF) activity. J Immunol Methods. 1988;115:61–9.

22. Korzeniewski C, Callewaert DM. An enzyme-release assay for natural cytotoxicity. J Immunol Methods. 1983;64:313–20.

23. Alley MC, Scudiero DA, Monks A, Hursey ML, Czerwinski MJ, Fine DL, et al. Feasibility of drug screening with panels of human tumor cell lines using a microculture tetrazolium assay. Cancer Res. 1988;48:589–601.

24. Campling BG, Pym J, Baker HM, Cole SP, Lam YM. Chemosensitivity testing of small cell lung cancer using the MTT assay. Br J Cancer. 1991;63:75–83.

25. Fisichella M, Dabboue H, Bhattacharyya S, Saboungi ML, Salvetat JP, Hevor T, et al. Mesoporous silica nanoparticles enhance MTT formazan exocytosis in HeLa cells and astrocytes. Toxicol In Vitro. 2009;23:697–703.

26. Silva GA. Introduction to nanotechnology and its applications to medicine. Surg Neurol. 2004;61:216–20.

27. Wang H, Cheng H, Wang F, Wei D, Wang X. An improved 3-(4,5-dimethyl-thiazol-2-yl)-2,5-diphenyl tetrazolium bromide (MTT) reduction assay for evaluating the viability of Escherichia coli cells. J Microbiol Methods. 2010;82:330–3.

28. Berridge MV, Herst PM, Tan AS. Tetrazolium dyes as tools in cell biology: new insights into their cellular reduction. Biotechnol Annu Rev. 2005;11:127–52.

29. Costa-Lotufo LV, Khan MT, Ather A, Wilke DV, Jimenez PC, Pessoa C, et al. Studies of the anticancer potential of plants used in Bangladeshi folk medicine. J Ethnopharmacol. 2005;99:21–30.

30. Kheiri Manjili H, Jafari H, Ramazani A, Davoudi N. Anti-leishmanial and toxicity activities of some selected Iranian medicinal plants. Parasitol Res. 2012;111:2115–21.

31. Ramazani A, Sardari S, Zakeri S, Vaziri B. In vitro antiplasmodial and phytochemical study of five Artemisia species from Iran and in vivo activity of two species. Parasitol Res. 2010;107:593–9.

32. Ramazani A, Zakeri S, Sardari S, Khodakarim N, Djadidt ND. In vitro and in vivo anti-malarial activity of Boerhavia elegans and Solanum surattense. Malar J. 2010;9:124.

33. Sangian H, Faramarzi H, Yazdinezhad A, Mousavi SJ, Zamani Z, Noubarani M, et al. Antiplasmodial activity of ethanolic extracts of some selected medicinal plants from the northwest of Iran. Parasitol Res. 2013;112:3697–701.

34. Mclaughlin JL, Rogers LL, Anderson JE. The use of biological assays to evaluate botanicals. Drug Inf J. 1998;32:513–24.

35. Insanu M, Anggadiredja J, Kayser O. Curcacycline A and B–new pharmacological insights to an old drug. Int J Appl Res Nat Prod. 2012;5:26–34.

36. Nunes BS, Carvalho FD, Guilhermino LM, Van Stappen G. Use of the genus Artemia in ecotoxicity testing. Environ Pollut. 2006;144:453–62.

37. Meyer BN, Ferrigni NR, Putnam JE, Jacobsen LB, Nichols DE, McLaughlin JL. Brine shrimp: a convenient general bioassay for active plant constituents. Planta Med. 1982;45:31–4.

38. Ashtari K, Khajeh K, Fasihi J, Ashtari P, Ramazani A, Vali H. Silica-encapsulated magnetic nanoparticles: enzyme immobilization and cytotoxic study. Int J Biol Macromol. 2012;50:1063–9.

39. Finney DJ. The adjustment for a natural response rate in probit analysis. Ann Appl Biol. 1949;36:187–95.

40. Padmaja R, Arun PC, Prashanth D, Deepak M, Amit A, Anjana M. Brine shrimp lethality bioassay of selected Indian medicinal plants. Fitoterapia. 2002;73:508–10.

41. Lyon DY, Fortner JD, Sayes CM, Colvin VL, Hughe JB. Bacterial cell association and antimicrobial activity of a C60 water suspension. Environ Toxicol Chem. 2005;24:2757–62.

42. Zhu S, Oberdorster E, Haasch ML. Toxicity of an engineered nanoparticle (fullerene, C60) in two aquatic species, Daphnia and fathead minnow. Mar Environ Res. 2006;62(Suppl):S5–9.

43. Zhu X, Zhu L, Li Y, Duan Z, Chen W, Alvarez PJ. Developmental toxicity in zebrafish (Danio rerio) embryos after exposure to manufactured nanomaterials: buckminsterfullerene aggregates (nC60) and fullerol. Environ Toxicol Chem. 2007;26:976–9.

44. Templeton RC, Ferguson PL, Washburn KM, Scrivens WA, Chandler GT. Life-cycle effects of single-walled carbon nanotubes (SWNTs) on an estuarine meiobenthic copepod. Environ Sci Technol. 2006;40:7387–93.

45. Hund-Rinke K, Simon M. Ecotoxic effect of photocatalytic active nanoparticles (TiO2) on algae and daphnids. Environ Sci Pollut Res Int. 2006;13:225–32.

46. Roberts AP, Mount AS, Seda B, Souther J, Qiao R, Lin S, et al. In vivo biomodification of lipid-coated carbon nanotubes by Daphnia magna. Environ Sci Technol. 2007;41:3025–9.

47. Smith CJ, Shaw BJ, Handy RD. Toxicity of single walled carbon nanotubes to rainbow trout, (Oncorhynchus mykiss): respiratory toxicity, organ pathologies, and other physiological effects. Aquat Toxicol. 2007;82:94–109.

48. Fraser TW, Reinardy HC, Shaw BJ, Henry TB, Handy RD. Dietary toxicity of single-walled carbon nanotubes and fullerenes (C60) in rainbow trout (Oncorhynchus mykiss). Nanotoxicology. 2011;5:98–108.

49. Ambrosone A, Marchesano V, Mazzarella V, Tortiglione C. Nanotoxicology using the sea anemone Nematostella vectensis: from developmental toxicity to genotoxicology. Nanotoxicology. 2014;8:508–20.

50. Cornejo-Garrido H, Kibanova D, Nieto-Camacho A, Guzman J, Ramirez-Apan T, Fernandez-Lomelin P, et al. Oxidative stress, cytoxicity, and cell mortality induced by nano-sized lead in aqueous suspensions. Chemosphere. 2011;84:1329–35.

51. Ates M, Daniels J, Arslan Z, Farah IO. Effects of aqueous suspensions of titanium dioxide nanoparticles on Artemia salina: assessment of nanoparticle aggregation, accumulation, and toxicity. Environ Monit Assess. 2013;185:3339–48.

52. Pretti C, Oliva M, Pietro RD, Monni G, Cevasco G, Chiellini F, et al. Ecotoxicity of pristine graphene to marine organisms. Ecotoxicol Environ Saf. 2014;101:138–45.

53. Hong W, Meier P, Deininger R. Estimation of a single probit line from multiple toxicity test data. Aquat Toxicol. 1988;12:193–202.

20

Molecular docking and inhibition studies on the interactions of *Bacopa monnieri*'s potent phytochemicals against pathogenic *Staphylococcus aureus*

Talha Bin Emran[1,2*], Md Atiar Rahman[2], Mir Muhammad Nasir Uddin[3], Raju Dash[1], Md Firoz Hossen[1], Mohammad Mohiuddin[1] and Md Rashadul Alam[1]

Abstract

Background: *Bacopa monnieri* Linn. (Plantaginaceae), a well-known medicinal plant, is widely used in traditional medicine system. It has long been used in gastrointestinal discomfort, skin diseases, epilepsy and analgesia. This research investigated the *in vitro* antimicrobial activity of *Bacopa monnieri* leaf extract against *Staphylococcus aureus* and the interaction of possible compounds involved in this antimicrobial action.

Methods: Non-edible plant parts were extracted with ethanol and evaporated *in vacuo* to obtain the crude extract. A zone of inhibition studies and the minimum inhibitory concentration (MIC) of plant extracts were evaluated against clinical isolates by the microbroth dilution method. Docking study was performed to analyze and identify the interactions of possible antimicrobial compounds of *Bacopa monnieri* in the active site of penicillin binding protein and DNA gyrase through GOLD 4.12 software.

Results: A zone of inhibition studies showed significant ($p < 0.05$) inhibition capacity of different concentrations of *Bacopa monnieri*'s extract against *Staphylococcus aureus*. The extract also displayed very remarkable minimum inhibitory concentrations (≥ 16 µg/ml) which was significant compared to that (≥ 75 µg/ml) of the reference antibiotic against the experimental strain *Staphylococcus aureus*. Docking studies recommended that luteolin, an existing phytochemical of *Bacopa monnieri*, has the highest fitness score and more specificity towards the DNA gyrase binding site rather than penicillin binding protein.

Conclusions: *Bacopa monnieri* extract and its compound luteolin have a significant antimicrobial activity against *Staphylococcus aureus*. Molecular binding interaction of an *in silico* data demonstrated that luteolin has more specificity towards the DNA gyrase binding site and could be a potent antimicrobial compound.

Keywords: *Bacopa monnieri* L, *Staphylococcus aureus*, Antibacterial activity, MIC, Molecular docking, GOLD, *in silico* drug discovery

* Correspondence: talhabmb@gmail.com
[1]Department of Pharmacy, BGC Trust University Bangladesh, Chittagong 4000, Bangladesh
[2]Department of Biochemistry and Molecular Biology, University of Chittagong, Chittagong 4331, Bangladesh
Full list of author information is available at the end of the article

Background

Effective therapeutic options to combat *Staphylococcus aureus* infection are still limited. And this makes a major burden to control *Staphylococcus aureus* [1]. *S. aureus* is a commensal Gram-positive bacterium, which colonizes in human nasal mucosa either permanently or transiently [2], causing severe infections eventually [3,4]. But the clinical symptoms are not visualized until the immune system is affected [5]. However, the major problem in controlling the *S. aureus* infection is the occurrence of multi-drug resistance produced mainly due to the misuse of antibiotics. This is also caused by the treatment of non-bacterial infections with antibiotics or inadequate compliance with the regulations for drug ingestion. Therefore, new therapeutic molecule is an urgence to be introduced as antibiotic in the treatment of multi-drug resistant *S. aureus*. Several studies have proposed that phytocompounds are the best alternative to develop therapies for multidrug resistant bacterial infections [6-8].

Bacopa monnieri (L.) Wellst. (Family: Plantaginaceae) is known as *Herpestis monniera*. It is a water hyssop or "Brahmi" and is reputed as Ayurvedic medicine. It is used for gastrointestinal discomfort, rejuvenation, promoting memory and intellect, skin disorders, epilepsy, pyrexia and analgesia [9]. Number of biologically active compounds has been isolated from this plant. GC-MS analysis of the leaf extract of this plant showed the presence of tetracyclic triterpenoids, saponin, bacosides A and B phytosterols, hersaponin, D-mannitol, flavonoids viz., luteolin-7-glucoside, apigenin-7-glucocronide, alkaloids such as nicotine and herpestine, betulic acid, β-sitosterol, stigma-sterol and its esters, aspartic acid, glutamic acid and serine [10]. Despite enormous possibilities of this plant, no compound-activity relationship study has been conducted yet to investigate the phytochemicals responsible for its antimicrobial action. This research evaluates the *in vitro* antimicrobial activity of *B. monnieri* against *S. aureus* establishing the interaction of existing phytocompounds involved in this antimicrobial activity through *an in silico* molecular docking analysis [11,12].

Methods

Media and chemicals

Mueller-Hinton broth and agar media (Hi media, India; final pH 7.3 ± 0.2 at 25°C), was used for the determination of MIC and antibacterial activity. Tetracycline (50 µg/disk) and ampicillin disks (50 µg/disk) were procured from Oxoid, England.

Collection and identification of plant materials

The plant *B. monnieri* was selected by Talha Bin Emran, Lecturer, Department of Pharmacy, BGC Trust University Bangladesh. Fresh leaves of *B. monnieri* were collected from the Chittagong University hilly forest on December 2013. The plant was identified by Dr. Shaikh Bokhtear Uddin, Taxonomist and Associate Professor, Department of Botany, University of Chittagong-4331, Bangladesh. A voucher specimen (Accession Number: 36285) containing the identification characteristics of the plant has been preserved in the Bangladesh National Herbarium for future reference.

Preparation of crude ethanol extract

The fresh leaves of *B. monnieri* were washed immediately after collection and chopped into small pieces, air dried and ground (Moulinex Blender AK-241, Moulinex, France) into powder (40-80 mesh, 500 g). The resulting powder was soaked in an Erlenmeyer flask of absolute ethanol (2.0 L, at room temperature) and left for seven days allowing occasional stirring of the flask. Filtrate obtained through cheesecloth and Whatman filter paper No. 1 was concentrated under reduced pressure at the temperature below 50°C using a rotatory evaporator (RE 200, Bibby Sterling Ltd., UK). The extracts (yield 4.4 - 5.6% w/w) were all placed in glass Petri dishes (90 × 15 mm, Pyrex, Germany) to allow an air-dry for complete evaporation of solvent.

Study of antibacterial activity

Bacterial strain

Gram-positive *Staphylococcus aureus* (ATCC6538) was used for screening the antibacterial effect of the plant extract. Bacterial strain was collected from the Microbiology Division of Bangladesh Council of Scientific and Industrial Research (BCSIR), Chittagong-4220, Bangladesh.

Preparation of sample solutions

Small amount (1, 2 and 3 mg) of solid sample was dissolved in a definite volume (1 ml) of DMSO to make a solution of 1 mg/ml. DMSO was chosen as solvent because it does not have any inhibitory effect on bacterial cultures and it has extraordinary capacity to dissolve solid sample completely.

Media preparation

The bacterial strain was grown and maintained on Standard Nutrient Agar (DIFCO) media (Hi media, India) at 37°C and pH 7.3 ± 0.2. The bacterium was sub-cultured overnight in nutrient agar broth which was further adjusted to obtain turbidity comparable to McFarland (0.5) standard when required. Test tube slants of nutrient agar medium were prepared for the maintenance of culture. Then a small amount of the collected microorganism was transferred to the test tubes with the help of sterilized needles. A number of test tubes were freshly cleaned for bacterial pathogen. The inoculated slants were inoculated at temperature below laboratory condition.

Antibacterial screening through disk diffusion technique

The antibacterial activity of the extract was determined by disk diffusion technique (National Committee for Clinical Laboratory Standards, NCCLS, 2002). The test microbes were taken from the broth culture with inoculating loop and transferred to test tubes containing 5.0 ml sterile distilled water. The inoculums were added until the turbidity was equal to 0.5 McFarland standards. Cotton swab was then used to inoculate the test tube suspension onto the surface of the Muller Hinton agar plate and the uniformly swabbed plates were then allowed to dry. On the dry inoculated surfaces prepared paper disks were placed as follows. Sterilized Whatman paper disks (6 mm in diameter) were prepared previously by punching the filter paper with the help of a punch machine. After that the disks were placed upon 0.5 ml of the desired solution (1, 2 and 3 mg/disk) of the extract. After each application the disks were allowed to the temperature 40°C (one minute) for drying purposes. The disks containing plant extract were placed with blunt-nosed thumb forceps on the inoculated plates at equidistance in a circle. These plates were kept for 4-6 h at a low temperature (<8°C) to allow for diffusion of the extract from the disk into the medium. The same was done for negative control (ethanol). The plates were incubated at 37°C for 24 h. The experiment was conducted in triplicates. Antimicrobial activity was determined by a measurement of the inhibition zone diameter (mm) around each test organism.

Minimum inhibitory concentration (MIC) determination

Minimum inhibitory concentration was determined by the microdilution method using serially diluted (2 folds) plant extract according to the National Committee for Clinical Laboratory Standards (NCCLS) (National Committee for Clinical Laboratory Standards, 2000). The MIC of the extract was determined by the dilution of *B. monnieri* extract with the concentrations of 0.0-25, 0.0-50, 0.0-75, 0.0-100, 0.0-125, and 0.0-150 µg/ml. Equal volume of each extract and nutrient broth was mixed in a test tube. Specifically 0.1 ml of standardized inoculum ($1\text{-}2 \times 10^7$ cfu/ml) was added in each tube. The tubes were incubated aerobically at 37°C for 18-24 h. Two control tubes were maintained for each test batch. These included antibiotic control (a tube containing extract and growth media without inoculum) and organism control (a tube containing the growth medium, saline and the inoculum). The lowest concentration (highest dilution) of the extract that produced no visible bacterial growth (no turbidity) was considered as MIC.

Statistical analysis

All data are presented as mean ± standard deviation (SD). The data were analyzed by a statistical software statistical package for social science (SPSS, version 18.0, IBM Corporation, NY, USA) using Tukey's multiple range *post hoc* tests. The values were considered significantly different at $p < 0.05$.

Docking approach

To have a better understanding about the inhibitory mechanism as well as the mode of interactions of the phytochemical compounds of the crude extract, docking analysis was accomplished using the GOLD 4.12 package. Two primary drug-target-pathways, i.e., penicillin-binding protein [13] and DNA gyrase [14] of *S. aureus* were subject to forecast the mechanism of plant derived compounds. Protein X-ray structure pdb ID: 3vsl and 3g7b was retrieved from protein data bank [15] and compared with standard inhibitor orientation in crystal structure. From the literature review, all compounds represented in Figure 1 were drawn in Symyx Draw 4.0 and to prepare for docking using the Sybyl 7.3 Molecular Modeling Suite of Tripos, Inc. Three dimensional (3D) conformations generated by using Concord 4.0 [16]; hydrogen atoms were added and charges were loaded using the Gasteiger and Marsili charge calculation method [17]. Basic amines were protonated and acidic carboxyl groups were de-protonated prior to charge calculation. The ligands were minimized with the Tripos Force Field prior to docking using the Powell method with an initial Simplex [18] optimization and 1000 interactions or gradient termination at 0.01 kcal/(mol*A). The input ligand file format was mol2 for all docking programs investigated. Three dimensional structure of standard drugs i.e., penicillin G and ciprofloxacin was occupied from zinc databases. The docking tool "GOLD" utilizes genetic algorithm to explore the rotational flexibility of receptor hydrogen's and ligand conformational flexibility [19]. Such GOLD docking was carried out using the wizard with default parameters population size (100); selection pressure (1.1); number of operations (10,0 00); number of islands (1); niche size (2); and operator weights for migrate (0), mutate (100), and crossover (100). The active site with a 10 Å radius sphere was defined by selecting an active site residue of protein. Default genetic algorithm settings were used for all calculations and a set of 10 solutions was saved for each ligand. GOLD was used by a GoldScore fitness function. GoldScore is a molecular mechanism like function and has been optimized for the calculation of binding positions of ligand. It takes into account for four terms:

$$\textbf{Fitness} = \textbf{S}_{(hb\_ext)} + \textbf{1.3750}*\textbf{S}_{(vdw\_ext)} + \textbf{S}_{(hb\_int)} + \textbf{1.0000}*\textbf{S}_{(int)}$$

$$\textbf{S}_{(int)} = \textbf{S}_{(vdw\_int)} + \textbf{S}_{(tors)}$$

Where, S $_{hb\_ext}$ is the protein-ligand hydrogen bonding

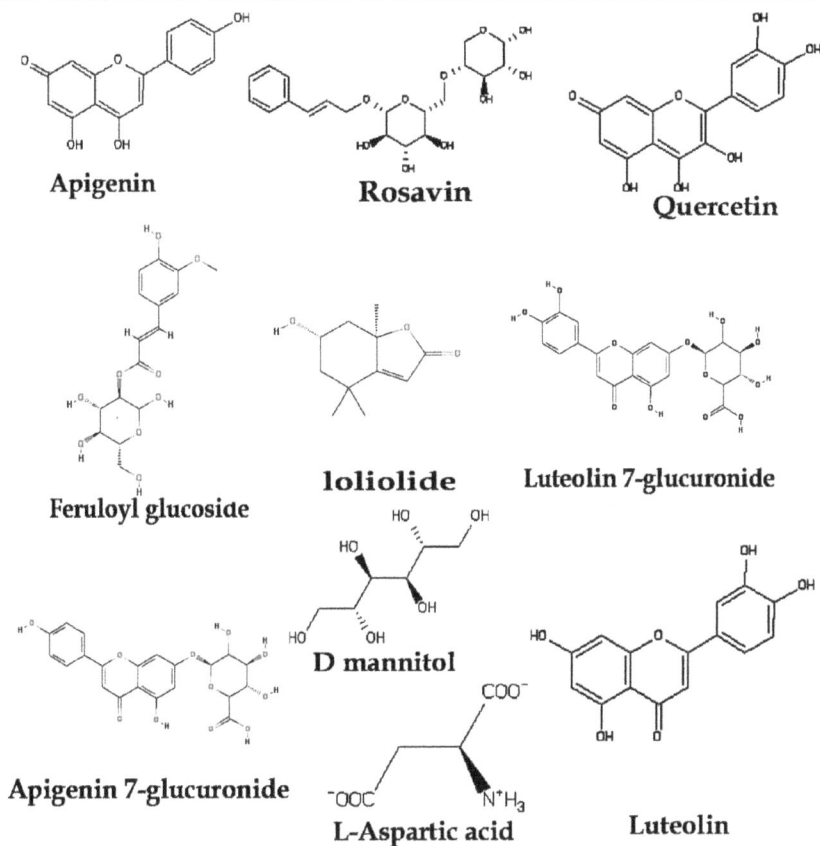

Figure 1 2D structure of all compounds of *B. monnieri*.

and s_{vdw_ext} are the Vanderwaals interactions between protein and ligand. S_{hb_int} are the intramolecular hydrophobic interactions whereas S_{vdw_int} is the contribution due to intramolecular strain in the ligand.

Results

In vitro antimicrobial assay

Results for the antibacterial activity of *B. monnieri* extract showed that the mean zone of inhibition (13.0-15.0 mm) produced by the extract was close to those produced by the reference antibiotics, i.e., tetracycline and ampicillin which had the zone of inhibitions between 16 to 20 mm. The extract of three different concentrations (1, 2 and 3 mg/disk) produced significant ($p < 0.05$) zone of inhibition against *S. aureus* and the values were 13.33 ± 2.08, 13.33 ± 2.08 and 15.33 ± 1.52 for 1, 2 and 3 mg/disk, respectively. The result of antibacterial activity of *B. monnieri* ethanol extract is shown in Table 1.

Minimum inhibitory concentration

The minimum inhibitory concentrations of *B. monnieri* leaf extract for different bacterial strains were ranged from 25 to 100 µl/ml (Table 2). The arbitrary MIC against the Gram-positive bacteria *S. aureus* was greater than or equal to 75 for the extract and 16 for the reference antibiotic tetracycline.

Docking experiments

Considering the results obtained in *in vitro* study, it was thought worthy to perform molecular docking studies which correlate both *in silico* and *in vitro* results. Docking studies are used at different stages of drug discovery such as to predict a ligand-receptor interaction and also to rank the compounds based on the binding energies or fitness score [20]. In our present study, docking of tested compounds with the primary drug pathway for *S. aureus* was performed, and the corresponding fitness score was also determined as shown in Table 3. The interacting energies followed the order of the best fitness core. Highest fitness scored compound was further subjected to compare its binding pattern and molecular interaction with the standard drug penicillin G and ciprofloxacin.

In the docking studies of DNA gyrase binding site, luteolin among the other tested compounds has the

Table 1 *in vitro* antibacterial activity of *B. monnieri* ethanol extract

Bacterial type	Test organism	Source ID (ATCC)	Diameter of zone of inhibition (mm)				
			Bacopa monnieri			Standard antibiotics	
Gram + ve			1 mg/disk	2 mg/disk	3 mg/disk	Tetracycline (50 µg/disk)	Ampicillin (50 µg/disk)
	Staphylococcus aureus	6538	13.33 ± 2.08^a	13.33 ± 2.08^b	15.33 ± 1.52^c	16.00 ± 3.54^d	20.00 ± 1.60^e

Data are shown as mean ± SD for triplicate of concentration. Different superscript letters (a-e) shown in the data indicate that the values are significantly different (Tukey's multiple range, *post hoc* test, $p < 0.05$) from each other.

highest fitness score 53.77 compared with the highest fitness score 46.48 of ciprofloxacin. Molecular binding pattern of ciprofloxacin revealed that it has two hydrogen bonds with ARG144 and GLY85 consisting of hydrogen bonding distances 2.634 Å and 2.476 Å shown in Figure 2. These two hydrogen bonding residues in luteolin are found to be similar with different hydrogen bonds viz. 2.641 Å for ARG144 and 2.520 Å for GLY85. Additionally, it also formed two other hydrogen bonds with ARG84 and ASP81 having a bonding distance of 2.932 Å and 2.956 Å.

For the most potent inhibitor of penicillin binding protein, luteolin showed the highest fitness score among the other tested compounds viz., 45.35 fitness score compared to its reference standard drug penicillin G 46.48. In context of different binding patterns, luteolin has formed the three hydrogen bonds SER429, THR621 and THR619 where bonding distances were 3.020, 2.798 and 2.331. On the other hand, reference drug penicillin G formed hydrogen bonds with ASN450, SER778, THR621 and GLN524 with corresponding hydrogen bonds 2.956 Å, 2.968 Å, 2.556 Å and 3.031 Å, respectively. Binding mode and related interactions are summarized in Figure 3.

The emergence of bacterial resistance to current clinical drugs has brought intention to develop novel antimicrobial agents for selectively inhibiting the constantly evolved bacterial targets which have been also continually promoted with challenges. Presently known target of *Staphyloccus* sp. includes PBP (penicillin binding protein) of peptidoglycan biosynthesis pathway where beta-lactam antibiotics were known to be effective against it [21]. A different prescribing drug i.e. Fluroquinolone, DNA Gyrase A enzyme which is essential for the replication and super-coiling of DNA, is the main target at this case. But according to Stephen *et al.*, a highly significant association between Levofloxacin and Ciprofloxacin

treatment and consequent isolation of MRSA is reported [22]. However, in this research, molecular docking analysis suggested that luteolin has the more specificity towards the DNA gyrase binding site than penicillin binding protein. Regarding the obtained results, luteolin could serve as an appropriate starting point for designing new chemical entities as potent *S. aureus* inhibitor.

Discussion

Plants have long been a very important source of drug and many plants have been screened whether they contain compounds with therapeutic activity. Therefore, it is vital to evaluate the antimicrobial activity of *B. monnieri*. The bacterial strain was chosen to be studied as it is an important pathogen and rapidly develop antibiotic resistance with its increased uses. In disk diffusion technique, the mean zone of inhibition produced by the commercial antibiotic, tetracycline and ampicillin, was larger than that produced by ethanol extract. It may be attributed to the fact that the plant extract being in crude form contains a smaller concentration of bioactive compounds. In classifying the antimicrobial activity it would be generally expected that a greater number would be active against Gram-positive than Gram-negative bacteria. Apart from this, the higher MIC value is an indication that either the plant extracts are less effective on bacteria or the organism has the potential to develop antibiotic resistance. On the contrary, the low MIC value for bacteria is an indication of the higher efficacy of the plant extracts.

Most of the pathogenic bacteria have developed resistance to currently available antibiotics due to their misuse or overuse. This situation has led to an urgent need to explore different sources of efficient, less toxic and cost-effective antimicrobial agents [23,24]. Medicinal plants play a major role and constitute the backbone of traditional medicine. According to the World Health Organization (WHO) estimate, 80% of populations in developing countries rely exclusively on traditional medicine for their healthcare need. Moreover, 20% of the available allopathic drugs have an active principal obtained from higher plants [25]. Recognizing the significance of indigenous medicinal plants WHO states in its 1997 guideline that locally available effective plants may

Table 2 Minimum inhibitory concentrations (MIC) of *B. monnieri* and tetracycline against *Staphylococcus aureus*

Test organism	MIC of *Bacopa monnieri* extract (µg/ml)	MIC of tetracycline (µg/ml)
Staphylococcus aureus	≥75	≥16

Table 3 Gold fitness score of B. monnieri's all compounds against DNA gyrase and penicillin binding protein

Compound name	DNA gyrase					Penicillin binding protein				
	Fitness score	S(hb_ext)	S(vdw_ext)	S(hb_int)	S(int)	Fitness Score	S(hb_ext)	S(vdw_ext)	S(hb_int)	S(int)
Apigenin	46.59	5.57	36.00	0.00	-8.48	41.73	7.29	30.70	0.00	-7.77
Rosavin	51.58	5.44	42.31	0.00	-12.03	41.96	8.88	31.27	0.00	-9.92
Quercetin	45.71	6.04	37.32	0.00	-11.64	40.14	9.37	30.55	0.00	-11.23
Feruloyl glucoside	49.23	8.14	42.78	0.00	-17.74	32.42	4.76	35.88	0.00	-21.68
Loliolide	29.61	0.10	23.41	0.00	-2.68	31.02	3.34	22.10	0.00	-2.71
Luteolin-7-glucoside	47.87	10.04	42.46	0.00	-20.56	43.85	2.46	42.08	0.00	-16.48
Apigenin-7- glucocronide	45.63	8.34	39.19	0.00	-16.59	43.35	8.74	37.80	0.00	-17.36
D-mannitol	32.55	9.88	23.13	0.00	-9.13	30.21	8.15	20.48	0.00	-6.11
L-asperatic acid	33.35	17.74	17.07	0.00	-7.86	28.29	14.01	16.69	0.00	-8.66
Luteolin	53.77	11.23	37.44	0.00	-8.94	45.35	7.81	41.67	0.00	-19.77
Penicillin G	-------	-------	-------	-------	-------	46.48	2.62	35.14	0.00	-4.46
Ciprofloxacine	46.48	0.21	42.47	0.00	-8.94	-------	-------	-------	-------	-------

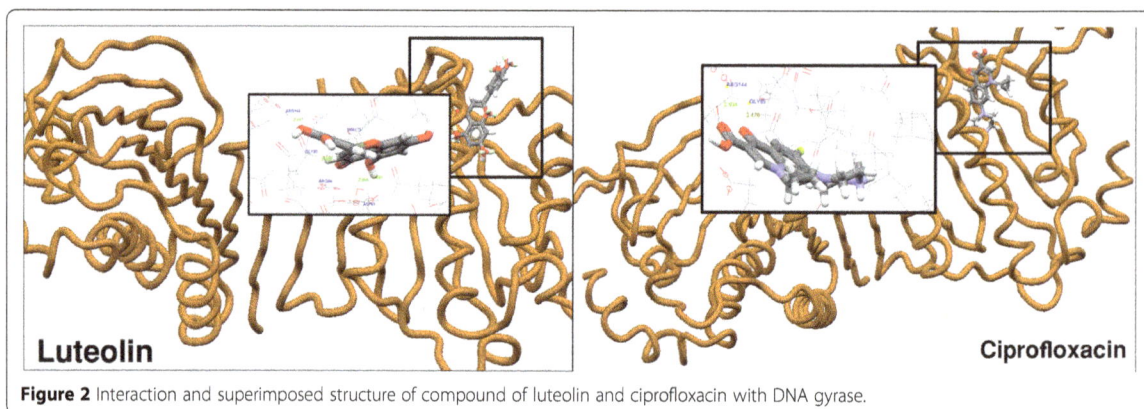

Figure 2 Interaction and superimposed structure of compound of luteolin and ciprofloxacin with DNA gyrase.

be used as substitutes for drugs. Research work on medicinal plants and exchange of obtained information will go a long way in scientific exploration of medicinal plants for the benefit of mankind. This will ultimately decrease our dependence on synthetic drugs [26]. Plant synthesizes natural products as its chemical weapon that arrests the growth of environmental microbes [27] and some plants inhibit the growth of potential human pathogens too. In the current study, *in vitro* MIC of *B. monnieri* leaf parts, prescribed in indigenous system of medicine, that are available in the local market or growing in Bangladesh and India were evaluated against local clinical bacterial isolate of *S. aureus*. Determination of MIC of this plant is important to find out the best plant that eradicates infectious agents (Table 2). Clinicians also select the antibiotic on the basis of their MIC value to treat infectious diseases. Plant extracts having MIC below 8000 µg/ml have been reported as therapeutically effective [28]. Our results for *B. monnieri* implicated a significant MIC value

(below or equal to 75 µg/ml) in this study. This significance suggests that we have identified antimicrobial activity of plant that is effective for arresting the growth of *S. aureus* causing hospital-,-acquired- and opportunistic-infections.

Conclusions

B. monnieri extract and its compound luteolin have a significant antimicrobial activity against *S. aureus*. Molecular binding interaction of *in silico* data demonstrated that luteolin has more specificity towards the DNA gyrase binding site and could be a potent antimicrobial compound. However several scientific reports manifested that lead-drug discovery projects on the basis of binding efficiency indices would afford bioactive compounds with better pharmacokinetic outcomes. Hence, isolated bioactive compounds should be employed for establishing more rational structure activity relationships in the era of antimicrobial drug development.

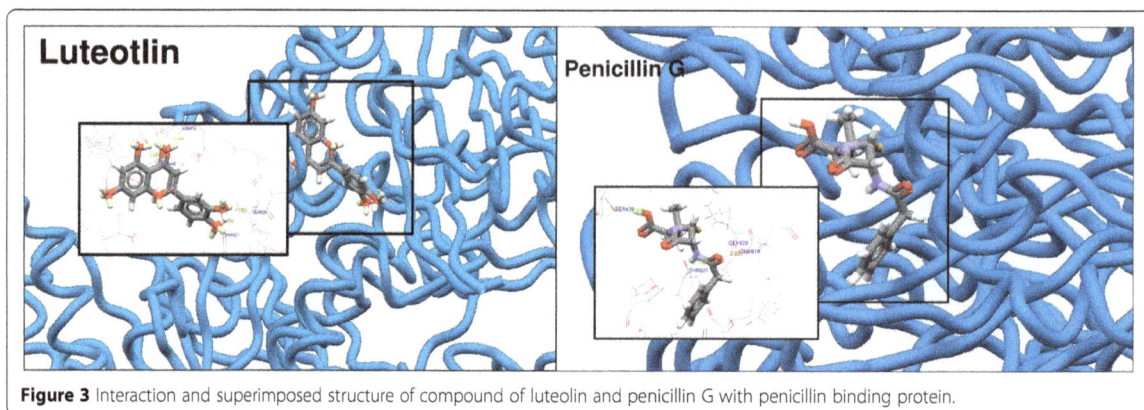

Figure 3 Interaction and superimposed structure of compound of luteolin and penicillin G with penicillin binding protein.

Competing interests

The authors declare that they have no competing interests.

Authors' contributions

TBE has designed the study, performed data analysis and interpretation and written the manuscript. MAR has revised the whole manuscript and also helped in the grammatical corrections. MMNU has modified the *in silico* sections. RD has performed data analysis and written the *in silico* sections. MFH and MM have participated in experiments, data collection and literature search. MRA has provided assistance in taxonomical identification and collections of voucher specimen's number of the plant. All authors read and approved the final version of the manuscript.

Acknowledgements

Authors are thankful to Dr. Shaikh Bokhtear Uddin, Taxonomist and Associate Professor, Department of Botany, University of Chittagong, Chittagong-4331, Bangladesh for identifying the plant sample. We are also grateful to Bangladesh Council of Scientific and Industrial Research (BCSIR), Chittagong-4220, Bangladesh for supplying the microbial strains.

Author details

[1]Department of Pharmacy, BGC Trust University Bangladesh, Chittagong 4000, Bangladesh. [2]Department of Biochemistry and Molecular Biology, University of Chittagong, Chittagong 4331, Bangladesh. [3]Department of Pharmacy, University of Chittagong, Chittagong 4331, Bangladesh.

References

1. Boucher HW, Talbot GH, Bradley JS, Edwards JE, Gilbert D, Rice LB, et al. Bad bugs, no drugs: no ESKAPE! An update from the Infectious Diseases Society of America. Clin Infect Dis. 2009;48(1):1–12.
2. Kluytmans J, van Belkum A, Verbrugh H. Nasal carriage of Staphylococcus aureus: epidemiology, underlying mechanisms, and associated risks. Clin Microbiol Rev. 1997;10(3):505–20.
3. Kuehnert MJ, Hill HA, Kupronis BA, Tokars JI, Solomon SL, Jernigan DB. Methicillin-resistant-*Staphylococcus aureus* hospitalizations, United States. Emerg Infect Dis. 2005;11(6):868–72.
4. Klevens RM, Morrison MA, Nadle J, Petit S, Gershman K, Ray S, et al. Invasive methicillin-resistant *Staphylococcus aureus* infections in the United States. Jama. 2007;298(15):1763–71.
5. Diefenbeck M, Mennenga U, Guckel P, Tiemann AH, Muckley T, Hofmann GO. Vacuum-assisted closure therapy for the treatment of acute postoperative osteomyelitis. Z Orthop Unfall. 2011;149:336–41.
6. Garo E, Eldridge GR, Goering MG, DeLancey PE, Hamilton MA, Costerton JW, et al. Asiatic acid and corosolic acid enhance the susceptibility of *Pseudomonas aeruginosa* biofilms to tobramycin. Antimicrob Agents Chemother. 2007;51(5):1813–7.
7. Coutinho HD, Costa JG, Lima EO, Falcao-Silva VS, Siqueira-Junior JP. Enhancement of the antibiotic activity against a multiresistant *Escherichia coli* by *Mentha arvensis* L. and chlorpromazine. Chemotherapy. 2008;4:328–30.
8. Coutinho HD, Costa JG, Lima EO, Falcao-Silva VS, Siqueira Jr JP. Herbal therapy associated with antibiotic therapy: potentiation of the antibiotic activity against methicillin–resistant Staphylococcus aureus by *Turnera ulmifolia* L. BMC Complement Altern Med. 2009;9(13):1472–6882.
9. Aguiar S, Borowski T. Neuropharmacological review of the nootropic herb *Bacopa monnieri*. Rejuvenation Res. 2013;16(4):313–26.
10. Chopra RNNL, Chopra IC. Glossary of Indian Medicinal Plants. New Delhi: Council of Scientific and Industrial Research; 1956. p. 32.
11. Ghosh S, Nie A, An J, Huang Z. Structure-based virtual screening of chemical libraries for drug discovery. Curr Opin Chem Biol. 2006;10(3):194–202.
12. Dash R, Emran TB, Uddin MM, Islam A, Junaid M. Molecular docking of fisetin with AD associated AChE, ABAD and BACE1 proteins. Bioinformation. 2014;10(9):562–8.
13. Yoshida H, Kawai F, Obayashi E, Akashi S, Roper DI, Tame JR, et al. Crystal structures of penicillin-binding protein 3 (PBP3) from methicillin-resistant *Staphylococcus aureus* in the apo and cefotaxime-bound forms. J Mol Biol. 2012;423(3):351–64.
14. Ronkin SM, Badia M, Bellon S, Grillot AL, Gross CH, Grossman TH, et al. Discovery of pyrazolthiazoles as novel and potent inhibitors of bacterial gyrase. Bioorg Med Chem Lett. 2010;20(9):2828–31.
15. Berman HM, Westbrook J, Feng Z, Gilliland G, Bhat TN, Weissig H, et al. The Protein Data Bank. Nucleic Acids Res. 2000;28(1):235–42.
16. Hevener KE, Zhao W, Ball DM, Babaoglu K, Qi J, White SW, et al. Validation of molecular docking programs for virtual screening against dihydropteroate synthase. J Chem Inf Model. 2009;49(2):444–60.
17. Hristozov DP, Oprea TI, Gasteiger J. Virtual screening applications: a study of ligand-based methods and different structure representations in four different scenarios. J Comput Aided Mol Des. 2007;21(10–11):617–40.
18. Osolodkin DI, Palyulin VA, Zefirov NS. Structure-based virtual screening of glycogen synthase kinase 3-beta inhibitors: analysis of scoring functions applied to large true actives and decoy sets. Chem Biol Drug Des. 2011;78(3):378–90.
19. Jones G, Willett P, Glen RC, Leach AR, Taylor R. Development and validation of a genetic algorithm for flexible docking. J Mol Biol. 1997;267(3):727–48.
20. Kitchen DB, Decornez H, Furr JR, Bajorath J. Docking and scoring in virtual screening for drug discovery: methods and applications. Nat Rev Drug Discov. 2004;3(11):935–49.
21. Hao H, Cheng G, Dai M, Wu Q, Yuan Z. Inhibitors targeting on cell wall biosynthesis pathway of MRSA. Mol Biosyst. 2012;8(11):2828–38.
22. Weber SG, Gold HS, Hooper DC, Karchmer AW, Carmeli Y. Fluoroquinolones and the risk for methicillin-resistant *Staphylococcus aureus* in hospitalized patients. Emerg Infect Dis. 2003;9(11):1415–22.
23. Russell AD. Bacterial resistance to disinfectants: present knowledge and future problems. J Hosp Infec. 1999;43(0):S57–68. Supplement 1.
24. Sheldon Jr AT. Antibiotic resistance: a survival strategy. Clin Lab Sci. 2005;18(3):170–80.
25. Gurib-Fakim A. Medicinal plants: traditions of yesterday and drugs of tomorrow. Mol Aspects Med. 2006;27(1):1–93.
26. Veerappan A, Miyazaki S, Kadarkaraisamy M, Ranganathan D. Acute and subacute toxicity studies of *Aegle marmelos* Corr., an Indian medicinal plant. Phytomedicine. 2007;14(2-3):209–15.
27. Gibbons S. Anti-staphylococcal plant natural products. Nat Prod Rep. 2004;21(2):263–77.
28. Fabry W, Okemo PO, Ansorg R. Antibacterial activity of East African medicinal plants. J Ethnopharmacol. 1998;60(1):79–84.

Effect of ethylene glycol dimethacrylate on swelling and on metformin hydrochloride release behavior of chemically crosslinked pH–sensitive acrylic acid–polyvinyl alcohol hydrogel

Muhammad Faheem Akhtar*⬤, Nazar Muhammad Ranjha and Muhammad Hanif

Abstract

Background: The present work objective was to prepare and to observe the effect of ethylene glycol dimethacrylate on swelling and on drug release behavior of pH-sensitive acrylic acid–polyvinyl alcohol hydrogel.

Methods: In the present work, pH sensitive acrylic acid–polyvinyl alcohol hydrogels have been prepared by free radical polymerization technique in the presence of benzoyl peroxide as an initiator. Different crosslinker contents were used to observe its effect on swelling and on drug release. Dynamic and equilibrium swelling studies of prepared hydrogels were investigated in USP phosphate buffer solutions of pH 1.2, 5.5, 6.5 and 7.5 with constant ionic strengths. Hydrogels were evaluated for polymer volume fraction, solvent interaction parameter, molecular weight between crosslinks, number of links per polymer chain, diffusion coefficient, sol–gel fraction and porosity. To demonstrate the release pattern of the drug, zero-order, first-order, higuchi and korsmeyer-peppas models were applied. Quality and consistency of hydrogels was examined by FTIR and surface morphology of hydrogels was examined by SEM.

Results: Decrease in swelling and in drug release was seen by increasing content of ethylene glycol dimethacrylate. A remarkable high swelling was observed at high pH indicating the potential of this hydrogel for delivery of drugs to intestine. By increasing the concentration of ethylene glycol dimethacrylate, porosity decreased. Order of release was observed first order in all cases and the mechanism was non–fickian diffusion. FTIR confirmed the formation of network. SEM results showed the incorporation of drug.

Conclusion: The prepared hydrogels can be suitably used for targeted drug delivery to the intestine.

Keywords: Acrylic acid–polyvinyl alcohol hydrogel, Ethylene glycol dimethacrylate, Glutaraldehyde, Metformin hydrochloride, Dynamic swelling, Drug release

Background

Hydrogel, three–dimensional crosslinked polymeric network, can swell and collapse reversibly in response to variables such as ionic strength, pH, electric field and temperature [1]. Hydrogels can be used as controlled release systems when they are in contact with any surface. This can happen through spaces inside the network and the matrix dissolution/disintegration effect [2].

Polyvinyl alcohol (PVA) is being extensively used in fields, such as: pharmaceutical (for the wound dressing systems); biomedical (as a scaffold supporting material for tissue engineering applications) and environmental (for the production of films for removal of heavy metal ions from water). Other applications comprise fuel cells, electrochemistry and agriculture. The –OH group on every second carbon atom on PVA backbone allows it to take part in many chemical crosslinking reactions, to interact with many other polymers by hydrogen bonding, and to form a hydrogel by the freeze thaw process. Excellent

* Correspondence: m_faheem1986@yahoo.com
Faculty of Pharmacy, Bahauddin Zakariya University, P.O.Box: 60800, Multan, Pakistan

biocompatibility, noncarcinogenicity, biodegradability and non-toxicity are supplementary attractive properties of PVA. PVA is also useful in the pharmaceutical industries, where it is being used as a polymer for the loading/encapsulation and the subsequent release of cells, enzymes, proteins and a range of drugs [3].

Acrylic acid (AA) is a superabsorbent and a common pH-sensitive electrolyte. Because gels can be prepared at varying concentrations, AA based materials present huge potential for biomedical applications. They may be easily converted to a broad range of shapes and sizes. Prior to gel formation, other materials may be included into AA. AA polymers exhibit high tolerance in living cells. In addition, a glycoprotein i.e. mucin secreted locally that coats the mucosal surfaces forms hydrogen bonds with carboxylic groups of AA. AA is a fine applicant for many drug delivery routes e.g. nasal, ocular and oral due to its bioadhesive property. As, carboxylic groups of AA intermingle with different groups, attachment sites are created for a variety of therapeutics [4].

In the synthesis of a large number of hydrogels, crosslinkers are used, which interconnect the lineal polymeric chains establishing a three-dimensional network of chemical bonds among them. It is necessary that the polymer has certain groups in its structure that can be used as anchor points in order to form the network. The choice of crosslinker depends on the selected monomers, must have at least two reactive groups in its structure, in order to be able to crosslink different polymeric chains, normally tetrafunctional and hexafunctional compounds, such as ethylene glycol dimethacrylate (EGDMA) and 1,1,1,trimethylolpropane trimethacrylate, although other crosslinking agents have also been used such as ethylenediaminetetraacetic dianhydride and pentaerythritol triacrylate [5]. Glutaraldehyde (GA) has been extensively used for crosslinking polymers containing hydroxyl groups [6]. Hydrogels containing ionic network structure show pH–dependent swelling behavior [7].

In the present work, ethylene glycol dimethacrylate and glutaraldehyde crosslinked pH–sensitive acrylic acid–polyvinyl alcohol hydrogels were synthesized for drug delivery to intestine. Different quantities of crosslinking agent were used in order to evaluate its effects on swelling and on drug release.

Methods
Materials
Polymer used was polyvinyl alcohol (Mol.wt. 72000; degree of hydrolysis ≥98 %; Merck, Germany). The monomer used was acrylic acid (Sigma-Aldrich, Netherland). Crosslinkers used were ethylene glycol dimethacrylate (Sigma-Aldrich, Germany) and glutaraldehyde (Scharlau, Spain). Benzoyl peroxide (Fisher Scientific, UK) was used as an initiator and HCl (Fluka, Switzerland) was used as

a catalyst. Distilled water was used as a solvent. Potassium dihydrogen phosphate was purchased from Merck, Germany. Metformin hydrochloride was gifted by Popular International (PVT) LTD., Karachi, Pakistan.

Synthesis of pH sensitive AA–PVA hydrogels
AA–PVA hydrogels were prepared by the free radical polymerization technique. The process of hydrogel preparation was analogous to that reported [8] but with some essential modifications due to the properties of ingredients. A 10 % w/v PVA solution was prepared at 80 °C using reflux condenser. Mixing was continued until heated solution cooled to room temperature and then HCl and GA were added with continuous stirring at slow speed. This solution was named as solution A. Benzoyl peroxide was dissolved in acrylic acid and then varying amounts of EGDMA were added to this solution. After stirring, this solution was named as solution B. Both solutions were mixed very slowly to prevent the formation of air bubbles [9] and distilled water was added to make the final weight of the solution 100 g. Immediately after mixing the solution [9], the mixture was poured into Pyrex glass tubes having 150 mm length and 16 mm internal diameter to start polymerization. Nitrogen bubbling was done for 10–15 min to prevent obstruction in normal polymerization process by oxygen [10]. Glass tubes after being capped were placed in the water bath at a temperature regime of 45 °C for 1 h, 50 °C for 2 h, 55 °C for 3 h, 60 °C for 4 h and 65 °C for 5 h. To avoid auto-acceleration and air bubbles formation, there was a gradual increase in temperature from 45 °C to 65 °C. Then the tubes were cooled down and cylindrical hydrogels were removed from the tubes. 7 mm length disks were cut from each cylinder. Extensive washing of these discs with freshly distilled water was done for the unreacted material removal. Drying of disks was done at room temperature and then in an oven to constant weight at 45 °C and stored in a desiccator for further use. Figure 1 is showing the possible chemical structure of synthesized acrylic acid–polyvinyl alcohol hydrogel. A list of different formulations of AA–PVA hydrogel is given in Table 1.

Buffer solutions preparation
pH 1.2, 5.5, 6.5 and 7.5 USP phosphate buffer solutions were prepared with potassium dihydrogen phosphate. 0.2 M HCl or NaOH solution was used to adjust the pH of these solutions. NaCl was used to keep the ionic strength of all the buffer solutions constant.

Dynamic and equilibrium swelling study
Dynamic and equilibrium swelling study was done in 100 ml pH 1.2, 5.5, 6.5 and 7.5 buffer solutions. Dried and weighed hydrogel was kept in a desired pH solution. For dynamic swelling study, the swollen gel was taken out of the buffer solution, blotted with tissue paper,

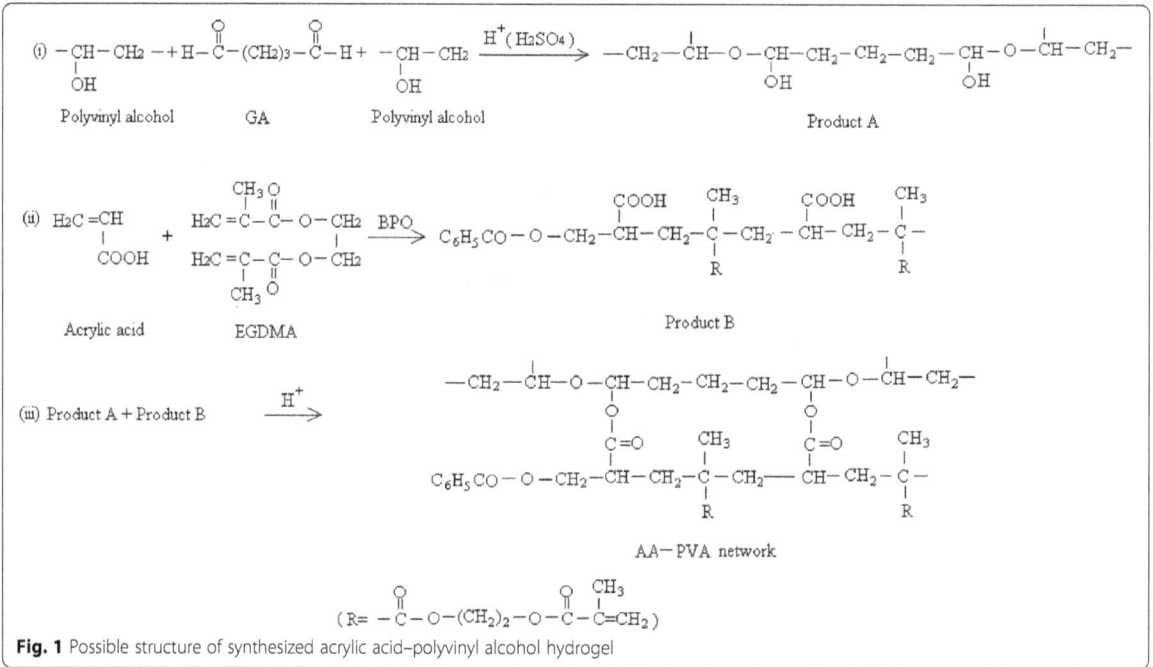

Fig. 1 Possible structure of synthesized acrylic acid–polyvinyl alcohol hydrogel

weighed and then placed back in the same buffer solution, at regular interval upto 8 h. Following equation was used to calculate the swelling ratio [11]:

$$q = W_t/W_d \qquad (1)$$

W_t is the swollen gel weight at time t and W_d is the dry gel initial weight. For equilibrium swelling, the swollen gels were weighed daily until they reach constant weight which took almost 2 weeks.

Network parameters of AA–PVA hydrogels
Polymer volume fraction
Polymer volume fraction ($v_{2,s}$) is the fluid amount that a hydrogel can absorb in the equilibrium swollen state. Following equation was used to calculate $v_{2,s}$ [12]:

v_p is the dried hydrogel volume and v_{gel} is the volume in swollen state.

Table 1 A list of different formulations of AA–PVA hydrogel

Sample code	AA	PVA	AA/PVA	EGDMA	GA
	(g/100 g solution)	(g/100 g solution)	(wt.%)	(g/100 g solution)	(g/100 g solution)
S_1	21	7.38	74/26	0.082	0.01
S_2	21	7.38	74/26	0.123	0.01
S_3	21	7.38	74/26	0.165	0.01

$$v_{2,s} = \left[\frac{v_p}{v_{gel}}\right] \qquad (2)$$

Solvent interaction parameter (χ)
Following equation was used to calculate χ values [13]:

$$X = \frac{1}{2} + \frac{v_{2,s}}{3} \qquad (3)$$

Molecular weight between crosslinks (M_c)
M_c was calculated by the following equation [12]:

$$M_c = \frac{Mr}{2X} \qquad (4)$$

where M_r is the polymer repeating unit molar mass and X is the degree of crosslinking.

M_r was calculated by the following equation [14]:

$$M_r = \frac{n_{PVA}M_{PVA} + n_{AA}M_{AA}}{n_{PVA} + n_{AA}} \qquad (5)$$

where n_{PVA} and n_{AA} are the number of moles of PVA and AA, respectively while M_{PVA} and M_{AA} are PVA and AA molar masses, respectively.

Table 2 Swelling coefficients (Dynamic and equilibrium) of AA–PVA hydrogels using EGDMA and GA as crosslinkers

Sample codes	Dynamic swelling coefficients				Equilibrium swelling coefficients			
	1.2 pH	5.5 pH	6.5 pH	7.5 pH	1.2 pH	5.5 pH	6.5 pH	7.5 pH
S_1	2.9	3.29	4.32	4.82	10.19	11.72	18.11	23.85
S_2	2.58	2.9	4.08	4.33	10.07	11.53	17.67	21.4
S_3	2.26	2.56	3.76	4	9.88	11.25	17.03	19.8

Number of links per polymer chain (N)

The equation used is given below [15]:

$$N = \frac{2M_c}{M_r} \qquad (6)$$

Diffusion coefficient

Usually, diffusion is the mechanism of drug release from hydrogels. Equation used to calculate water diffusion coefficient is given below [16]:

$$D = \pi \left(\frac{h.\theta}{4.Q_{eq}} \right)^2 \qquad (7)$$

where D is the hydrogel diffusion coefficient, θ is the swelling curve linear part slope, Q_{eq} is the equilibrium swelling ratio and h is the sample thickness before swelling.

Sol–gel fraction

To remove uncrosslinked polymer, hydrogel unwashed samples were cut into 3–4 mm diameter pieces, dried in an oven at 45 °C to constant weight (W_o), and subjected to soxhlet extraction with deionized water for 4 h. Extracted gels were dried again at 45 °C in an oven to constant weight (W_1). Following equations were used to calculate gel fraction [17]:

$$\text{Sol fraction}(\%) = \left[\frac{W_o - W_1}{W_o} \right] X100 \qquad (8)$$

$$\text{Gel fraction}(\%) = 100 - \text{sol fraction} \qquad (9)$$

Porosity measurement

Solvent replacement method was used for porosity measurement. Dried and weighed hydrogel was soaked in absolute ethanol over night and weighed after blotting excess ethanol from the surface and the porosity was calculated by the following equation [18]:

$$Porosity = \frac{(M_2 - M_1)}{\rho V} \times 100 \qquad (10)$$

M_1 and M_2 are the hydrogel masses before and after immersion in ethanol, respectively: ρ is the absolute ethanol density and V is the hydrogel final volume.

Loading of metformin hydrochloride into crosslinked AA–PVA hydrogels

Weighed and dried hydrogel samples were placed in 1 % w/v solution of metformin hydrochloride. Metformin hydrochloride solution was prepared by dissolving the drug in USP phosphate buffer solution of pH 7.5. After attaining the equilibrium swelling, hydrogel samples were dried first at room temperature and then in an oven at 45 °C to constant weight.

Determination of metformin hydrochloride loading

Three methods were applied. Following equation was used to determine drug loading by the first method:

$$\text{Amount of drug} = W_D - W_d \qquad (11)$$

Weights of dried hydrogels before and after immersion in drug solution are W_d and W_D, respectively. In the second method, drug entrapped was calculated by repeatedly extracting the weighed quantity of loaded gels using USP phosphate buffer solution (pH 7.5). Each time fresh 50 ml USP phosphate buffer solution (pH 7.5) was used until drug exhaustion. Drug concentration was determined spectrophotometrically. Drug present in all portions of the extracts was considered as the drug amount loaded. Weighed gel disk was placed in drug solution up to equilibrium swelling, in the third method.

Table 3 Metformin amount loaded in different samples of AA–PVA hydrogel

Sample code	Amount of metformin loaded		
	(g/g of dry gel)		
	Swelling method	Extraction method	Weight method
S_1	0.2194	0.22	0.2157
S_2	0.2065	0.2093	0.2029
S_3	0.1999	0.1995	0.1921

Table 4 Effect of pH on dug release after 12 h drug release study

Sample	Time (hours)	pH 1.2	pH 5.5	pH 7.5
S_1	12	26.02 %	49.77 %	80.42 %
S_2	12	25.48 %	47.48 %	75.95 %
S_3	12	22.81 %	45.27 %	71.76 %

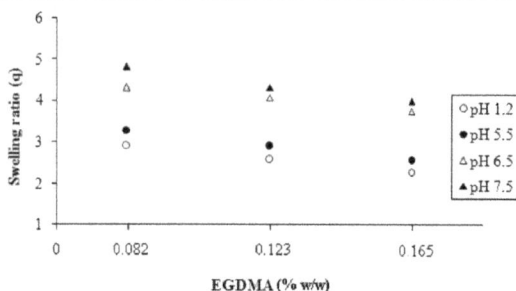

Fig. 2 Swelling behavior after 8 h of AA–PVA hydrogel with different EGDMA content

Loaded gel was weighed again after blotting with filter paper. Difference in weight before and after swelling is the weight of drug solution. Dividing the weight of drug solution with the density of drug solution gave us the volume of drug solution. So, amount of drug was easily calculated from the volume of drug solution [4].

Metformin release studies
The weighed hydrogel disks were immersed separately in 500 ml 0.05 M USP phosphate buffer solutions of pH 1.2, 5.5 and 7.5 at 37 °C and dissolution medium was stirred at a rate of 100 rpm for maintaining a uniform drug concentration (Dissolution apparatus, Pharmatest; PT–Dt 7, Germany). Metformin HCl release study was conducted at 218 nm up to 12 h (UV–VIS spectrophotometer, IRMECO, UV–VIS U2020) [4].

Analysis of drug release pattern
For the analysis of release of metformin hydrochloride, zero-order [19], first-order [20], higuchi [21] and korsmeyer-peppas [22] models were applied. To get an insight into the solute release mechanism, the release profile was analyzed using the peppas semi-empirical power equation [22]. Following equations were used for release calculations.

$$\text{Zero-order kinetics}: \quad F_t = K_o t \tag{12}$$

where F represents the fraction of drug release in time t and K_o is the zero-order release constant.

$$\text{First-order kinetics}: \quad \ln(1\text{-}F) = -K_1 t \tag{13}$$

where F represents the fraction of drug release in time t and K_1 is the first-order release constant.

$$\text{Higuchi model}: \quad F = K_2 t^{1/2} \tag{14}$$

where F represents the fraction of drug release in time t and K_2 is the higuchi constant.

$$\text{Korsmeyer-peppas model}: \quad M_t/M^\infty = K_3 t^n \tag{15}$$

M_t is the mass of water absorbed at any time t; M^∞ is the amount of fluid intake at equilibrium; K_3 is the kinetic constant and n is the swelling exponent.

FTIR spectroscopic analysis
The crushed hydrogel samples were mixed with potassium bromide (Merck IR spectroscopy grade) in 1:100 proportions and dried at 45 °C. The mixtures were compressed to a 12 mm semitransparent disk by a pressure of 65 kN (Pressure gauge, Shimadzu) for 1 min. The FTIR spectra were recorded over the wavelength range 4,000–400 cm^{-1} using FTIR spectrometer (FTIR 8400 S, Shimadzu).

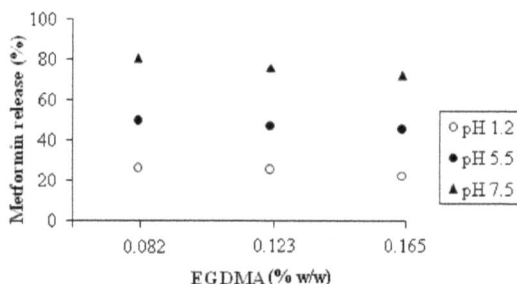

Fig. 3 Effect of EGDMA content on metformin HCl release after 12 h from AA–PVA hydrogel

Table 5 Network parameters of AA–PVA hydrogels

Sample code	$v_{2,s}$	X	M_C	M_r	N	D (cm²/sec.)	Gel fraction (%)	Porosity (%)
S_1	0.041929	0.513976	208.8924	97.35177	4.291497	162.78	98.1	18.22
S_2	0.046729	0.515576	181.6807	97.35177	3.732457	158.61	98.9	14.2
S_3	0.050505	0.516835	143.1054	97.35177	2.939966	154.45	99.35	11.21

Scanning electron microscopy (SEM)

The morphology of AA–PVA hydrogel and drug loaded AA–PVA hydrogel was observed using scanning electron microscope JSM–6480.

Results and discussion

pH impact on swelling and on drug release behavior of AA–PVA hydrogels

The polymer chains absorb water in the presence of an aqueous solution, and the association/dissociation of various ions to polymer chains cause the IPN (Interpenetrating polymeric network) to swell. Ionic hydrogels are those hydrogels which have ionizable functional groups. Anionic gels swell at basic pH values and collapse at acidic pH values. The pKa of AA is 4.26. Carboxylic groups of the network ionize and attract cations to replace the H^+ ions, as the pH of the environmental solution is above its pKa. This successfully increases the concentration of free ions inside the gel. So, the ionic swelling pressure will increase and so does the swelling. Additionally, the carboxylate anions cause more hydrophilicity and electrostatic repulsion to the polymer segments in the hydrogel. So, by the increase in pH, the AA–PVA hydrogels swelled speedily due to more swelling driving force caused by the electrostatic repulsion between the ionized carboxylate groups [23–25]. Manifestation of the swelling ratios (dynamic and equilibrium) of AA–PVA hydrogels is given in Table 2. Table 3 is showing metformin amount loaded in various samples. To see the pH effect on drug release behavior, dissolution profiles were obtained in buffer solutions (pH 1.2, 5.5 and 7.5). Drug release increased as the medium pH increased, in all samples. Table 4 is showing the effect of pH on dug release after 12 h drug release study. Drug release can be correlated with the AA–PVA hydrogel samples swelling behavior where the swelling increased when the medium pH increased.

Effect of EGDMA content on swelling and on drug release behavior of AA–PVA hydrogel

The swelling of three hydrogel samples (S_1–S_3) was studied at different pH values as a function of different feed EGDMA concentrations. Fig. 2 is showing EGDMA content effect on the dynamic swelling coefficient keeping PVA and AA contents constant. A clear picture can be seen that the swelling ratio decreased by increasing the amount of EGDMA. This was due to the fact that as the crosslinker content increased, there was a decrease in the network mesh size and an increase in the stability of the network resulting in lower swelling [26, 27].

By increasing EGDMA concentration, a decrease in drug release at all pH values was observed. It can be correlated with the swelling behavior. The effect of EGDMA content on drug release is shown in Fig. 3.

Network parameters of AA–PVA hydrogels

The key parameters to characterize crosslinked swollen network are M_C and $v_{2,s}$ because M_C is a gauge of degree of crosslinking of the polymer while $v_{2,s}$ evaluates the liquid amount retained by the network. During mathematical modeling, equilibrium swelling data of pH 7.5 was used. Values of $v_{2,s}$, χ, M_C, M_r, N and D are elaborated in Table 5.

Table 6 Effect of EGDMA concentration on release kinetics of AA–PVA hydrogel at different pH

Sample code	EGDMA content (% w/w)	pH	Zero order kinetics		First order kinetics		Higuchi Model	
			K_0 (h⁻¹)	r	K_1 (h⁻¹)	r	K_2 (h⁻¹)	r
S_1	0.082	1.2	2.221	0.976	0.026	0.983	0.104	0.995
		5.5	4.016	0.992	0.058	0.999	0.186	0.998
		7.5	5.833	0.976	0.137	0.997	0.274	0.996
S_2	0.123	1.2	2.179	0.983	0.025	0.988	0.102	0.997
		5.5	3.953	0.99	0.056	0.997	0.183	0.998
		7.5	5.47	0.966	0.116	0.993	0.259	0.993
S_3	0.165	1.2	2.028	0.98	0.023	0.984	0.094	0.994
		5.5	3.852	0.99	0.053	0.997	0.179	0.997
		7.5	5.407	0.963	0.108	0.988	0.256	0.99

Table 7 Effect of EGDMA concentration on release mechanism of AA–PVA hydrogel

Sample code	EGDMA content (%w/w)	pH	r	Release exponent (n)	Order of release
S₁	0.082	1.2	0.983	0.991	non-fickian
		5.5	0.996	0.875	non-fickian
		7.5	0.995	0.665	non-fickian
S₂	0.123	1.2	0.987	0.989	non-fickian
		5.5	0.994	0.929	non-fickian
		7.5	0.99	0.689	non-fickian
S₃	0.165	1.2	0.989	0.999	non-fickian
		5.5	0.996	0.991	non-fickian
		7.5	0.985	0.741	non-fickian

Because of the high molar mass of the components involved, only a very small positive $v_{2,s}$ value can be tolerated. The higher the value of x, weaker is the interaction between solvent and polymer, and stronger is the interaction among polymer chains. The polymer-solvent interaction parameter (x) has values that increased by increasing the content of crosslinker. For many systems, x was found to increase by increasing the polymer content for a given polymer volume fraction, smaller the value of x, greater the rate at which the free energy of the solution decreased by the solvent addition. As a result, liquids with the smallest x values are the best solvents for a polymer. When there is an increase in swelling ratio, $v_{2,s}$ and x

values are decreased. When there is a decrease in swelling ratio, the mesh size decreased leading to a decrease in M_C and the rate of diffusion of solute would also be expected to decrease [15, 28–34].

By increasing the content of EGDMA, the gel fraction increased while the sol fraction decreased. This can be credited to the development of intermolecular crosslinks. Table 5 is elaborating the effects of EGDMA contents on the gel fraction of AA–PVA hydrogel. As by increasing crosslinker concentration, there will be more crosslinking which will ultimately increase the gel fraction [4, 8, 35–37].

Due to the porous structure, hydrogels take in more water via capillary action and transfer the drug into the pores. Table 5 is elaborating the effects of crosslinking agent on porosity. By increasing the concentration of EGDMA, porosity decreased. As a result of increased amount of EGDMA, there was an increase in crosslinking density, decrease in hydrogel mesh size which resulted in decreased porosity [4, 8, 38–40].

Drug release mechanism

When penetrant gets into the polymer network, the water soluble drug loaded in hydrogel is dissolved and drug diffusion occurs through the aqueous pathways to the surface of the device. The drug release was strongly linked to the swelling characteristics of the hydrogel which is a key parameter of structural design of the hydrogel. The method that best fits the release data was evaluated

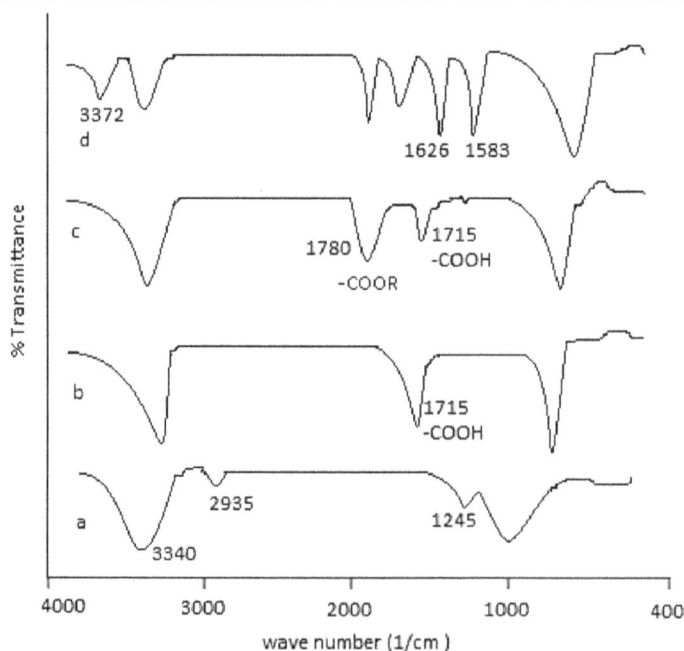

Fig. 4 FTIR spectra of PVA (**a**), acrylic acid (**b**), AA–PVA unloaded hydrogel (**c**) and drug loaded AA–PVA hydrogel (**d**)

by the regression coefficient (r). Criterion for selecting the most appropriate model was based on the ideal fit indicated by the values of regression coefficient (r) near to 1.

Values of regression coefficient (r) for zero order, first order and higuchi models obtained from drug loaded AA–PVA hydrogels at varying content of EGDMA are given in Table 6. For the most of samples, the values of regression coefficient (r) obtained for first order release rate constants were found higher than those of zero order.

It is attributed to the fact that drug release from the samples of varying degree of crosslinking are according to first order release. In higuchi model, r values at different crosslinker compositions indicated that the drug release mechanism is diffusion controlled [41].

Effect of EGDMA content on release exponent (n) is given in Table 7. The n value for the metformin HCl release was evaluated from the slope and intercept of the plot ln M_t/M_∞ versus ln t and the results showed that

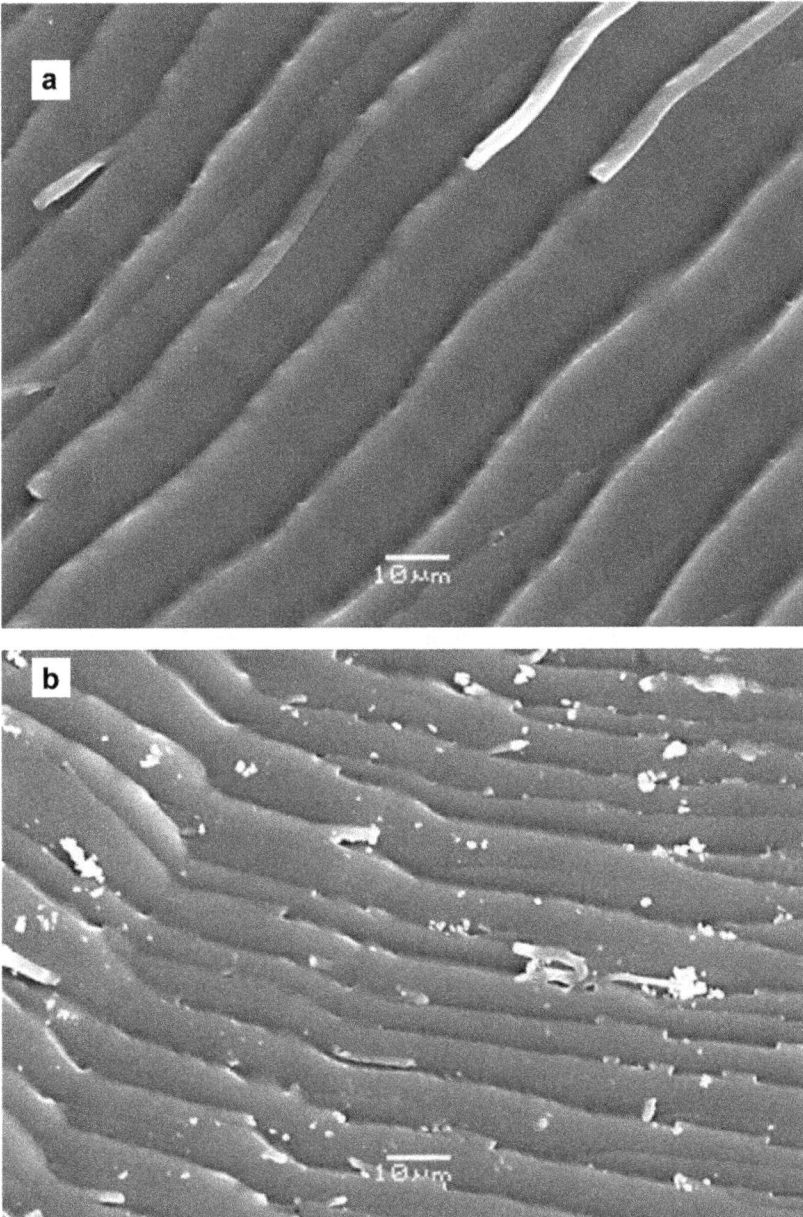

Fig. 5 SEM images of S_1 sample (**a**) and drug loaded S_1 sample (**b**)

the 'n' values are between 0.5 and 1.0 which indicated a non-fickian diffusion mechanism. It also clarified that the rate of drug diffusion from the hydrogels and the rate of polymer chain relaxation are interrelated [42].

FTIR spectroscopy
Comparative FTIR spectra of PVA, AA, AA–PVA hydrogel without drug and drug loaded AA–PVA hydrogel are shown in Fig. 4. The characterstic peak at 3340 cm^{-1} was due to the O–H stretching vibration of PVA and due to aliphatic C–H stretching vibration, a peak at 2935 cm^{-1} was observed. Due to C–O–C symmetrical stretching of the PVA backbone, a peak at 1245 cm^{-1} was seen. Peak at 1715 cm^{-1} was due to –COOH group of AA. A peak at 1780 cm^{-1} appeared for ester group in AA–PVA hydrogel representing the reaction between the –OH group of PVA with the –COOH group of AA [25]. In drug loaded AA–PVA hydrogel, a peak at 3372 cm^{-1} appeared representing N–H stretching of C = NH group of metformin and peaks at 1626 cm^{-1} and 1583 cm^{-1} appeared indicating C = N stretching of metformin [43].

Scanning electron microscopy
SEM images showed the voids present on the surface that will assist in drug incorporation. Fig. 5b is showing drug particles in hydrogel.

Conclusion
Chemically crosslinked pH–sensitive AA–PVA hydrogels were synthesized in the presence of EGDMA&GA as crosslinkers and proved to be a good candidate for drug delivery to intestine. By increasing the content of EGDMA, a decrease in swelling and in drug release was noted due to more crosslinking. Gel fraction was found to increase by increasing the EGDMA concentration. Porosity was found to decrease by increasing the EGDMA content. Drug release followed first order and the mechanism was non-fickian diffusion in all cases. The FTIR confirmed the formation of graft polymer. SEM image of the drug loaded hydrogel showed incorporation of drug in the hydrogel along with the voids present on the hydrogel surface. S_1–S_3 samples can be effectively used as carriers for targeted drug delivery to intestine.

Competing interests
The authors declare that they have no competing interests.

Authors' contributions
MFA performed the work and drafted the manuscript. NMR participated in its design and in sequence alignment. He also helped acquisition and interpretation of data. MH also helped acquisition and interpretation of data. All authors read and approved the final manuscript.

Acknowledgement
This work was financially supported by Faculty of Pharmacy, Bahauddin Zakariya University, Multan, Pakistan.

References
1. Liewen L, Hangbo Y, Yingde C. Crosslink polymerization kinetics and mechanism of hydrogels composed of acrylic acid and 2-acrylamido-2-methylpropane sulfonic acid. Chin J Chem Eng. 2011;19(2):285–91.
2. Lowman AM, Peppas NA. Hydrogels. In: Mathowitz E, editor. Encyclopedia of controlled drug delivery, vol. 2. New York: John Wiley & Sons; 1999. p. 397–418.
3. Cozzolino CA, Blomfeldt TOJ, Nilsson F, Piga A, Piergiovanni L, Farris S. Dye release behavior from polyvinyl alcohol films in a hydro-alcoholic medium: influence of physicochemical heterogeneity. Colloids surf. A: Physicochem Eng Asp. 2012;403:45–53.
4. Ranjha NM, Ayub G, Naseem S, Ansari MT. Preparation and characterization of hybrid pH-sensitive hydrogels of chitosan-co-acrylic acid for controlled release of verapamil. J Mater Sci Mater Med. 2010;21:2805–16.
5. Blanco MD, Olmo RM, Teijo'n JM. Hydrogels. In: Swarbrick J, editor. Encyclopedia of pharmaceutical technology, vol. 3. New York: Informa Healthcare; 2007. p. 2022.
6. Rana V, Rai P, Tiwary AK, Singh RS, Kennedy JF, Knill CJ. Modified gums: Approaches and applications in drug delivery. Carbohydr Polym. 2011;83:1031–47.
7. Kikuchi A, Okano T. Temperature-responsive polymers as on-off switches for intelligent biointerfaces. In: Okano T, editor. Biorelated polymers and gels. Boston: Academic; 1998. p. 1–28.
8. Ranjha NM, Mudassir J, Sheikh ZZ. Synthesis and characterization of pH-sensitive pectin/acrylic acid hydrogels for verapamil release study. Iran Poly J. 2011;20(2):147–59.
9. Juntanon K, Niamlang S, Rujiravanit R, Sirivat A. Electrically controlled release of sulfosalicylic acid from crosslinked poly (vinyl alcohol) hydrogel. Int J Pharm. 2008;356(1–2):1–11.
10. Omidian H, Park K. Experimental design for the synthesis of polyacrylamide superporous hydrogels. J Bioact Compat Polym. 2002;17:433–50.
11. Peppas NA, Barr-Howel BD. Characterization of the crosslinked structure of hydrogels. In: Peppas NA, editor. Hydrogels in medicine and pharmacy, vol. 1. Florida: CRC Press: Boca Raton; 1987. p. 22–56.
12. Peppas NA, Huang Y, Lugo MT, Ward JH, Zhang J. Physicochemical foundations and structural design of hydrogels in medicine and biology. Annu Rev Biomed Eng. 2000;2:9–29.
13. Pourjavadi A, Barzegar S. Smart pectin based superabsorbent hydrogel as a matrix for ibubrofen as an oral Non-steroidal anti inflammatory drug delivery. Starch/Strake. 2009;61:173–87.
14. Shukla S, Bajpai AK. Preparation and characterization of highly swelling smart grafted polymer networks of poly (vinyl alcohol) and poly (acrylic acid-co-acrylamide). J Appl Polym Sci. 2006;102:84–95.
15. Peppas NA, Hilt JZ, Khademhosseini A, Langer R. Hydrogels in biology and medicine: From molecular principles to bionanotechnology. Adv Mater. 2006;18:1345–60.
16. Crank J. The mathematics of diffusion. Claredon press: Oxford; 1975. p. 244.
17. Alla SGA, El-Din HMN, El-Naggar AWM. Structure and swelling-release behaviour of poly(vinyl pyrrolidone) (PVP) and acrylic acid (AAc) copolymer hydrogels prepared by gamma irradiation. Eur Polym J. 2007;43:2987–98.
18. Yin L, Fei L, Cui F, Tang C, Yin C. Superporous hydrogels containing poly(acrylicacid-co-acrylamide)/O-carboxymethyl chitosan interpenetrating polymer networks. Biomaterials. 2007;28:1258–66.
19. Najib N, Suleiman M. The kinetics of drug release from ethyl cellulose solid dispersions. Drug Dev Ind Pharm. 1985;11:2169–89.
20. Desai SJ, Singh P, Simonelli AP, Higuchi WI. Investigation of factors influencing release of solid drug dispersed in wax matices. Quantitative studies involving polyethylene plastic matrix. J Pharm Sci. 1966;55:1230–4.
21. Higuchi T. Mechanism of sustained action medication. Theoretical analysis of rate of release of solid drugs dispersed in solid matrices. J Pharm Sci. 1963;50:1145–9.
22. Peppas NA. Analysis of Fickian and non-Fickian drug release from polymers. Pharm Acta Helv. 1985;60:110–1.
23. Yun J, Kim H. Preparation of poly (vinyl alcohol)/poly (acrylic acid) microcapsules and microspheres and their pH-responsive release behavior. J Ind Eng Chem. 2009;15:902–6.

24. Kurkuri MD, Aminabhavi TM. Poly (vinyl alcohol) and poly (acrylic acid) sequential interpenetrating network pH-sensitive microspheres for the delivery of diclofenac sodium to the intestine. J Control Release. 2004;96:9–20.
25. Ray D, Gils PS, Mohanta GP, Manavalan R, Sahoo PK. Comparative delivery of diltiazem hydrochloride through synthesized polymer: hydrogel and hydrogel microspheres. J Appl Polym Sci. 2010;116:959–68.
26. Hussain T, Ranjha NM, Shahzad Y. Swelling and controlled release of tramadol hydrochloride from a pH-sensitive hydrogel. Des Monomers Polym. 2011;14:233–49.
27. Ranjha NM, Mudassir J, Akhtar N. Methyl methacrylate-co-itaconic acid (MMA-co-IA) hydrogels for controlled drug delivery. J Sol–gel. Sci Technol. 2008;47:23–30.
28. Li X, Wu W, Wang J, Duan Y. The swelling behaviour and network parameters of guar gum/poly (acrylic acid) semi-interpenetrating polymer network hydrogels. Cabohydr Polym. 2006;66:473–9.
29. Mellott MB, Searcy K, Pishko V. Release of protein from highly cross-linked hydrogels of poly (ethylene glycol) diacrylate fabricated by UV polymerization. Biomaterials. 2001;22:929–41.
30. Savas H. Gu¨ven O. Investigation of active substance release from poly (ethylene oxide) hydrogels. Int J Pharm. 2001;224:151–8.
31. Xue W, Champ S, Huglin MB. Network and swelling parameters of chemically crosslinked thermoreversible hydrogels. Polymer. 2001;42:3665–9.
32. Davis TD, Huglin MB, Yip DCF. Properties of poly (N-vinyl-2-pyrrolidone) hydrogels crosslinked with ethyleneglycol dimethacrylate. Polymer. 1988;29:701–6.
33. Orwoll RA, Arnold PA. Polymer-solvent interaction parameter x. In: Mark JE, editor. Physical properties of polymers handbook. New York: AIP Press; 1996. p. 177–96.
34. Ekenstein GORAV, Meyboom R, Ikkala GTBO. Determination of the Flory-Huggins interaction parameter of styrene and 4-vinylpyridine using copolymer blends of poly (styrene-co-4-vinylpyridine) and polystyrene. Macromolecules. 2000;33:3752–6.
35. Alla SGA, Sen M, El-Naggar AWM. Swelling and mechanical properties of superabsorbent hydrogels based on Tara gum/acrylic acid synthesized by gamma radiation. Carbohydr Polym. 2012;89:478–85.
36. El-Rehim HAA, Diaa DA. Radiation-induced eco-compatible sulfonated starch/acrylic acid graft copolymers for sucrose hydrolysis. Carbohydr Polym. 2012;87:1905–12.
37. Amin MCIM, Ahmad N, Halib N, Ahmad I. Synthesis and characterization of thermo- and pH-responsive bacterial cellulose/acrylic acid hydrogels for drug delivery. Carbohydr Polym. 2012;88:465–73.
38. Rafat M, Rotenstein LS, You JO, Auguste DT. Dual functionalized PVA hydrogels that adhere endothelial cells synergistically. Biomaterials. 2012;33:3880–6.
39. Juby KA, Dwivedi C, Kumar M, Kota S, Misra HS, Bajaj PN. Silver nanoparticle-loaded PVA/gum acacia hydrogel: Synthesis, characterization and antibacterial study. Carbohydr Polym. 2012;89:906–13.
40. Singh B, Sharma V. Design of psyllium-PVA-acrylic acid based novel hydrogels for use in antibiotic drug delivery. Int J Pharm. 2010;389:94–106.
41. Mishra RK, Datt M, Banthia AK. Synthesis and characterization of pectin/PVP hydrogel membrnes for drug delivery system. AAPS PharmSciTech. 2008;9(2):395–403.
42. Singh B, Bala R, Chauhan N. Invitro release dynamics of model drugs from psyllium and acrylic acid based hydrogels for the use in colon specific drug delivery. J Mater Sci Mater Med. 2008;19:2271–80.
43. Gunasekaran S, Natarajan RK, Renganayaki V, Natarajan S. Vibrational spectra and thermodynamic analysis of metformin. Indian J Pure Appl Phys. 2006;44:495–500.

22

Can donepezil facilitate weaning from mechanical ventilation in difficult to wean patients? An interventional pilot study

Saeed Abbasi[1], Shadi Farsaei[2*], Kamran Fazel[3], Samad EJ Golzari[4] and Ata Mahmoodpoor[5]

Abstract

Background: Management of difficult to wean patients is a dilemma for health care system. Recently published studies demonstrated efficacy of donepezil to counteract respiratory depression in sleep apnea. However, to the best of our knowledge, pharmaceutical interventions with donepezil to facilitate weaning have not been tested so far. Therefore in the present study, we evaluated the efficacy of using donepezil on weaning course in difficult to wean patients.

Methods: In this non-randomized interventional clinical study, difficult to wean patients with prior inappropriately depressed respiratory responses were included from two referral intensive care units (ICU) in Iran. Patients with another potentially reasons of weaning failure were excluded from the study. Donepezil was started for eligible patients at dose of 10 mg daily for 2–4 weeks. For the primary outcomes, arterial blood gas (ABG) parameters were also measured before and after intervention to evaluate the possible effects of donepezil on them. In addition, weaning outcomes of patients were reported as final outcome in response to this intervention.

Results: Twelve out of 16 studied patients experienced successful results to facilitate weaning with donepezil intervention. The mean duration of donepezil treatment until outcome measurement was 12 days. There were not any significant differences in ABG parameters among patients with successful and failed weaning trial on day of donepezil initiation. However after donepezil intervention, mean of PCO_2 and HCO_3 decreased in patients with successful weaning trial and mean of PCO_2 increased in those with weaning failure.

Conclusions: Reduced central respiratory drive was infrequently reason of failed weaning attempts but it must be considered especially in patients with hypercapnia secondary to inefficient gas exchange and slow breathing. Our results in the clinical setting suggest that, the use of donepezil can expedite weaning presumably by stimulation of respiratory center and obviate the need to re-intubation in cases of respiratory drive problem in difficult to wean patients. We suggest decrease PCO_2 and HCO_3 during donepezil steady could be valuable predictors for positive response to donepezil intervention.

Background

Difficult weaning is a common problem of patients in whom weaning trials were attempted [1]. Since, 26% of medical and surgical patients were considered difficult-to-wean in a prospective cohort study [2]. Similarly, another prospective cohort study found that the incidence of difficult weaning was 39% among patients who needed mechanical ventilaion for more than 12 hours [3].

Both prolonged weaning and duration of mechanical ventilation are associated with increased risk of mortality. Therefore, difficult weaning is an important challenge for critically ill patients with mechanical ventilation support [4]. Management of patients who are difficult-to-wean is based on identification and correction of potential causes related to ventilator dependency [5].

Although impaired respiratory drive is an uncommon cause of weaning failure, but its important role should be highlighted if any definite reason is not found for weaning failure [1]. Therefore, treatment targeting the respiratory drive can be helpful in facilitating weaning of

* Correspondence: farsaei@pharm.mui.ac.ir
[2]Department of Clinical Pharmacy and Pharmacy Practice, Isfahan University of Medical Sciences, Isfahan, Iran
Full list of author information is available at the end of the article

difficult-to-wean patients [6]. Respiratory stimulants such as caffeine, aminophylline and doxapram have been used effectively to increase central respiratory drive and subsequently weaning from mechanical ventilation and avoiding post-extubation apnea in preterm infants [7-9]. In addition, some studies showed beneficial effects of cholinergic drugs like donepezil to stimulate respiratory drive [10,7].

Some advances in understanding the role of central cholinergic modulation in the process of respiration provide a pharmacological basis for explaining beneficial effects of cholinergic drugs as therapeutic agents for disorders related to neural control of breathing [10]. Donepezil is cholinergic drug which reversibly and noncompetitively inhibits centrally-active acetyl cholinesterase [11]. It was first introduced for Alzheimer treatment but many studies showed efficacy and safety of donepezil for different clinical problems such as cognitive impairment resulting from severe traumatic brain injury [12-14]. Nausea, diarrhea, insomnia and infection were reported the most prevalent adverse reactions of donepezil with prevalence of less than 20% in high doses of donepezil [15].

Moreover, findings of conducted animal studies indicated the beneficial effect of systemically administered donepezil to counteract respiratory depression in anesthetized rabbits [16,17]. Recently published clinical studies showed donepezil may improve sleep apnea [18,19]. As a result, it seems donepezil is safe and may be effective medication to stimulate respiratory drive. To the best of our knowledge, pharmaceutical interventions with donepezil in difficult-to-wean patients have not been tested so far. Therefore, in the present study we hypothesized that using donepezil could facilitate weaning course in difficult-to-wean patients.

Methods

This is an interventional non-randomized clinical study approved by medical ethics committee of Isfahan University of Medical Sciences (Code Number: 292232) and conducted in the intensive care units (ICUs) of two referral hospitals in Iran (Alzahra and Imam reza hospitals).

Intubated patients who failed the first spontaneous breathing trial (SBT) on weaning trial and required up to three SBTs or 7 days to pass a SBT were defined as difficult-to-wean. Difficult-to-wean patients with prior inappropriately depressed respiratory responses when removed from the ventilator were considered eligible to enter in this study.

According to clinical judgment of intensivist, when other possible reasons of weaning failure such as electrolytes and acid–base disorders were ruled out, depressed respiratory response could be considered the cause of this failure.

Since electrolytes and acid–base imbalances (in particular metabolic alkalosis from volume depletion which promoted hypoventilation) could interfere in weaning process, we did

our best to control and maintain normal ranges of serum electrolytes and nutritional support in this study and preserve the pH less than 7.45 during the time of active weaning [20].

Patients with unconsciousness and need for sedation or hypothyroidism were excluded from this study.

A continuous electrocardiograms (ECG), heart rate, mean arterial blood pressure, and oxygen saturation were also monitored during SBT. Therefore, patients with weaning-related myocardial ischemia or hemodynamic instability were excluded from the study to omit the potentially negative effects of these confounding factors on weaning failure [21]. Treatment with other potentially respiratory stimulants such as doxapram and medroxyprogesterone was additional criterion to exclude patients from this study.

Donepezil was started for eligible patients according to inclusion and exclusion criteria at dose of 10 mg daily. Because time to steady state for donepezil was expected 15 days [22], donepezil administration was continued at least for 2 weeks and patients were followed up daily during this period and evaluated for readiness of weaning and other endpoints of the study. If weaning was failed during first two weeks, patients would be assessed again for another potential barrier to extubation. In cases with strong clinical suspicion of central respiratory drive problem during weaning, donepezil was continued for another two weeks until 4-week duration of donepezil treatment [23].

For the primary outcomes of the study, oxygenation variables such as partial pressures of oxygen (PO2) and carbon dioxide (PCO2), pH and hemoglobin oxygen saturation (SO2) were measured on day of donepezil initiation and on day of outcome evaluation. Moreover, weaning outcomes of patients were reported as final outcome in response to this intervention. Thereafter for statistical analysis patients were categorized in two groups: patients with successful or failure weaning and then oxygenation variables mentioned above were compared between two groups.

Statistical analysis: Descriptive and statistical analyses were performed. The distribution of continuous variables was assessed by the Kolmogrov-Smirnov test, and continuous data were expressed as mean ± SD. The Mann–Whitney U test and independent sample t-tests were used to assess differences in quantitative data of patients' characteristics for nonparametric and parametric variables, respectively. For categorical data expressed as percentage, chi-squared test was applied.

Results

Eighteen difficult-to-wean patients with suspicion of depressed respiratory response (62 ± 18 years old) were included in this study and finally 16 patients completed the study for outcome measurement. Two patients of enrolled subjects died before any evaluations, therefore data were not applicable to evaluate weaning outcome of them (Figure 1). Characteristics of the patients were summarized in Table 1.

The study patients had been on mechanical ventilation for 32 ± 21 days prior to study enrollment. In addition, more than 80% of patients had been failed weaning trial more than 2 times before enter to study. Among 16 studied patients, 13 patients had pneumonia, whereas; 30% of them experienced concomitant acute exacerbation of COPD. Pulmonary edema was also reported in 3 patients (Table 1).

The results showed 12 out of 16 patients experienced successful weaning during donepezil intervention. However, in one of the successful weaning trial, re-intubation was occurred during 24 hours and therefore considered as final unsuccessful weaning outcome.

Therefore, 11 patients were categorized as successful weaning and remained patients were classified in unsuccessful weaning group. In comparison of these two groups of patients (successful or failure weaning), there were not any significant differences in age, duration of mechanical ventilation and number of failed weaning trial before donepezil initiation (p-value > 0.05) (Table 2).

The effects of donepezil on arterial blood gas (ABG) were also evaluated on day of donepezil initiation and on day of outcome measurement. Variations in arterial PH, PO2, PCO2, HCO3 and oxygen saturation were demonstrated in part A, B, C, D and E of Figure 2 respectively. Results showed patients had no evidence of primary metabolic alkalosis at weaning time.

According to independent sample t-test, there were not any significant differences in ABG parameters between successful and unsuccessful weaning patients on day of donepezil initiation (p-value > 0.05). In patients with successful weaning trial, paired sample analyses revealed

mean of PCO2 and HCO3 decreased, whereas mean of PO2 and PO2 saturation increased after donepezil intervention. Although, in those with failed weaning, mean of PCO2 increased after donepezil intervention. However none of these statistical analyses were significant (Table 3).

Discussion

This present study was performed in difficult-to-wean patients with potential respiratory drive problems which caused repeatedly failing spontaneous breathing attempts. Donepezil administration in our study enabled successful SBT and weaning in nearly 70% of patients. Our patients manifested hypercapnia and hypopnea when removed from the ventilator in prior weaning trials which promoted the probability of reduced ventilator central drive before donepezil initiation. Since, we initially could find neither reversible causes for repeated failure to prior weaning trials, nor any contraindication for the use of donepezil, we empirically used donepezil to facilitate weaning in these patients.

According to recent systematic review and meta-analysis, 10 mg donepezil was well tolerated without any life threatening effect [24]. In addition, regarding to the long half-life of donepezil (70 hours) it is unlikely that adverse reactions of donepezil occurs in first days of its initiation [25]. Therefore, deaths of two patients in the initial days of donepezil intervention might be related to poor clinical condition of them not donepezil adverse reactions. Also it should be mentioned that no related adverse reaction of donepezil was reported during follow up of our study.

Etiologies of failures upon removal from the ventilator in spite of donepezil treatment in our study were not readily clear. Although it seems patients apparently had a depressed ventilatory drive initially, but possible inadequate resolution of the illness that had caused mechanical ventilation and/or progress of new problem could incorporate to weaning failure in few patients.

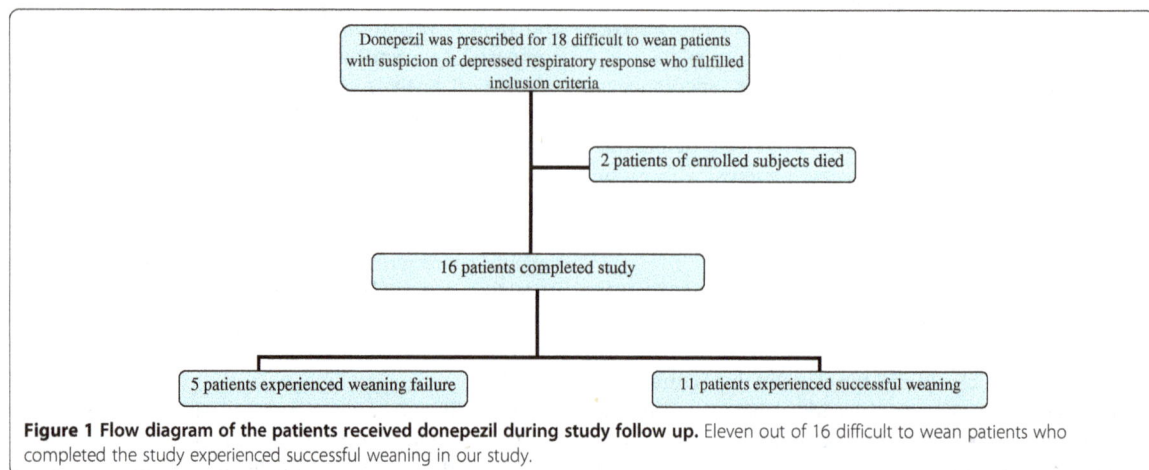

Figure 1 Flow diagram of the patients received donepezil during study follow up. Eleven out of 16 difficult to wean patients who completed the study experienced successful weaning in our study.

Table 1 Demographic and clinical characteristics of the patients with donepezil intervention to facilitate weaning

Patient	Age	Sex	Diagnosis	Number of failed weaning trial[a]	Duration of MV[a]	Days of donepezil treatment*	Outcome of weaning	ICU outcome
1	73	M	COPD exacerbation, pneumonia, pulmonary edema	2	10	28	S but re-intubated	D
2	26	M	Opioid intoxiction, seizure	2	30[#]	6	S	A
3	55	M	COPD exacerbation, PTE, pneumonia	2	5	4	S	A
4	73	M	COPD exacerbation, Pneumonia	2	5	8	S	D
5	72	M	Brain tumor, PTE, pneumonia	2	10	15	F'	D
6	64	F	Abdominoplasty, PTE	2	19	9	S	A
7	80	F	PTE, dyspnea, pneumonia, pulmonary edema	1	18	8	S	A
8	68	M	Arrest, pneumonia	3	60[#]	6	S	A
9	41	F	Arnoldikiary, pneumonia	2	25[#]	13	S	A
10	81	F	cholecystectomy	2	32[#]	10	S	A
11	78	M	COPD exacerbation, pneumonia	3	33[#]	17	F'	A
12	68	M	CVA, pneumonia	3	65[#]	27	S	A
13	67	M	PTE, dyspnea, pneumonia	3	60[#]	4	S	A
14	81	M	Massive pleural effusion, pneumonia, pulmonary edema	3	57[#]	15	F'	A
15	24	M	Multiple trauma, pneumonia	1	57[#]	21	S	A
16	46	M	Cerebral tumor, pneumonia, PTE	1	33[#]	15	F'	A

[a]Before donepezil initiation.
*From initial donepezil treatment until outcome measurement.
[#]Tracheostomy tube used for mechanical ventilation.
A, alive; COPD, chronic obstructive pulmonary disease; CVA, cerebrovascular accident; D, died; F, female; F', failure; MV, mechanical ventilation; M, male; NA, not applicable and excluded; PTE, pulmonary thromboembolism; S, success.

Muscle fatigue is one of the frequent causes of weaning failure manifested ultimately by rising in PCO_2 [26]. Weaning failure in our study might be contributed to muscle fatigue during donepezil intervention. Because as mentioned in results, mean PCO_2 rose in patients with unsuccessful weaning in this period. If fatigue developed during donepezil treatment, further stimulation of the respiratory muscles with donepezil would have inevitably made the fatigue worse and patients would have weaning failure or required re-intubation.

In addition, in a patient with cervical tumor, phrenic nerve was involved and patient had also peripheral neuropathy. Since, diaphragm muscle is primarily innervated by the phrenic nerve, partial damage of that in surgical removal of cervical tumor could be a reason for failed response to donepezil intervention.

Moreover, metabolic alkalosis may be another causative factor for re-intubation of the first patient in our study because compensatory hypoventilatory response to metabolic alkalosis disposed patient to weaning failure or re-intubation [27]. Some studies maintained pH less than 7.4 during the time of active weaning [28].

Most of patients had history of pneumonia in our study which justified extubation failure and predisposition of them in difficult-to-wean condition. Pneumonia at the initiation of ventilation was one of the best predictors of extubation failure for patients following a successful SBT [29].

Cholinergic stimulation to develop respiratory coordination [30], increasing neuromuscular transmission and improving the effectiveness of upper airways muscles are some reasons which donepezil can accelerate weaning [31].

Table 2 Comparison of clinical parameters in patients with successful and unsuccessful weaning trial

Parameters	Successful weaning (N = 11)	Unsuccessful weaning (N = 5)	p-value *
Age (Mean ± SD)	58.8 ± 20.1	70.0 ± 14.0	0.22
duration of mechanical ventilation (Mean ± SD)	34.2 ± 22.6	28.6 ± 19.6	0.83
duration of donepezil treatment (Mean ± SD)	10.6 ± 7.3	18.0 ± 5.7	0.03

*Mann–Whitney U test was performed.

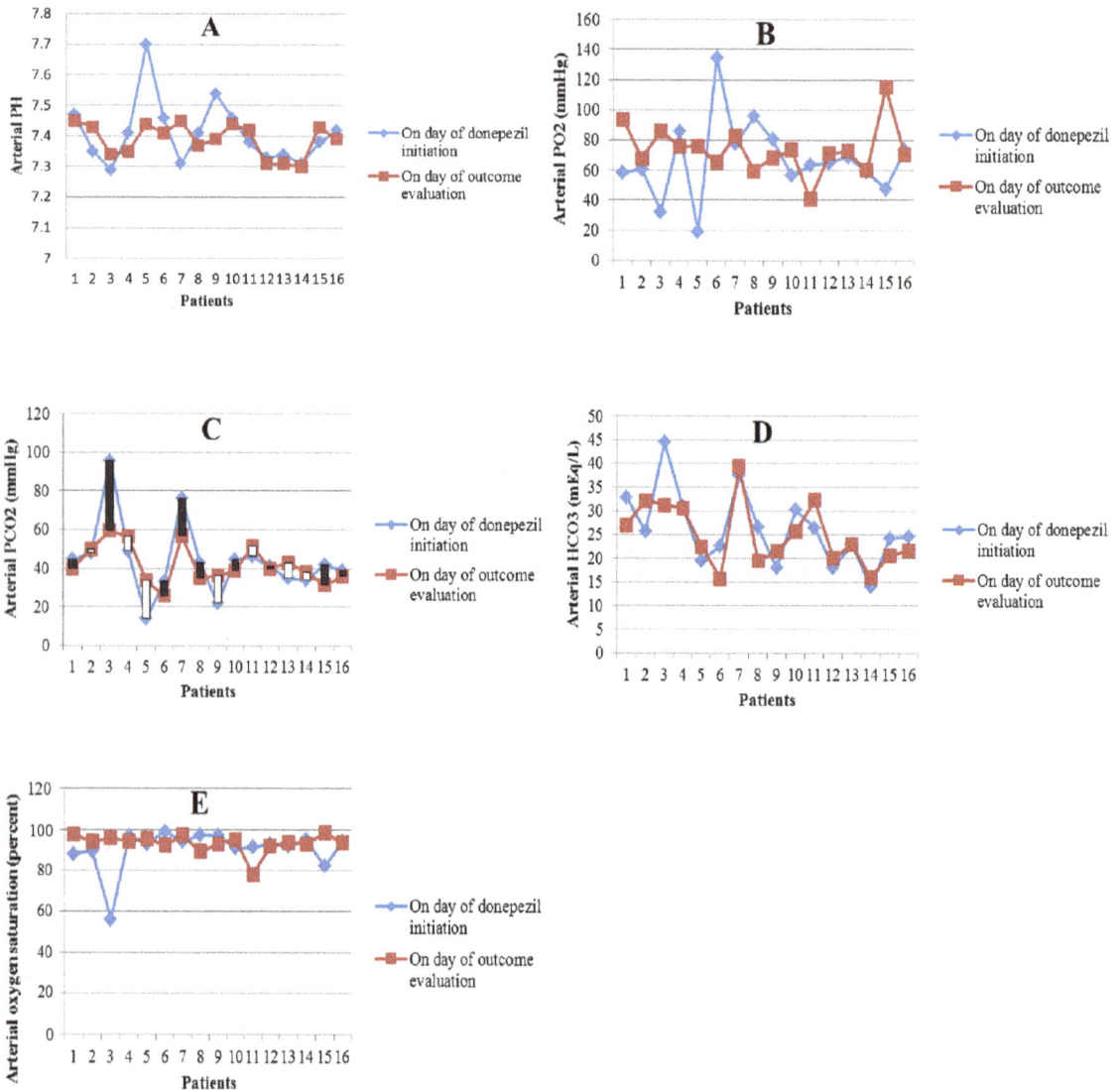

Figure 2 Variation of Arterial blood gas during donepezil treatment. Variations in arterial PH, PO2, PCO2, HCO3 and oxygen saturation were demonstrated in part **A**, **B**, **C**, **D** and **E** respectively. For each patient the first reported parameter was related to donepezil initiation day and the last one demonstrated that parameter on weaning day or until donepezil treatment was continued in cases of weaning failure. Patients with number 5, 11, 14 and 16 had unsuccessful attempts for weaning.

Not only cholinergic drugs can increase chemoreflex response to hypoxia by acting upon carotid body and stimulate respiratory center, but also play an important role in the neural control of respiration [31-33]. In addition, beneficial effects of cholinergic drugs to increase saliva secretion can reduce collapsibility of upper airways and contribute in this result [34]. Although different mechanisms can explain the beneficial effect of donepezil to expedite weaning but the exact mechanism is not clear.

By considering these mechanisms, donepezil facilitated the weaning of most patients in our study. We conclude

that ABG parameters can be valuable factors to predict patient response to donepezil intervention. As our results also showed, decrease of PCO2 and HCO3 during donepezil steady state would give us good news about positive response of donepezil and possibly successful weaning trial in near future. Conversely, increase or unchanged PCO2 during steady state of donepezil could promote clinicians to seek for other reasons of weaning failure such as muscle fatigue. However, because of small sample size analyzed in this study differences in ABG parameters between two groups

Table 3 Arterial blood gas parameters before and after donepezil intervention

	ABG parameters	Group	Mean ± SD	p-value
Successful weaning (N = 11)	PH	Before	7.39 ± .076	0.96
		After	7.38 ± .047	
	PO2	Before	73.2 ± 27.1	0.84
		After	75.5 ± 15.3	
	PCO2	Before	48.2 ± 20.6	0.23
		After	42.8 ± 11.3	
	HCO3	Before	27.4 ± 8.0	0.19
		After	25.1 ± 7.4	
	PO2 saturation	Before	89.9 ± 12.1	0.29
		After	94.49 ± 2.4	
Unsuccessful weaning or re-intubation (N = 5)	PH	Before	7.46 ± 0.15	0.19
		After	7.40 ± 0.06	
	PO2	Before	54.7 ± 20.9	0.67
		After	68.2 ± 19.6	
	PCO2	Before	35.5 ± 13.0	0.192
		After	39.8 ± 7.0	
	HCO3	Before	23.5 ± 7.1	0.132
		After	23.9 ± 6.1	
	PO2 saturation	Before	92.4 ± 2.7	0.99
		After	91.7 ± 7.8	

PCO2: carbon dioxide, PO2: Partial pressures of oxygen, SO2: hemoglobin oxygen saturation and SD: standard deviation.

(successful and failure weaning) were not statistically significant.

Various pharmacokinetic parameters in population study and contribution of different factors in weaning process might be the reasons of diverse time needed for donepezil treatment to achieve its response goal during the study. As expected, mean duration of donepezil until successful weaning was 12 days which was parallel to the time required for donepezil to receive its steady state [20]. However, clinical benefit of donepezil may occur before or after steady state of donepezil. Therefore we suggest if weaning is not facilitated during 2 weeks of donepezil initiation and clinician do not find any other factor for this failure, patient may benefit from 4 weeks therapy. This study protocol justify the significant higher duration of donepezil treatment in patients who failed weaning trial compared to those with successful weaning outcomes.

Finally, potential limitations of the present study should be mentioned. First, however patients ruled out for other potential barriers of weaning in our study but other reasons of weaning failure might not be completely resolved or some new barriers evolved during the study. So, outcome of weaning failure in our population is not necessarily or primarily related to respiratory drive problem which is discussed in patients with unsuccessful weaning trial. Another limitation which should be pointed out is that relatively small number of studied patients. Despite more than 1 year study duration and inclusion of consecutive patients in two centers; only limited number of patients entered the study according to inclusion and exclusion criteria. A non-randomized design of this study without control group is the third limitation. Therefore, these results require further confirmation with larger controlled clinical trials to clarify and establish donepezil role in the management of difficult-to-wean patients. Additional studies should be conducted to compare the efficacy of donepezil with other respiratory center stimulants such as doxapram or cholinergic drugs to facilitate weaning in difficult-to-wean patients with respiratory drive problem. Moreover, the effect of donepezil on weaning of patients with different diagnoses can be evaluated in future studies.

Conclusion

According to safety consideration and previous study in obstructive sleep apnea (OSA) we evaluated 10 mg of donepezil during 2–4 weeks in our study [19]. In accordance with our findings, donepezil also supported breathing regulation in OSA patients [19]. To the best of our knowledge, this is the first study in which donepezil was given as respiratory drive stimulant in difficult-to-wean patients in order to expedite the weaning.

However ventilator drive failure uncommonly exists on the list of reversible causes of weaning problem, but it may prolong mechanical ventilation and lead impaired weaning. We think this condition may be overlooked by the other factors which contribute to weaning failure and may remain unrecognized. Our results showed donepezil could be considered as useful treatment option in this condition.

Competing interests
The authors declare that they have no competing interests.

Authors' contributions
SA carried out patient assessment for inclusion and exclusion criteria, donepezil prescription and patient follow up to evaluate outcome of donepezil intervention in Alzahra hospital. He is also participated in design of study and revising the manuscript. SF conceived of the study, and participated in its design and coordination and participated in sequence alignment and drafted the manuscript. She also helped acquisition and interpretation of data and statistical analysis. KF carried out patient assessment for inclusion and exclusion criteria, donepezil prescription and patient follow up to evaluate outcome of donepezil intervention in Alzahra hospital and helped acquisition of data. SEJG and AM carried out patient assessment for inclusion and exclusion criteria, donepezil prescription and patient follow up to evaluate outcome of donepezil intervention in Imam reza hospital. SEJG also helped acquisition of data. All authors read and approved the final manuscript.

Acknowledgements
This work was financially supported by anesthesiology and critical care research center of Isfahan University of Medical Sciences, Iran.

Author details
[1]Anesthesiology and Critical Care Research Center, Isfahan University of Medical Sciences, Isfahan, Iran. [2]Department of Clinical Pharmacy and Pharmacy Practice, Isfahan University of Medical Sciences, Isfahan, Iran. [3]Department of Anesthesia and Critical Care Medicine, Bagiatalla University of Medical Sciences, Tehran, Iran. [4]Medical Education Research Center, Tabriz University of Medical Sciences, Tabriz, Iran. [5]Cardiovascular Research Center, Tabriz University of Medical Sciences, Tabriz, Iran.

References
1. Heunks LM, van der Hoeven JG. Clinical review: the ABC of weaning failure–a structured approach. Crit Care. 2010;14:245.
2. Funk GC, Anders S, Breyer MK, Burghuber OC, Edelmann G, Heindl W, et al. Incidence and outcome of weaning from mechanical ventilation according to new categories. Eur Respir J. 2010;35:88–94.
3. Penuelas O, Frutos-Vivar F, Fernandez C, Anzueto A, Epstein SK, Apezteguia C, et al. Characteristics and outcomes of ventilated patients according to time to liberation from mechanical ventilation. Am J Respir Crit Care Med. 2011;184:430–7.
4. Thille AW, Cortes-Puch I, Esteban A. Weaning from the ventilator and extubation in ICU. Curr Opin Crit Care. 2013;19:57–64.
5. Grasso S, Pisani L. Weaning and the heart: from art to science*. Crit Care Med. 2014;42:1954–5.
6. Durbin Jr CG, Blanch L, Fan E, Hess DR. Respiratory care year in review 2013: airway management, noninvasive monitoring, and invasive mechanical ventilation. Respir Care. 2014;59:595–606.
7. Bancalari E, Claure N. Strategies to accelerate weaning from respiratory support. Early Hum Dev. 2013;89 Suppl 1:S4–6.
8. Parnell H, Quirke G, Farmer S, Adeyemo S, Varney V. The successful treatment of hypercapnic respiratory failure with oral modafinil. Int J Chron Obstruct Pulmon Dis. 2014;9:413–9.
9. Kim DW, Joo JD, In JH, Jeon YS, Jung HS, Jeon KB, et al. Comparison of the recovery and respiratory effects of aminophylline and doxapram following total intravenous anesthesia with propofol and remifentanil. J Clin Anesth. 2013;25:173–6.
10. Shao XM, Feldman JL. Central cholinergic regulation of respiration: nicotinic receptors. Acta Pharmacol Sin. 2009;30:761–70.
11. Seltzer B. Donepezil: a review. Expert Opin Drug Metab Toxicol. 2005;1:527–36.
12. Hansen RA, Gartlehner G, Webb AP, Morgan LC, Moore CG, Jonas DE. Efficacy and safety of donepezil, galantamine, and rivastigmine for the treatment of Alzheimer's disease: a systematic review and meta-analysis. Clin Interv Aging. 2008;3:211–25.
13. Ballesteros J, Guemes I, Ibarra N, Quemada JI. The effectiveness of donepezil for cognitive rehabilitation after traumatic brain injury: a systematic review. J Head Trauma Rehabil. 2008;23:171–80.
14. Foster M, Spiegel DR. Use of donepezil in the treatment of cognitive impairments of moderate traumatic brain injury. J Neuropsychiatry Clin Neurosci. 2008;20:106.
15. Donepezil. In: Lexi-Comp Online™, Lexi-Drugs Online™. Hudson (OH): Lexi-Comp, Inc.; Accessed via UpToDate 2014 Dec 9.
16. Sakuraba S, Tsujita M, Arisaka H, Takeda J, Yoshida K, Kuwana S. Donepezil reverses buprenorphine-induced central respiratory depression in anesthe-tized rabbits. Biol Res. 2009;42:469–75.
17. Tsujita M, Sakuraba S, Kuribayashi J, Hosokawa Y, Hatori E, Okada Y, et al. Antagonism of morphine-induced central respiratory depression by donepezil in the anesthetized rabbit. Biol Res. 2007;40:339–46.
18. Moraes W, Poyares D, Sukys-Claudino L, Guilleminault C, Tufik S. Donepezil improves obstructive sleep apnea in Alzheimer disease: a double-blind, placebo-controlled study. Chest. 2008;133:677–83.
19. Sukys-Claudino L, Moraes W, Guilleminault C, Tufik S, Poyares D. Beneficial effect of donepezil on obstructive sleep apnea: a double-blind, placebo-controlled clinical trial. Sleep Med. 2012;13:290–6.
20. Gruber PC, Gomersall CD, Leung P, Joynt GM, Ng SK, Ho KM, et al. Randomized controlled trial comparing adaptive-support ventilation with pressure-regulated volume-controlled ventilation with automode in weaning patients after cardiac surgery. Anesthesiology. 2008;109:81–7.
21. Routsi C, Stanopoulos I, Zakynthinos E, Politis P, Papas V, Zervakis D, et al. Nitroglycerin can facilitate weaning of difficult-to-wean chronic obstructive pulmonary disease patients: a prospective interventional non-randomized study. Crit Care. 2010;14:15.
22. Liptzin B, Laki A, Garb JL, Fingeroth R, Krushell R. Donepezil in the prevention and treatment of post-surgical delirium. Am J Geriatr Psychiatry. 2005;13:1100–6.
23. Rogers SL, Cooper NM, Sukovaty R, Pederson JE, Lee JN, Friedhoff LT. Pharmacokinetic and pharmacodynamic profile of donepezil HCl following multiple oral doses. Br J Clin Pharmacol. 1998;46 Suppl 1:7–12.
24. Tan CC, Yu JT, Wang HF, Tan MS, Meng XF, Wang C, et al. Efficacy and safety of donepezil, galantamine, rivastigmine, and memantine for the treatment of Alzheimer's disease: a systematic review and meta-analysis. J Alzheimers Dis. 2014;41:615–31.
25. Prvulovic D, Schneider B. Pharmacokinetic and pharmacodynamic evaluation of donepezil for the treatment of Alzheimer's disease. Expert Opin Drug Metab Toxicol. 2014;10:1039–50.
26. Laghi F, D'Alfonso N, Tobin MJ. A paper on the pace of recovery from diaphragmatic fatigue and its unexpected dividends. Intensive Care Med. 2014;40:1220–6.
27. Lian JX. Using ABGs to optimize mechanical ventilation: three case studies illustrate how arterial blood gas analyses can guide appropriate ventilator strategy. Dimens Crit Care Nurs. 2013;32:204–9.
28. Haake RE, Saxon LA, Bander SJ, Haake RJ. Depressed central respiratory drive causing weaning failure. Its reversal with doxapram. Chest. 1989;95:695–7.
29. Frutos-Vivar F, Ferguson ND, Esteban A, Epstein SK, Arabi Y, Apezteguia C, et al. Risk factors for extubation failure in patients following a successful spontaneous breathing trial. Chest. 2006;130:1664–71.
30. Haxhiu MA, Cherniack NS, Mitra J, van Lunteren E, Strohl KP. Nonvagal modulation of hypoglossal neural activity. Respiration. 1992;59:65–71.
31. Hedner J, Kraiczi H, Peker Y, Murphy P. Reduction of sleep-disordered breathing after physostigmine. Am J Respir Crit Care Med. 2003;168:1246–51.

32. Bellingham MC, Ireland MF. Contribution of cholinergic systems to state-dependent modulation of respiratory control. Respir Physiol Neurobiol. 2002;131:135–44.
33. Gilman S, Chervin RD, Koeppe RA, Consens FB, Little R, An H, et al. Obstructive sleep apnea is related to a thalamic cholinergic deficit in MSA. Neurology. 2003;61:35–9.
34. Proctor GB, Carpenter GH. Salivary secretion: mechanism and neural regulation. Monogr Oral Sci. 2014;24:14–29.

23

Characterization and pharmacological potential of *Lactobacillus sakei* 1I1 isolated from fresh water fish *Zacco koreanus*

Vivek K. Bajpai[1†], Jeong-Ho Han[2†], Gyeong-Jun Nam[1], Rajib Majumder[1], Chanseo Park[2], Jeongheui Lim[2*], Woon Kee Paek[2], Irfan A. Rather[1] and Yong-Ha Park[1*]

Abstract

Background: There are still a large variety of microorganisms among aquatic animals which have not been explored for their pharmacological potential. Hence, present study was aimed to isolate and characterize a potent lactic acid bacterium from fresh water fish sample *Zacco koreanus*, and to confirm its pharmacological potential.

Methods: Isolation of lactic acid bacteria (LAB) from fresh water fish samples was done using serial dilution method. Biochemical identification and molecular characterization of selected LAB isolate 1I1, based on its potent antimicrobial efficacy, was accomplished using API kit and 16S rRNA gene sequencing analysis. Further, 1I1 was assessed for α-glucosidase and tyrosinase inhibitory potential as well as antiviral efficacy against highly pathogenic human influenza virus H1N1 using MDCK cell line in terms of its pharmacological potential.

Results: Here, we first time report isolation as well as biochemical and molecular characterization of a lactic acid bacterium *Lactobacillus sakei* 1I1 isolated from the intestine of a fresh water fish *Z. koreanus*. As a result, *L. sakei* 1I1 exhibited potent antimicrobial effect in vitro, and diameter of zones of inhibition of 1I1 against the tested pathogens was found in the range of 13.32 ± 0.51 to 23.16 ± 0.32 mm. Also *L. sakei* 1I1 at 100 mg/ml exhibited significant ($p < 0.05$) α–glucosidase and tyrosinase inhibitory activities by 60.69 and 72.59 %, in terms of its anti-diabetic and anti-melanogenic potential, respectively. Moreover, *L. sakei* 1I1 displayed profound anti-cytopathic effect on MDCK cell line when treated with its ethanol extract (100 mg/ml), confirming its potent anti-viral efficacy against H1N1 influenza virus.

Conclusions: These findings reinforce the suggestions that *L. sakei* 1I1 isolated from the intestine of fresh water fish *Z. koreanus* might be a candidate of choice for using in pharmacological preparations as an effective drug.

Keywords: Fish microbiota, Lactic acid bacteria, α-glucosidase inhibitory activity, Anti-viral activity, Anti-tyrosinase activity

Background

Microflora of the intestinal tract is an integral part of the whole living organism. A huge number of endogenous and exogenous factors influence determination of composition of microbe populations and affect physiological and biochemical features of the microorganisms.

Lactic acid bacteria (LAB) are widely distributed in the intestinal tract of various animals [1], and some of them have played an important role in beneficial functions for industrial animals as probiotics [2]. There have been several reports on LAB occurring among the major microbial populations in animal intestine [2, 3]. It is well established that some LAB improve the intestinal microflora and promote the growth and health of animals [2].

LAB are characterized as Gram-positive, usually non-motile, non-sporulating bacteria that produce lactic acid as a major or sole product of fermentative metabolism which have been classified based on their morphology, physiology and molecular characteristics [4]. Although

---

* Correspondence: jeongheuilim@gmail.com; peter@ynu.ac.kr
†Equal contributors
[2]National Science Museum, Ministry of Science, ICT and Future Planning, Daejeon 32143, Republic of Korea
[1]Department of Applied Microbiology and Biotechnology, Microbiome Laboratory, Yeungnam University, Gyeongsan, Gyeongbuk 712-749, Republic of Korea

LAB from food and their current taxonomical status have been reviewed previously [5], taxonomic studies on LAB from animal origin are rare [5]. Moreover, LAB exhibit various medicinal and pharmacological properties against number of microorganisms, including food spoilage and pathogenic bacteria as well as variety of viruses [6].

Consequences of diabetes mellitus type 2 stage are associated with postprandial hyperglycemia due to imbalanced acute secretion of insulin after food intake [7]. Digestive enzymes such as glucosidases are well-known for their ability to break down the larger carbohydrate molecules into simple monosaccharide molecules. Excess production of monosaccharide and less uptake of sugars by the body may result in the development of diabetic complications. Inhibitors of glucosidase enzymes have potent ability to delay the absorption of carbohydrates and reduce the digestion rate of carbohydrates into simple monosaccharides. These features of glucosidase inhibitors allow them to act as anti-diabetic substances because they reduce postprandial blood glucose level thereby preventing the incidences of type-2 diabetes [8].

Tyrosinase, a copper-containing polyphenol oxidase, plays a highly critical role in forming melanin pigments [9]. Previous reports have shown that tyrosinase might also be involved in neuromelanin production and be associated with Parkinson's disease [10]. Therefore, inhibiting tyrosinase activity is applicable to skin-lightening and in preventing neurodegeneration [11]. Although a broad spectrum of tyrosinase inhibitors are available [12], there is a still need to explore the microbial world for inventing more effective classes of tyrosinase inhibitors from LAB due to their Generally Recognized as Safe "GRAS" status.

Influenza A (H1N1) is the sub-type of influenza A virus that is known as the most common cause of human influenza. Consequences of influenza viruses result in the development of a contagious respiratory disease influenza, also called flu. It has been confirmed that every year over 220,000 hospitalizations and approximately 36,000 annual deaths are reported by influenza viruses in the USA [13]. Current scenario on emergence of life threatening viruses has resulted in enormous attention on finding anti-viral drugs of natural origin due to less potential of currently available anti-viral vaccines [14], in addition to their limited applications [15] against influenza viruses. This has resulted in the increasing need on the development of un-conventional measurements against influenza viruses.

A number of reports have confirmed that LAB are normal flora in gastrointestinal tract of healthy animals like mammals and aquaculture animals including fish [16] with no harmful effects [17]. Probiotics improve

intestinal microflora with health beneficial efficacy protecting them against infections by stimulating the immune system, as well as alleviate lactose intolerance, reduce blood cholesterol levels, improve weight gain and feed conversion ratio [18–21]. Isolation of LAB from variety of samples has raised debate over the safety of probiotic bacteria and whether or not the bacteria are actually infectious [22]. Fish viscera are not only rich in different biomolecules but are also rich in beneficial LAB with probiotics properties [23]. Since LAB are reported to be very effective in recovery of biomolecules from fish industry waste [24–26], isolation of LAB from fish industry waste itself becomes all the more important.

Against this background, the main objective of present study was to isolate, and characterize a native LAB strain *L. sakei* 1I1 from intestinal microbiota of fresh water fish *Zacco koreanus*, and to confirm its various pharmacological properties such as antimicrobial, α-glucosidase inhibitory effect, tyrosinase inhibitory effect and antiviral properties against influenza virus H1N1 in terms of its bio-preservative, anti-diabetic, anti-melonogenic and anti-viral potential in order to explore LAB for simultaneous recovery of bioactive compounds of pharmacological significance.

Methods
Media and reagents
The Bromocresol Purple (BCP) agar medium was purchased from Sigma-Aldrich (Sigma, MO, USA). The de Man, Rogosa and Sharpe (MRS) agar medium was purchased from Difco (USA). Kojic acid, acarbose, yeast α-glucosidase, p-nitrophenyl-α-D-glucopyranoside, mushroom tyrosinase, and 3,4-dihydroxy-L-phenylalanine (DOPA) were obtained from Sigma (MO, USA). Other chemicals and reagents used were of very pure and high analytical grade.

Microbial strains
The following microorganisms as pathogenic bacteria were used in this study for preliminary screening including *Staphylococcus aureus* (KCTC 1621), *Escherichia coli* O157:H7, *Salmonella enterica* ATCC 4731, *Bacillus subtilis* KCTC 1021, and *Listeria monocytogenes* KCTC 3569. The bacterial pathogens were obtained from the American Type Culture Collection and Korean Type Culture Collection, respectively and maintained on nutrient agar (NA) medium at 4 °C.

Collection and sampling of fish samples
A total of 64 fresh water fish samples, belonging to different species were collected from five different rivers and different locations in Korea, supplied by Daejeon National Science Museum, Daejeon. Fish sampling was

conducted in the five major river watersheds of Korea (34–42°N, 124–130°E): the Han River, the Nakdong river, the Geum river, the Yeongsan river, and the Sumjin river watersheds during the year 2014. In total, 16 sites consisting of first- through fourth-order streams [27] were sampled for the five major river watersheds; 3 sites in the Han river, 4 sites in the Nakdong river, 3 sites in the Geum river, 3 sites in the Yeongsan river and 3 sites in the Sumjin river. The sampling approach was followed by a modified protocol of the Ohio environmental protection agency (EPA) method [28]. Sampling gears used were casting nets (mesh size, 7 × 7 mm; 1.5 m × 1.5 m × 3.14 m) and kick nets (mesh size, 4 × 4 mm, 1.8 m × 0.9 m), the most common sampling gears used for wading streams. Casting net was applied to habitats with unobstructed open water, viz. riffles, pools, and slow runs, and kick net was used in sites subject to fast current regime and with obstructions, where it is difficult to use a casting net. All sampling procedures and/or experimental manipulations were reviewed following catch per unit effort (CPUE) methods [29], and the collected samples were transported in ice-packed boxes to the Microbiome laboratory, Yeungnam University and stored at –20 °C for further analysis. In addition, this study did not involve any endangered or protected species, hence no specific permissions and ethics were required to collect the fish samples. However, national ethical approval was obtained for fish samples on "Animal Care and Use" by the ethical committee of Daejeon National Science Museum, Daejeon, Korea. All fish samples were of different feeding nature such as insectivore, omnivore, herbivore, and carnivore. Taxonomic identification of the fish species was conducted by the fish expert at the National Science Museum of Korea according to the methods of species identification [30]. A detailed description on variety of fish samples has been given in Table 1.

Isolation, sub-culturing and maintenance of LAB from fish samples

For isolation of lactic acid bacteria (LAB) from fresh water fish samples, a previously developed standard serial dilution method was adopted [31]. In brief, scarification of experimental fish was done in a sterilized clean bench using sterilized knife and forces. To isolate LAB from fresh water fish samples, dissected fish tissues such as stomach, gill and intestine were used since these are known major reservoirs of microbial community in fish. Each fish sample was dissected, and stomach, gill and intestine were collected separately. Each part was weighed and homogenized using a pestle-mortar followed by serial dilution in phosphate buffer saline (PBS) using Bromocresol Purple (BCP) agar medium. Each homogenized sample was put in 1 ml of PBS and vortexed vigorously in order to make a uniform inoculum size followed by

its serial dilution to the maximum serial dilution factor from 10^{-1} to 10^{-9}. Finally an inoculum of 100 μl was spread on BCP agar plates, and plates were sealed using paraffin and incubated at 37 °C for 24 h. Identification of LAB isolates was based on the clear zone around the colony on BCP agar plates [21]. Each set was prepared in triplicate and positive results were confirmed. Representative colonies were picked from plates and well-isolated colonies were inoculated into fresh MRS broth for stock preparation. For long term storage, stock cultures were maintained at –20 °C in MRS broth. A detail of number of LAB strains isolated from variety of fish samples has been summarized in Table 2.

Screening of LAB strains on the basis of anti-pathogenic assay

To confirm the bio-preservative and pharmacological potential of LAB strains isolated from variety of fresh water fish samples, anti-pathogenic assay was performed in vitro using different pathogenic microorganisms including *Staphylococcus aureus* KCTC 1621, *Escherichia coli* O157:H7, *Salmonella enterica* ATCC 4731, *Bacillus subtilis* KCTC 1021, and *Listeria monocytogenes* KCTC 3569. The agar well diffusion method [32] was used for anti-pathogenic assay. Petri plates were prepared by pouring 20 ml of nutrient broth (NB) medium (BD Difco™) and allowed to solidify. Plates were dried, and a 24 h grown culture (200 μl) of each test organism of standardized inoculum suspension (10^7 CFU/ml) was poured and uniformly spread, and the inoculum was allowed to dry for 5 min. The wells were made by using sterilized borer where 100 μl cell free supernatant of isolated LAB strains was poured in each well against each of the tested pathogen. Negative controls were prepared using the same solvent employed to dissolve the samples. Antibacterial activity was evaluated by measuring the diameter of inhibition zones against the tested bacteria. Each assay in this experiment was replicated three times.

Morphological and biochemical identification of LAB isolate

Morphological identification of one of the selected isolates 1I1, based on its potential efficacy in anti-pathogenic assay, was conducted by observing colony shape on BCP agar plates, Gram-staining, and cell morphology using microscope. Selected isolate was biochemically identified using API 50CH strips with API 50CHL medium at species level based on the instructions of manufacturer (API 50 CHL, BioMerieux, France). In brief, freshly-grown bacterial colony of the selected LAB isolate was picked-up and inoculated in MRS medium at 36 °C for 24 h, and then the bacterial culture was serially diluted to prepare desired concentration of 10^8 CFU/ml [33]. From this, aliquot (2 ml) was inoculated into APL 50 CHL medium

Table 1 Isolation of lactic acid bacteria (LAB) from fresh water fish sample collected from different locations in Korea

Fish samples	Number of LAB isolates		
	Stomach	Intestine	Gill
Tridentiger bifasciatus	–	–	–
Acanthogobius flavimanus	–	–	1
Tribolodon hakonensis	3	–	–
Pseudobagrus koreanus	–	–	–
Coreoleuciscus splendidus	13	–	–
Plecoglossus altivelis	–	1	3
Misgurnus anguillicaudatus	1	4	–
Carassius auratus	1	1	–
Pseudorasbora parva	–	–	–
Zacco platypus	1	5	3
Rhinogobius giurinus	–	–	–
Zacco koreanus	–	–	–
Zacco temminckii	–	–	1
Tridentiger obscurus	2	–	–
Zacco koreanus	1	2	3
Odontobutis platycephala	2	2	1
Rhynchocypris oxycephalus	3	1	1
Zacco koreanus	1	3	2
Zacco temminckii	2	2	2
Rhynchocypris oxycephalus	3	3	2
Squalidus gracilis	5	5	2
Microphysogobio yaluensis	4	3	1
Hemibarbus longirostris	2	4	2
Zacco platypus	2	–	2
Odontobutis interrupta	1	2	2
Rhinogobius brunneus	1	1	1
Pseudogobio esocinus	2	–	1
Opsariichthys uncirostris	2	1	1
Zacco koreanus	3	3	4
Rhynchocypris oxycephalus	1	1	1
Odontobutis platycephala	1	1	1
Pungtungia herzi	1	1	2
Zacco platypus	2	2	2
Odontobutis platycephala	3	5	2
Zacco koreanus	3	3	2
Carassius cuvieri	2	2	2
Carassius auratus	3	2	3
Micropterus salmoides	2	3	2
Hemibarbus longirostris	1	1	2
Lepomis macrochirus	3	2	2
Pseudogobio esocinus	3	1	2
Zacco platypus	2	1	2
Squalidus chankaensis	2	2	2
Rhynchocypris oxycephalus	4	1	5
Microphysogobio yaluensis	3	2	2
Rhinogobius brunneus	3	2	2
Zacco temminckii	–	3	3
Odontobutis platycephala	2	2	2
Misgurnus anguillicaudatus	2	3	–
Zacco koreanus	2	3	4
Hemibarbus labeo			
Pungtungia herzi	2	3	2
Zacco platypus	3	2	1
Microphysogobio yaluensis	3	2	1
Odontobutis platycephala	3	1	1
Pseudogobio esocinus	1	3	2
Squalidus gracilis	4	–	2
Zacco temminckii			
Microphysogobio yaluensis	1	–	3
Squalidus gracilis			
Pungtungia herzi			
Zacco platypus	–	2	1
Pseudogobio esocinus	–	–	3
Odontobutis platycephala	–	–	–
Total	117	99	96

(10 ml), and mixed by gentle inversion. Then, a bacterial suspension (120 µl) was inoculated into API 50 CH strips that were pre-overlaid with mineral oil followed by further incubation for 48 h before measuring the color change abilities. Finally, strips were processed for analyzing the API profiles using computer APILAB Plus Version.

Molecular characterization of LAB isolate

Molecular methods are important for bacterial identification [34], and possibly more accurate for LAB than conventional phenotypic methods. In this study, LAB isolate 1I1 showing profound antimicrobial efficacy against pathogenic bacteria was characterized by 16S rRNA gene sequencing analysis. The gene sequences were compared in the National Center for Biotechnology Information (NCBI) for homology using BLAST and multiple-aligned with 16S rRNA gene sequences of different strains for similarity using ClustalW program coupled with MEGA 5. A neighbor-joining method was employed to construct the phylogenic tree using MEGA 5 software.

Pharmacological evaluation of *L. sakei* 1I1

Extraction and sample preparation

Selection of an accurate methodology is highly recommended for better metabolite extraction and high amount of yield recovery. Selective use of solvents has always been recommended for the extraction of specific category of metabolites such as polar and/or non-polar or less polar substances based on the solubility of compounds. Since ethanol can significantly extract majority of biologically active secondary metabolites from variety of microbial (outer and inner environment of bacterial cell) extract samples [35], in this study, ethanol solvent system was selected for extraction purposes. Briefly, to obtain ethanol extract, *L. sakei* 1I1 was grown in MRS broth for 36 h at 37 °C, and then double volume of ethanol was added to the culture broth followed by shaking for 4 h to kill the culture. After that, mixture was centrifuged at 8,000 rpm for 20 min. The upper solution containing ethanol extract was collected, vacuum evaporated and freeze-dried. The yield of ethanol extract of LAB strain *L. sakei* 1I1 was found as 19.34 %. Different test concentrations of freeze-dried ethanol extract of 1I1 were prepared in triple-distilled sterilized water.

Determination of α-glucosidase inhibitory activity

It is not known whether LAB colonizing the human gut possess inhibitory potential against digestive enzymes glucosidases. Hence, this study was undertaken to evaluate α-glucosidase inhibitory potential of 1I1 in order to confirm its type II anti-diabetic efficacy according to the chromogenic method with minor modifications as described previously [36]. Briefly, 50 μl of various concentrations (100, 50, 25, 5 and 1 mg/ml) of 1I1 ethanol extract and 100 μl of α-glucosidase dissolved in 0.1 M phosphate buffer (pH 6.9), were mixed in a 96-well microplate and incubated at 25 °C for 10 min. After pre-incubation, 50 μl of p-nitrophenyl-α-D-glucopyranoside (5 mM) in the same buffer (pH 6.9) as a substrate solution was added to each well. The reaction mixture was incubated at 25 °C for 5 min. Absorbance was recorded using a microplate reader (Tecan, Infinite M200, Mannedorf, Switzerland) at 405 nm before and after incubation with p-nitrophenyl-α-D-glucopyranoside solution and compared to that of control, having 50 μl of buffer solution instead of test solution. Acarbose at various concentrations (0.3125, 0.625, 1.25, 2.5 and 5 μg/ml) was used as a standard drug. Experiments were performed in triplicate, and enzyme inhibitory effect of the samples was calculated by the formula:

$$Inhibition\ (\%) = (Control\ absorbance - Sample\ absorbance / Control\ absorbance) \times 100$$

Table 2 Biochemical characterization of *Lactobacillus sakei* (1I1) based on carbohydrate interpretation using API 50 CHL kit

Active ingredient	Result	Active ingredient	Result
Glycerol	–	Salicin	+
Erythritol	–	D-cellobiose	+
D-arabinose	–	D-maltose	+
L-arabinose	+	D-lactose (bovine origin)	+
D-ribose	+	D-melibiose	+
D-xylose	+	D-saccharose	+
L-xylose	–	D-trehalose	+
D-adonitol	–	Inulin	–
Methyl-β-D-xylopyranoside	–	D-melezitose	+
D-galactose	+	D-raffinose	–
D-glucose	+	Amidon (starch)	–
D-fructose	+	Glycogen	–
D-mannose	+	Xylitol	–
L-sorbose	–	Gentiobiose	+
L-rhamnose	+	D-turanose	+
Dulcitol	–	D-lyxose	–
Inositol	–	D-tagatose	+
D-mannitol	+	D-fucose	–
D-sorbitol	+	L-fucose	–
Methyl-α-D-glucopyranoside	–	D-arabitol	–
N-acetylglucosamine	+	Potassium gluconate	+
Amygdalin	+	Potassium 2-ketogluconate	–
Arbutin	+	Potassium 5-ketogluconate	–
Esculin	–		

(–): The bacterium does not use this carbohydrate; (+): The bacterium uses this carbohydrate

Determination of tyrosinase inhibitory activity

Tyrosinase inhibitory activity of ethanol extract of *L. sakei* 1I1 was measured based on the method reported by Fawole et al. [37] with slight modifications. Briefly, 100 μl of different concentrations (100, 50, 25, 5 and 1 mg/ml) of 1I1 ethanol extract were mixed with 0.175 M sodium phosphate buffer (600 μl) (pH 6.8). After that, 200 μl of L-DOPA solution (10 mM) was added to each well, followed by addition of 200 μl of tyrosinase (110 units/ml in 0.175 M sodium phosphate buffer) into the reaction mixture, and incubated at 37 °C for 2 min. Further, the amount of dopachrome produced in the reaction mixture was measured at 475 nm using an ELISA reader. Kojic acid (15.63, 31.25, 62.5, 125 and 250 μg/ml) was used as a positive control. All the steps in the assay were conducted at room temperature. Experiments were performed in triplicate, and enzyme inhibitory effect of the samples was calculated as follows:

$$\text{Inhibition } (\%) = (\text{Control absorption–Sample absorption})/$$
$$\text{Control absorption} \times 100$$

Determination of antiviral effect
Harvesting of H1N1 virus from embryonated egg
A pathogenic H1N1 influenza virus (A/ Korea/01/2009) was procured from Korea Centers for Disease Control and Prevention, South Korea. Propagation of influenza virus (H1N1) was maintained on MDCK cell-line for 72 h at 37 °C, in a carbon dioxide (4 %) environment, and allantoic fluid was stored at –80 °C before use. Harvesting of virus H1N1 was accomplished from infected MDCK cell by centrifugation (1,500 rpm) for 5 min. The H1N1 titer was determined as $10^{6.5}$ median embryo infection dose $(EID_{50})/0.1$ ml as reported by Rather et al. and Reed and Muench [6, 38].

Assay test against H1N1 virus on MDCK cells
MDCK cell-line was cultured and maintained on DMEM medium with 10 % (v/v) fetal bovine serum (FBS), 1 % (v/v) penicillin (100 U/mol), and streptomycin (100 µg/ml) solution. After filter sterilization, ethanol extract (200 ~ 12.5 mg/ml) of L. sakei 1l1 was serially diluted in DMEM solution with FBS (2 %, v/v), 1 % (v/v) penicillin (100 U/mol), and streptomycin (100 µg/ml) solution. The H1N1 influenza virus was treated with a two-fold dilution of test sample of 1l1 in sterilized distilled water at 37 °C, under 5 % carbon dioxide for 1 h. Further, this reaction mixture was injected into MDCK cell-line, followed by incubation in DMEM solution with FBS (2 %, v/v) at 37 °C in a humidified chamber under 5 % carbon dioxide for 48 h. Confirmation of antiviral activity was made by observing the plates after 72 h for cytopathic effect (CPE). No CPE confirmed the presence of antiviral activity [6, 39].

Statistical analysis
Each experiment was performed in triplicate to calculate mean ± SD, and data were analyzed using one-way ANOVA to find statistical significance at $p < 0.05$.

Results and discussion
Isolation of LAB strains from fish samples
As presented in Table 1, a total of 312 LAB strains were isolated on BCP media from different tissues samples such as stomach, intestine and gills of 54 fresh water fish samples. Among three samples utilized for isolation of LAB isolates, stomach tissue showed higher number of LAB isolates (116) followed by intestine (99) and gills (96). Interestingly, 13 LAB strains were isolated from stomach tissue of one of the fish samples Coreoleuciscus splendidus. Surprisingly, no LAB strain was isolated from any fish tissue samples (stomach, intestine and gill)

of Tridentiger bifasciatus, Pseudobagrus koreanus, Pseudorasbora parva, Rhinogobius giurinus, Zacco koreanus, Hemibarbus labeo, Zacco temminckii, Squalidus gracilis, Pungtungia herzi and Odontobutis platycephala. In this study, a higher number of LAB were isolated from stomach tissue sample of a fresh water fish Coreoleuciscus splendidus. Also one of the fish samples Zacco platypus possessed higher number of LAB isolates in its stomach, intestine and gill microbiota as compared to other fish samples (Table 1).

Nair et al. [40] also reported distribution of different genera of LAB in fresh and frozen fish and prawn. They observed that from the cultures, 60 in fresh fish, 65 in fresh prawn and 80 % each in frozen fish and prawn belonged to the Lactobacillus genus. It is interesting to note that majority of the Lactobacillus spp. that have been isolated from fresh and frozen fish/prawns were those species which were commonly found on meat, animals and humans [41].

Anti-pathogenic potential of L. sakei 1l1
All the LAB strains isolated from various parts (stomach, intestine and gill) of fresh water fish samples were named accordingly coded with initial character of their respective tissue origin. Further, each LAB isolate was grown in MRS medium at 37 °C for 24 h. The culture was centrifuged at 12,000 rpm for 15 min to obtain cell free supernatant (CFS). Filter sterilize supernatant was further subjected to evaluate antimicrobial efficacy against pathogenic microorganisms using agar well diffusion assay. In each instance, diameter of inhibition zone was quantified against each bacterial species, and some of the tested strains of LAB showed remarkable antimicrobial activity against the tested pathogenic bacteria (data not shown). It was found in this study that the LAB isolated from the gill and intestine samples exhibited higher anti-pathogenic effect compared to LAB strains isolated from stomach samples. The findings of this study confirmed that the LAB strains isolated from the fresh water fish samples have potent therapeutic and biological potential to develop natural and novel types of antibiotics to combat against pathogenic microorganism causing severe diseases in humans and animals. Based on the result of aforementioned test, one of the strains Lactobacilli sakei 1l1, isolated from fresh water fish Zacco koreanus, showing highest antimicrobial activity against the tested pathogens (Fig. 1) was chosen as an active LAB isolate and was subjected to biochemical and molecular identification. Further, L. sakei 1l1 was assessed for its various pharmacological activities including anti-diabetic, anti-melanogenic and anti-viral efficacy.

Morphological and biochemical identification
Morphological identification of LAB isolate 1l1 was carried out as per the schemes outlined in the Bergey's

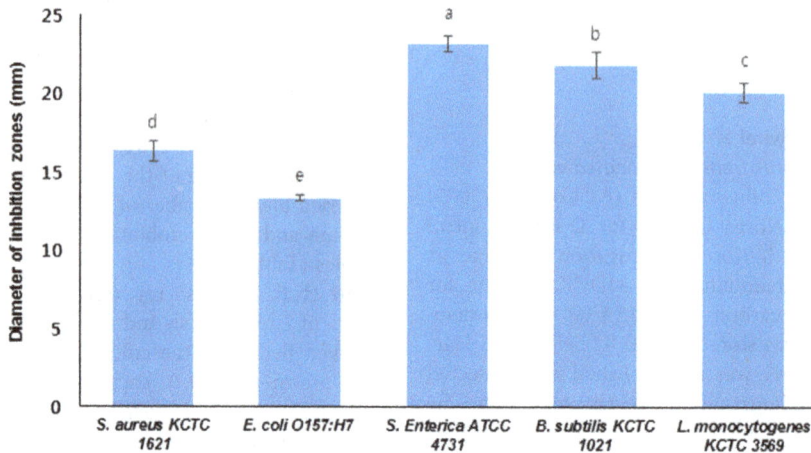

Fig. 1 Diameters of inhibition zones of cell free supernatant of *L. sakei* 1I1 against test pathogens in anti-pathogenic assay. Data are expressed as mean ± SD (*n* = 3). Values with different superscripts are significantly different (*p* < 0.05)

manual of Systematic Bacteriology [42]. Small yellow colonies of similar sizes that appeared on BCP agar using pour-plating method confirmed the presence of *Lactobacillus* strain as also reported previously [43]. The efficiency of detection of other Bifidobacterium such as *B. infantis* on BCP was very low, while *B. bifidum* did not grow on BCP even under anaerobic conditions [43]. Although plate count agar with Bromocresol Purple is a recommended medium for enumeration of LAB from variety of samples, it does not support the differentiation of each LAB in a mixed culture. It is known that BCP agar also prevents formation of colonies by concomitant bacteria and hence widely considered specific medium for the selective enumeration of LAB as also reported by others [44].

Further, biochemical analysis of 1I1 was done by using API50 strip kit and selected strain was identified as a Gram-positive and rod-shaped isolate which was found most closely associated to *L. sakei* (Table 2). The API web software confirmed that strain 1I1 showed typical utilization of carbohydrates that included L-arabinose, D-ribose, D-xylose, D-galactose, D-glucose, D-fructose, D-mannose, L-rhamnose, D-mannitol, D-sorbitol, N-acetylglucosamine, amygdalin, arbutin, salicin, D-cellobiose, D-maltose, D-lactose, D-melibiose, D-saccharose, D-trehalose, D-melezitose, gentiobiose, D-turanose, D-tagatose, and potassium gluconate (Table 2). Color change from violet to yellow in the strip capsule indicated complete fermentation of 1I1. Recently Casaburi et al. [45] also phenotypically and biochemically identified *Lactobacillus* species with the use of API50 kit isolated from fermented sausage.

Molecular characterization of *L. sakei* 1I1

Molecular identification of 1I1 was based on using 16S rRNA gene sequencing analysis. As a result, on the basis of molecular analysis with 16S rDNA gene sequencing, selected strain showed 99.9 % similarity with different *L. sakei* spp. (Fig. 2). The sequence was submitted in GenBank with nucleotide accession number KT372706. Thus, the strain was finally confirmed as *L. sakei* 1I1. Jini et al. [46] also isolated two potential isolates of LAB such as *Enterococcus faecalis* and *Pediococcus acidilactici* from fresh water fish microbiota having anti-pathogenic effect against human pathogens. Zapata [21] studied intestinal microflora of *Oreochromis niloticus* fish to isolate and identify LAB as new probiotics with a possibility to use them in aquaculture. It is known that the microbiota of fish is affected by nutritional, physiological and environmental factors, and it is also expected that the microbial population of fish vary among species [47]. Nevertheless, some authors have considered that seasonal change could be a decisive factor [48], indicating that it is very likely that feeding habits did not have a significant influence on fish LAB composition, when the fish species were grown in the same conditions. Consistent with these findings, our results showed that all species collected in different months had a different LAB composition, represented by various number and variety of LAB species.

α-Glucosidase inhibitory activity

In this study, anti-diabetic efficacy of *L. sakei* 1I1 was confirmed in α-glucosidase inhibition assay. The α-glucosidase inhibitory activity of ethanol extract of 1I1 was determined using p-nitrophenyl-α-D-glucopyranoside (pNPG) as a substrate and compared with standard compound acarbose. Higher blood glucose levels result in the development of a chronic metabolic disorder called diabetes mellitus. Prevention and control of after-meal blood glucose levels are considered preventive

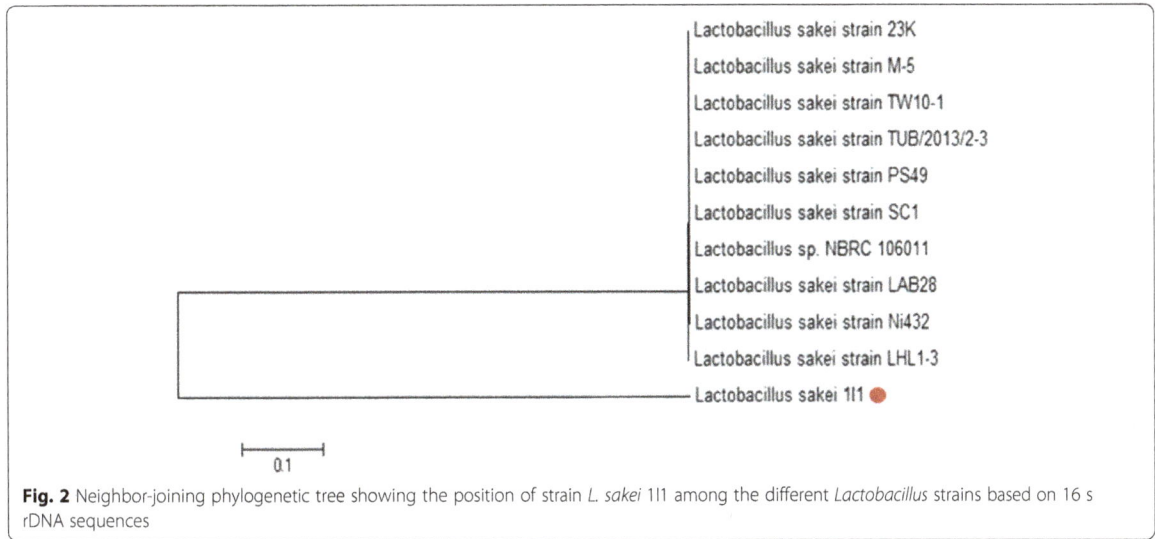

Fig. 2 Neighbor-joining phylogenetic tree showing the position of strain *L. sakei* 1I1 among the different *Lactobacillus* strains based on 16 s rDNA sequences

measures to treat diabetes at early stage which may result in the reduction of carbohydrate absorption from food by the inhibitory effect of α-glucosidase-like digestive enzymes [49]. Though commercial drugs as inhibitors of α-glucosidase enzymes are available, an approach on the development of new types of effective alternative measures is needed for inhibiting the action of these digestive enzymes to meet drug cost potential and to reduce the adversary side effects of chemical-based enzyme inhibitors. Moreover, glucosidases may play an active role in the carbohydrate metabolism of beneficial and pathogenic LAB species. Glucosidase activity is widespread among LAB and β-glucosidases release a wide range of plant secondary metabolites from their β-D-glucosylated precursors [50]. Plant metabolite deglycosylation has been shown to improve the flavour or fragrance of fermented products. It also increases the bioavailability of health-promoting, antioxidative plant metabolites [50]. For instance, soybeans contain high concentrations of β-glucosides genistin and daidzin which are hydrolyzed by β-glucosidase activities of LAB during soy milk fermentations. Fermentations with LAB could also increase the concentrations of bioactive isoflavones in traditional oriental herbal medicine formulas [50]. Cassava contains high concentrations of toxic cyanogenic glucoside linamarin, and LAB contribute to linamarin degradation by β-glucosidase activities [50]. In addition, there is considerable interest in the α- and β-glucosidase activities of LAB that conduct the malolactic fermentation of wine. The main volatile constituents of the primary wine aroma are terpenoid compounds derived from the grapes. As these can be released from glycosylated precursors, β-glucosidase activities of malolactic bacteria are of interest due to their impact on the aroma profile of wines [50].

The α-glucosidase inhibitory activity of ethanol extract of 1I1 was found to be in a concentration-dependent manner (Fig. 3a). The ethanol extract of 1I1 at different concentrations of 1, 5, 25, 50 and 100 mg/ml showed the inhibition of α-glucosidase by 9.34, 12.53, 21.54, 36.32 and 60.69 %, respectively (Fig. 3a). On the other hand, acarbose as a standard drug at various concentrations (0.3125, 0.625, 1.25, 2.5 and 5 μg/ml) displayed α-glucosidase inhibitory activities by 31.84, 42.07, 54.99, 68.59, and 80.32 %, respectively which were also found in a concentration-dependent manner (Fig. 3b).

Similarly, Ramchandran and Shah [51] reported α-glucosidase inhibitory activity of some selected LAB strains, isolated from yogurt starter culture and it was found that all selected strains such as *L. casei*, *L. acidophilus*, *L. delbrueckii* ssp. *bulgaricus*, and *Bifidobacterium longum* exhibited considerable amount of α-glucosidase inhibitory activity, being very high (>80 %). Recently Panwar et al. [52] also reported that LAB strains present in the human gut showed α- and β-glucosidase inhibitory activities as well as reduced blood glucose responses in vivo. Lastly, the inhibitory activity of whole culture ethanol extract of 1I1 observed was clearly in a concentration-dependent, indicating that intracellular cytoplasmic contents or products of bacterial metabolism may be responsible for this activity. Yet this LAB strain, isolated from fish microbiota has not been studied, and it appears that this organism may have some anti-diabetic properties along with its probiotic nature.

Tyrosinase inhibitory activity

Melanin is a color-determinant naturally found in animals, plants, and microorganisms. Production of various types of melanins is a process of number of enzymatic

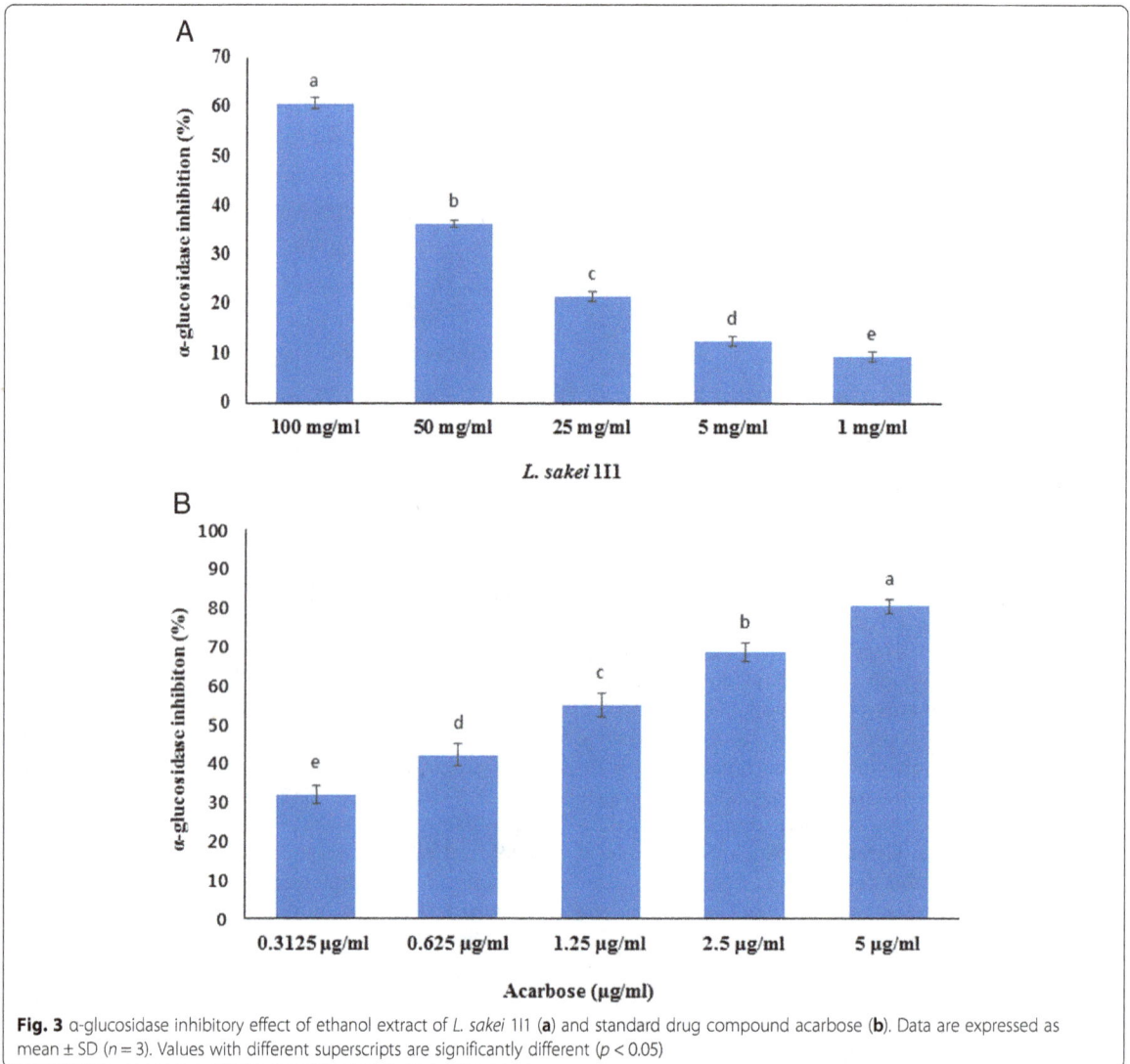

Fig. 3 α-glucosidase inhibitory effect of ethanol extract of *L. sakei* 1I1 (**a**) and standard drug compound acarbose (**b**). Data are expressed as mean ± SD (*n* = 3). Values with different superscripts are significantly different (*p* < 0.05)

and non-enzymatic oxidation steps and polymerization reactions. Due to its color reaction and solubility in alkaline medium, it can be divided in two sub-categories eumelanin and pheomelanin [53]. Mechanism of tyrosinase inhibition could be an important factor in the skin whitening and inhibition of browning reaction [53]. During melanin biosynthesis, L-DOPA substrate converts into L-dopaquinone through various enzymatic oxidation processes resulting in the formation of polymerized melanin [53].

The inhibitory effect of *L. sakei* 1I1 ethanol extract on the tyrosinase using a mushroom tyrosinase is demonstrated in Fig. 4. In this assay, ethanol extract of 1I1 (1, 5, 25, 50 and 100 mg/ml) showed inhibition of tyrosinase by 9.36, 15.33, 22.44, 39.34 and 72.59 %, respectively (Fig. 4a). Whereas, mushroom tyrosinase inhibitory effect of kojic acid (15.63, 31.25, 62.5, 125 and 250 µg/ml)

was found to be 76.60, 85.52, 91.17, 93.94 and 95.90 %, respectively (Fig. 4b). Kim et al. [54] reported that ethanolic extract of *Cortex radicis* bio-transformed by *Leuconostoc paramesenteroides* PR effectively enhanced the tyrosinase inhibitory activity by 6.5-fold in in vitro. Also Usuki et al. [55] demonstrated that LAB and/or their derivatives have wide range of application in the development of skin-whitening and cosmetic products with antioxidant potential that could directly inhibit tyrosinase enzyme activity. Herein this study, ethanol extract of 1I1 also exerted dose-dependent tyrosinase activity. It has been found that inhibitors of tyrosinase play a crucial role to maintain the imbalance of melanin biosynthesis through inhibition of conversion of tyrosine to DOPA, dopaquinone and subsequent formation of melanin [53].

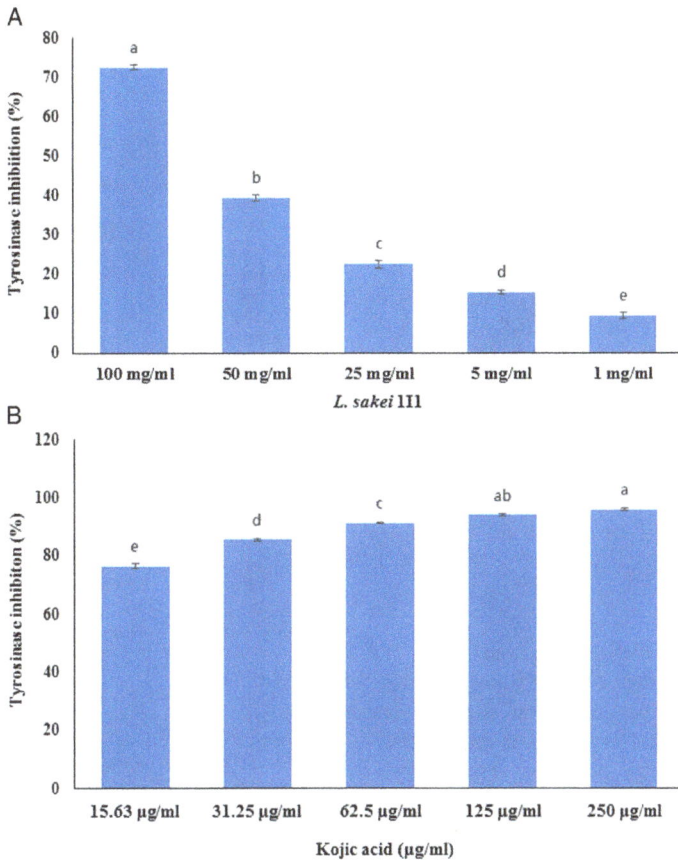

Fig 4 Tyrosinase inhibitory effect of ethanol extract of *L. sakei* 1I1 (**a**) and standard drug compound kojic acid (**b**). Data are expressed as mean ± SD ($n = 3$). Values with different superscripts are significantly different ($p < 0.05$)

Antiviral effect against H1N1 influenza virus using MDCK cells

To further confirm the pharmacological potential of 1I1, ethanol extract of 1I1 was tested for its potent antiviral efficacy against H1N1 influenza virus on MDCK cell-line. It was found that H1N1 when used alone caused cytopathic effect (CPE) in MDCK cell-line (Fig. 5a). However, the same CPE was not observed in control MDCK cells (Fig. 5b). Further observations based on microscopic analysis confirmed that MDCK cells treated

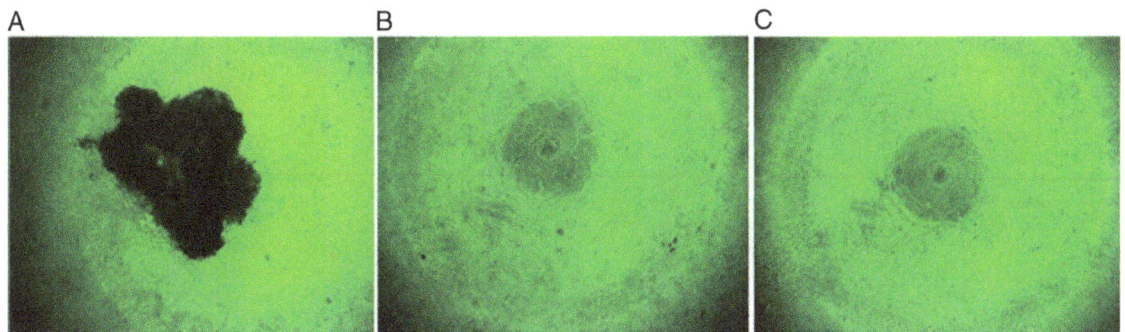

Fig. 5 Visualization of cytopathogenic effects of H1N1 virus infection in MDCK cells. Cytopathogenic effect in MDCK cells treated with H1N1 virus (**a**); control MDCK cells without any treatment (**b**); and anti-cytopathic effect in MDCK cells treated with *Lactobacillus sakei* 1I1 and H1N1 (**c**). Pictures were taken under fluorescence microscope at a magnification of 40×

with H1N1 and ethanol extract of *L. sakei* 1I1 (100 mg/ml) revealed similar morphological pattern as did by the control MDCK cells (no treatment) even after 72 h of the viral injection as shown in Fig. 5c. These findings suggested that 1I1 could be a potential anti-viral candidate to control CPE in MDCK cell-line. Recently we also reported that LAB strain isolated from different sources such a Korean traditional fermented food "Kimchi" exhibited potent antiviral effect against H1N1 influenza virus [6]. Tomosada et al. [56] also observed that it is possible to beneficially modulate the respiratory defense against respiratory syndrome virus (RSV) by using immunobiotics from *Lactobacillus* strains. Oh et al. [57] observed that oral administration of *L. gasseri* might protect a host animal from influenza virus (IFV) infection. Recently Kiso et al. [58] evaluated prophylactic efficacy of *Lactobacillus pentosus* b240 against lethal influenza A (H1N1) virus infection in a mouse model, suggesting it to be an effective candidate in anti-viral therapy.

Conclusions

This study confirmed that LAB isolate *L. sakei* 1I1, first time isolated from the intestine of fresh water fish *Zacco koreanus* exhibited inhibitory effect on α-glucosidase and tyrosinase enzymes in terms of its potent anti-diabetic and anti-melanogenic activities, respectively as well as exhibited anti-viral effect against influenza virus H1N1 on MDCK cells. These findings reinforce the suggestion that *L. sakei* 1I1 having a broader spectrum of pharmacological activities could be a novel candidate for using in health-care, food system and/or as dietary drug therapies in the treatment of various infectious diseases. Although this study ends with the development of an effective anti-diabetic, anti-melanogenic and anti-influenza candidate *L. sakei* 1I1, in vivo studies using live cultures of 1I1 in animal models should be undertaken to better understand the source of bioactivities.

Competing interests
The authors declare that they have no competing interests.

Authors' contributions
Conceived and designed the experiments: VKB JHH IAR GJN RM YHP. Performed the experiments: GJN RM. Analyzed the data: VKB IAR. Contributed reagents/materials/analysis tools: JHH CP JL WKP. Wrote the paper: VKB. All authors read and approved the final manuscript.

Acknowledgement
This work was supported by National Research Foundation of Korea (2013M3A9A5047052, 2008–2004707 and 2012–0006701).

References
1. Devriese LA, Kerckhove A, Kilpper-Balz R, Schleifer KH. Characterization and identification of *Enterococcus* sp. isolated from the intestines of animals. Int J Syst Bacteriol. 1987;37:257–9.
2. Perdigon G, Alvarez S, Rachid M, Aguero G, Gobbato N. Immune system stimulation by probiotics. J Dairy Sci. 1995;78:1597–606.
3. Mitsuoka T. A Color Atlas of Anaerobic Bacteria. 1st ed. Tokyo: Tokyo University Press; 1980. p. 20–9.
4. Kandler O, Weiss N. Microbiology of Mesu a Traditional Fermented Bamboo Shoot Product. In: Sneath PHA, Mair NS, Sharpe ME, Holt JG, editors. Bergey's Manual of Systematic Bacteriology. Baltimore: Williams and Wilkins; 1986. p. 1209–34.
5. Huber I, Spanggaard B, Appel KF, Rossen L, Neilson T, Gram L. Phylogenetic analysis and *in situ* identification of the intestinal microbial community of rainbow trout (*Oncorhynchus mykiss* Walbaum). J Appl Microbiol. 2004;96:117–32.
6. Rather IA, Choi KH, Bajpai VK, Park YH. Antiviral mode of action of *Lactobacillus plantarum* YML009 on influenza virus. Bang J Pharmacol. 2014;9:475–82.
7. Bajpai VK, Park YH, Na MK, Kang SC. α-Glucosidase and tyrosinase inhibitory effects of an abietane type diterpenoid taxoquinone from Metasequoia glyptostroboides. BMC Complement Altern Med. 2015;15:e84.
8. Liu L, Deseo MA, Morris C, Winter KM, Leach DN. Investigation of α-glucosidase inhibitory activity of wheat bran and germ. Food Chem. 2011;126:553–61.
9. Ozer O, Mutlu B, Kivcak B. Anti-tyrosinase activity of some plant extracts and formulations containing ellagic acid. Pharma Biol. 2007;45:519–24.
10. Chen YS, Liou HC, Chan CF. Tyrosinase inhibitory effect and antioxidative activities of fermented and ethanol extracts of *Rhodiola rosea* and *Lonicera japonica*. Sci World J. 2013;13:1–5.
11. Kwon SH, Hong SI, Kim JA. The neuroprotective effects of *Lonicera japonica* THUNB against hydrogen peroxide-induced apoptosis via phosphorylation of MAPKs and PI3K/Akt in SH-SYSY cells. Food Chem Toxicol. 2011;49:1011–9.
12. Kim YJ, Uyama H. Tyrosinase inhibitors from natural and synthetic sources: structure, inhibition mechanism and perspective for the future. Cell Mol Life Sci. 2005;62:1707–23.
13. Thompson WW, Shay DK, Weintraub E, Brammer L, Bridges CB, Cox NJ, Fukuda K. Influenza-associated hospitalizations in the United States. JAMA. 2004;292:1333–40.
14. Hancock K, Veguilla V, Lu X, Zhong W, Butler EN. Cross-reactive antibody responses to the 2009 pandemic H1N1 influenza virus. N Engl J Med. 2009; 361:1945–52.
15. Beigel J, Bray M. Current and future antiviral therapy of severe seasonal and avian influenza. Antiviral Res. 2008;78:91–102.
16. Nikoskelainen S, Salminen S, Bylund G, Ouwehand A. Characterization of the properties of human- and dairy-derived probiotics for prevention of infectious diseases in fish. J Appl Environ Microbiol. 2001;67:2430–5.
17. Ringø E, Gatesoupe FJ. Lactic acid bacteria in fish: A review. Aquaculture. 1998;160:177–203.
18. Axelsson L. Acid lactic bacteria: classification and physiology. In: Salminen S, Wright AV, Ouwehand A (eds) Lactic Acid Bacteria: Microbiological and Functional Aspects. New York: Marcel Dekker Inc; 2004 pp 1–66.
19. Lara-Flores M, Aguirre-Guzman G. The use of probiotic in fish and shrimp aquaculture. A review. In: Perez-Guerra N. & Pastrana-Castro L. (Eds), Probiotics: Production, evaluation and uses in animal feed, Kerala, India: Research Signpost; 2009;75–89.
20. Lara-Flores M. The use of probiotic in aquaculture: an overview. Int Res J Microbiol. 2011;2:471–8.
21. Zapata AA. Antimicrobial Activities of Lactic Acid Bacteria Strains Isolated from Nile Tilapia Intestine (*Oreochromis niloticus*). J Biol Life Sci. 2013;4:164–71.
22. Ishibashi N, Yamazaki S. Probiotics and safety. Am J Clin Nutr. 2001;73:465–70.
23. Balcazar JL, Venderll D, de Blas I, Ruiz-Zarzuela I, Muzquiz JL, Girones O. Characterization of probiotic properties of lactic acid bacteria isolated from intestinal microbiota of fish. Aquaculture. 2008;278:188–219.
24. Healy M, Green A, Healy A. Bioprocessing of Marine Crustacean Shell Waste. Acta Biotechnol. 2003;23:151–60.
25. Ennouali M, Elmoualdi L, Labioui H, Ouhsine M, Elyachioui M. Biotransformation of the fish waste by fermentation. Afr J Biotechnol. 2006;5:1733–7.
26. Amit KR, Swapna HC, Bhaskar N, Halami PM, Sachindra NM. Effect of fermentation ensilaging on recovery of oil from fresh water fish viscera. Enzyme Microb Technol. 2010;46:9–13.
27. Strahler AN. Quantitative analysis of watershed geomorphology. Trans Am Geophys. 1957;38:913–20.
28. Rankin ET. The qualitative habitat evaluation index (QHEI): Rationale, methods, and application. Columbus: Division of Water Quality Planning and Assessment. Ecological Assessment Section; 1989.

29. United State Environmental Protection Agency - USEPA. Working paper on regional nonpoint source guidance and supporting tables for section 319(h). Washington: U.S. Environmental Protection Agency, Office of Water; 1993.

30. Kim IS, Park JY. Freshwater Fishes of Korea. Seoul: Kyohak; 2002.

31. Cho YH, Hong SM, Kim CH. Isolation and characterization of lactic acid bacteria from Kimchi, Korean traditional fermented food to apply into fermented dairy products. Korean J Food Sci Anim Res. 2013;33:75–82.

32. Murray PR, Baron EJ, Pfaller MA, Tenover FC, Yolke RH. Manual Clinical Microbiology. 6th ed. Washington: ASM; 1995.

33. Shin SY, Bajpai VK, Kim HR, Kang SC. Antibacterial activity of bioconverted eicosapentaenoic (EPA) and docosahexaenoic acid (DHA) against foodborne pathogenic bacteria. Int J Food Microbiol. 2007;113:233–6.

34. Heilig HGHJ, Zoetendal EG, Vaughan EE, Marteau P, Akkermans ADL, de Vos WM. Molecular diversity of Lactobacillus ssp. and other lactic acid bacteria in the human intestine as determined by specific amplification of 16S ribosomal DNA. Appl Environ Microbiol. 2002;68:114–23.

35. Meyer H, Weidmann H, Lalk M. Methodological approaches to help unravel the intracellular metabolome of Bacillus subtilis. Microb Cell Fact. 2013;12:e69.

36. Yuan T, Wan C, Liu K, Seeram NP. New maplexin FI and phenolic glycosides from red maple (Acer rubrum) bark. Tetrahedron. 2012;68:959–64.

37. Fawole OA, Makunga NP, Opara UL. Antibacterial, antioxidant and tyrosinase-inhibition activities of pomegranate fruit peel methanolic extract. BMC Comp Alt Med. 2012;12:202–11.

38. Reed LJ, Muench H. A simple method of estimating fifty percent endpoints. Am J Hyg. 1938;27:493–7.

39. Seo BJ, Rather IA, Kumar VJR, Choi UH, Moon MR, Lim JH, Park YH. Evaluation of Leuconostoc mesenteroides YML003 as a probiotic against low-pathogenic avian influenza (H9N2) virus in chickens. J Appl Microbiol. 2012;113:163–71.

40. Nair PS, Surendran PK. Biochemical characterization of lactic acid bacteria isolated from fish and prawn. J Cult Collect. 2005;4:48–52.

41. Kandler O, Weiss N. In: Sneath PHA, Mair NS, Sharpe ME, Holt JG, editors. Bergey's Manual of Systematic Bacteriology. Baltimore: Williams and Wilkins; 1986. p. 1209–34.

42. Holt JG, Krieg NR, Sneath PHA, Staley JT, Williams ST. Bergey's manual of determinative bacteriology. 9th ed. MD: William and Wikkins; 1994. p. 559–64.

43. Ashraf R, Shah NP. Selective and differential enumerations of Lactobacillus delbrueckii subsp. bulgaricus, Streptococcus thermophilus, Lactobacillus acidophilus, Lactobacillus casei and Bifidobacterium spp. in yoghurt - a review. Int J Food Microbiol. 2011;149:194–208.

44. Bielecka M, Biedrzycka E, Majkowska A, Biedrzycka E. Method of Lactobacillus acidophilus viable cell enumeration in the presence of thermophilic lactic acid bacteria and bifidobacteria. Food Biotechnol. 2000;17:399–404.

45. Casaburi A, Di Martino V, Ferranti P, Picariello L. Technological properties and bacteriocins production by Lactobacillus curvatus 54 M16 and its use as starter culture for fermented sausage manufacturer. Food Control. 2016;59:31–45.

46. Jini R, Swapna HC, Rai AK, Vrinda R, Halami PM, Sachindra NM, Bhaskar N. Isolation and characterization of potential lactic acid bacteria (LAB) from freshwater fish processing wastes for application in fermentative utilization of fish processing waste. Braz J Microbiol. 2011;42:1516–25.

47. Sica MG, Olivera NL, Brugnoni LI, Marucci PL, López Cazorla AL, Cubitto MA. Isolation, identification and antimicrobial activity of lactic acid bacteria from the Bahía Blanca Estuary. Revis Biol Marin Oceanograf. 2010;45:389–97.

48. Hagi T, Tanaka D, Iwamura Y, Hoshino T. Diversity and seasonal changes in lactic acid bacteria in the intestinal tract of cultured freshwater fish. Aquaculture. 2004;234:335–46.

49. Lebovitz HE. Effect of postprandial state on non-traditional risk factors. Am J Cardiol. 2001;88:20–5.

50. Michlmayr H, Kneifel W. β-Glucosidase activities of lactic acid bacteria: mechanisms, impact on fermented food and human health. FEMS Microbiol Lett. 2014;352:1–10.

51. Ramchandran L, Shah NP. Proteolytic profiles and angiotensin-I converting enzyme and alpha-glucosidase inhibitory activities of selected lactic acid bacteria. J Food Sci. 2008;3:75–81.

52. Panwar H, Calderwood D, Grant IR, Grover S, Green BD. Lactobacillus strains isolated from infant faeces possess potent inhibitory activity against intestinal alpha- and beta-glucosidases suggesting anti-diabetic potential. Eur J Nutr. 2014;53:1465–74.

53. An BJ, Kwak JH, Park JM, Lee JY, Park TS, Lee JT, Son JH, Jo C, Byun MW. Inhibition of enzyme activities and the anti-wrinkle effect of polyphenol isolated from the Persimmon leaf (Diospyros kaki folium) on human skin. Dermatol Surg. 2005;31:848–54.

54. Kim JS, You HJ, Kang HY, Ji GE. Enhancement of the tyrosinase inhibitory activity of Mori Cortex radicis extract by biotransformation using Leuconostoc paramesenteroides PR. Biosci Biotechnol Biochem. 2012;76:1425–30.

55. Usuki A, Ohashi A, Sato H, Ochiai Y, Ichihashi M, Funasaka Y. The inhibitory effect of glycolic acid and lactic acid on melanin synthesis in melanoma cells. Exp Dermatol. 2003;12:43–50.

56. Tomosada Y, Chiba E, Zelaya H, Takahashi T, Tsukida K, Kitazawa H, Alvarez S, Villena J. Nasally administered Lactobacillus rhamnosus strains differentially modulate respiratory antiviral immune responses and induce protection against respiratory syncytial virus infection. BMC Immunol. 2013;14:40e.

57. Oh MH, Lee SG, Paik SY. Antiviral activity of Lactobacillus spp. and polysaccharide. J Bacteriol Virol. 2010;40:145–50.

58. Kiso M, Takano R, Sakabe S, Katsura H, Shinya K, Uraki R, Watanabe S, Saito H, Toba M, Kohda N, Kawaoka Y. Protective efficacy of orally administered, heat-killed Lactobacillus pentosus b240 against influenza A virus. Sci Rep. 2013;3:1563e.

Improved anticancer delivery of paclitaxel by albumin surface modification of PLGA nanoparticles

Mehdi Esfandyari-Manesh[1,2], Seyed Hossein Mostafavi[2,3,4], Reza Faridi Majidi[4], Mona Noori Koopaei[2], Nazanin Shabani Ravari[1,2], Mohsen Amini[5], Behrad Darvishi[1,4], Seyed Nasser Ostad[6], Fatemeh Atyabi[1,2] and Rassoul Dinarvand[1,2]*

Abstract

Background: Nanoparticles (NPs) play an important role in anticancer delivery systems. Surface modified NPs with hydrophilic polymers such as human serum albumin (HSA) have long half-life in the blood circulation system.

Methods: The method of modified nanoprecipitation was utilized for encapsulation of paclitaxel (PTX) in poly (lactic-co-glycolic acid) (PLGA). Para-maleimide benzoic hydrazide was conjugated to PLGA for the surface modifications of PLGA NPs, and then HSA was attached on the surface of prepared NPs by maleimide attachment to thiol groups (cysteines) of albumin. The application of HSA provides for the longer blood circulation of stealth NPs due to their escape from reticuloendothelial system (RES). Then the physicochemical properties of NPs like surface morphology, size, zeta potential, and in-vitro drug release were analyzed.

Results: The particle size of NPs ranged from 170 to 190 nm and increased about 20–30 nm after HSA conjugation. The zeta potential was about -6 mV and it decreased further after HSA conjugation. The HSA conjugation in prepared NPs was proved by Fourier transform infrared (FT-IR) spectroscopy, faster degradation of HSA in Differential scanning calorimetry (DSC) characterization, and other evidences such as the increasing in size and the decreasing in zeta potential. The PTX released in a biphasic mode for all colloidal suspensions. A sustained release profile for approximately 33 days was detected after a burst effect of the loaded drug. The in vitro cytotoxicity evaluation also indicated that the HSA NPs are more cytotoxic than plain NPs.

Conclusions: HSA decoration of PLGA NPs may be a suitable method for longer blood circulation of NPs.

Keywords: PLGA, Surface modified nanoparticles, Drug delivery, Albumin, Paclitaxel

Background

Different scientists including pharmaceutics, chemists, biologist, and nanotechnologist have been working indefatigably to defeat cancer. A major interest in this area is to improve drug targeting towards tumor cells and decrease the unwilling effects of chemotherapeutics [1-3]. Nanotechnology is very promising in this field and increases the efficacy of targeting by introducing passive and active targeting [4,5].

The interest on utilizing NPs formulated from biodegradable and biocompatible polymers such as the most commonly used PLGA are rising rapidly [6]. These NPs are broadly studied as anticancer delivery systems since it has special characteristics such as controlled release and biocompatibility [6].

A new approach to evade the short half-life of the conventional drug and allow targeted delivery to tumor cells is drug targeting achieved by size engineering and surface modification [7,8]. Vasculatures in tumor presents several irregularities in contrast with normal vessels resulting in enhanced permeation and retention (EPR) effect [9,10] and this will cause the nanoparticles with diameters less than 100 nm being selectively taken up by

* Correspondence: dinarvand@tums.ac.ir
[1]Nanotechnology Research Centre, Faculty of Pharmacy, Tehran University of Medical Sciences, Tehran, Iran
[2]Novel Drug Delivery Lab, Department of Pharmaceutics, Faculty of Pharmacy, Tehran University of Medical Sciences, Tehran, Iran
Full list of author information is available at the end of the article

tumor Vasculatures [8,11]. However, the drug bio-distribution profile of the cytotoxic drugs change massively while they are incorporated with NPs, because the modified particles are swiftly opsonised and massively cleared by mono nuclear phagocytes system (MPS) [10-12]. Surface modification of particles with hydrophilic polymers like polyethylene glycol (PEG) and albumin leading to the development of long-circulating and stealth particles for delivery of anticancer drugs [13,14]. Furthermore, the lack of lymph vessels and higher interstitial fluid pressure in the most tumors than normal ones causes inefficient removal of interstitial fluid and soluble macromolecules [15]. Therefore, the NPs mount up in the interstitium which retards their uptake (EPR effect), unless those particles are degraded [16,17].

The HSA coated NPs were prepared in two ways. First, non-covalent interactions where HSA molecules only saturate the surface without any covalent linkage [11] and second, albumin conjugated particles were synthesised via reaction between ξ-amino groups of lysine residues and the protein ligand with aldehyde functional or carboxylic acid [18,19]. The second method is more common.

Accordingly, we have developed a novel strategy that benefit from high efficiency and selectivity of the thiol. In this study we did a site-specific conjugation on the HSA that in spite of the fact that it minimize a loss in biological activity of it but meanwhile decrease immunogenicity. It happens because reagents that specifically react with the thiol group of cysteines, and the number of free cysteines on the surface of a protein is much less [15]. HSA conjugation to surface of NPs was done through the disulphide bonds between the HSA and the paramaleimido benzoic hydrazid (PMBH) derivative of PLGA. The encapsulation efficiency (EE), drug release, and morphology of nanoparticles were then investigated. At last cyto-toxicity of PTX loaded NPs was studied using 3-(4,5-dimethyathiazol-2-yl)-2,5-diphenyltetrazoliumbromide (MTT) assay.

Materials and methods

Materials

PLGA (50:50, M_W: 48000 g/mol) with carboxyl end group and HSA were purchased from Sigma company. N, N'-dicyclohexylcarbodiimide (DCC), N-hydroxysuccinimide (NHS), and 3-(4,5-dimethyathiazol-2-yl)-2,5-diphenyltetrazoliumbromide (MTT) were purchased from Sigma-Aldrich (St. Louis, MO, USA). PMBH, Na_3PO_4, NaH_2PO_4, NaOH, sodium bicarbonate and also NaCl was obtained from Merck. PTX purchased from Cipla Company. Dulbecco's modified eagle's medium (DMEM), penicillin, streptomycin antibiotic mixture and fetal bovine serum (FBS) were obtained from Life technologies (grand Island, NY, USA). Polyvinyl alcohol (PVA) was acquired from Acros (Geel, Belgium). 2-(N-morpholino

ethane sulfonic acid) (MES) was purchased from Fluka (St. Louis, MO, USA). All other solvents and reagents which are not stated were from Merck (Darmstadt, Germany).

Methods

Synthesis of PLGA with functional group of maleimide

Maleimide-functionalized copolymer PLGA was synthesized using the conjugation between paramaleimido benzoic hydrazid (PMBH) and PLGA–COOH. PLGA–COOH (5 g, 0.1 mmol) in 10 ml of methylene chloride was changed to PLGA–NHS with surfeit of N-hydroxysuccinimide (NHS, 135 mg, 1.1 mmol) in the presence of N, N'-dicyclohexylcarbodiimide (230 mg, 1.1 mmol). Then, 0.42 mol PMBH was added to the solution of activated PLGA and the reaction was allowed to proceed overnight on magnetic stirrer. The mixture was evaporated using rotary evaporator and the prepared film of PLGA-PMBH polymer was washed properly using de-ionized water and dried naturally for about two weeks. The synthesized polymer was assessed using H-NMR and FT-IR spectroscopy.

Preparation of PTX-loaded NPs

The method of modified nanoprecipitation was utilized for the preparation of drug encapsulated into particles of PLGA-PMBH [20-22]. In brief, 20 mg of polymer and 1.4 mg of PTX were dissolved in 4 ml of acetone and then injected (rate = 0.5 ml/min) into 16 ml of aqueous phase containing 0.5% PVA as surfactant and emulsified by probe sonication (Misonix, USA) for 5 min with amplitude of 10. Subsequently, the organic solution was evaporated gently on magnetic stirrer (600 rpm) for 9 hours. The NPs were washed and recovered using centrifuge process 25,000 rpm for 30 min (Sigma 3K30, Germany) and then lyophilized at – 40°C for 48 h (Christ Alpha 1–4; Germany). It should be mentioned that during the procedure, Several parameters in NPs preparation such as surfactant concentration, ratio of organic to aqueous, ratio of drug to polymer, and applied external energy witch have critical effects on the eventual size of NPs and drug loading were assessed in this experiment to obtain optimize situation.

HSA conjugation on the surface of PLGA NPs

5 mg of NPs was dispersed in 4 ml of degassed deionized water using bubbling nitrogen. HSA (10 mg/ml) were dissolved in 5 ml of degassed deionized water which have NaCl 0.15 M (pH 6.2–6.5) instantly before injecting it into the suspension. 1 ml of degassed solution contained ethylene diamine tetra acetic acid (EDTA) 4 mM and NaCl 0.3 M (pH 6.2–6.5) then were added to the suspension under the nitrogen pressure. The mixture was put a side overnight for the conjugation to perform

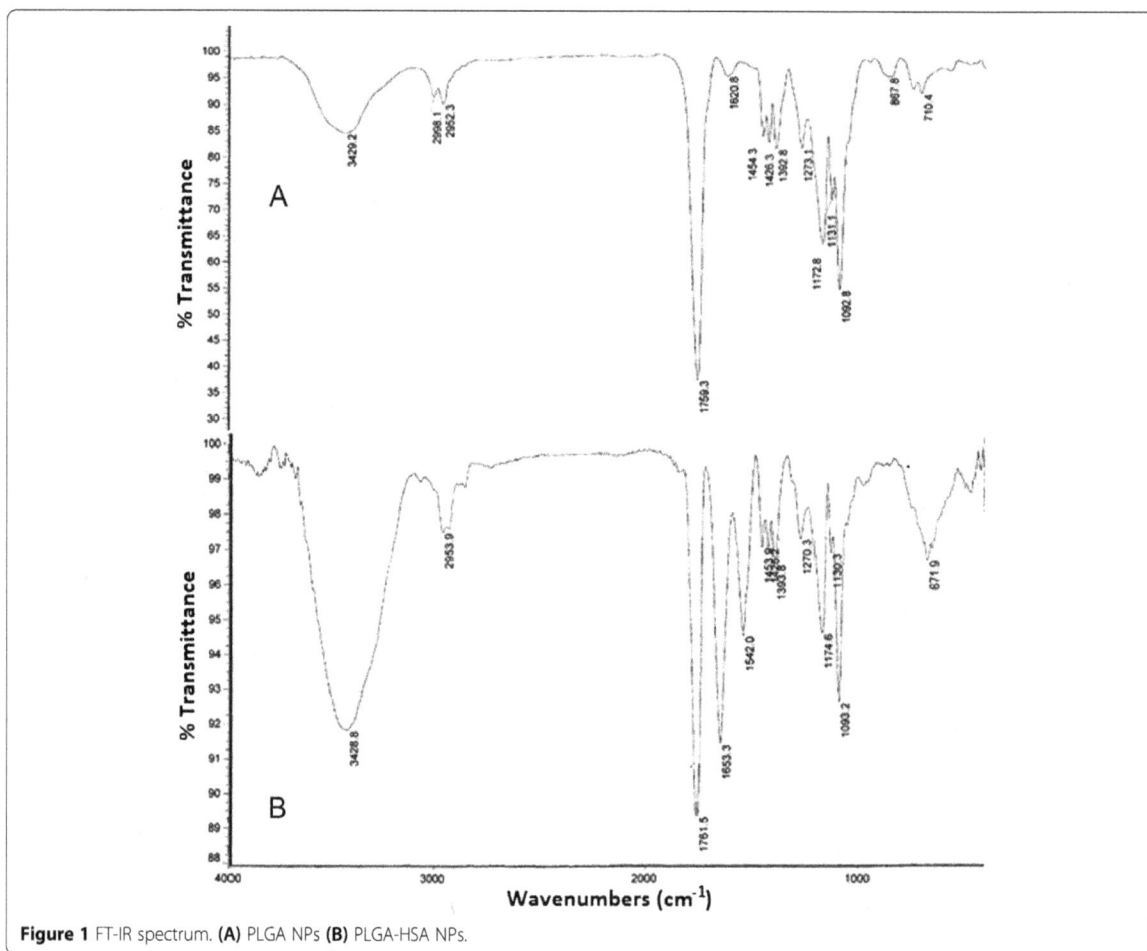

Figure 1 FT-IR spectrum. **(A)** PLGA NPs **(B)** PLGA-HSA NPs.

on the stirrer. The HSA conjugated PLGA NPs was purified and the unreacted HSA was removed using centrifuge (18000 rpm, 30 min, 3 times).

Measurement of size and zeta potential of NPs

Nearly 1 mg of NPs was suspended in 2 ml deionized water using bath sonicator. Mean size and polydispersity index (PDI) of NPs were evaluated using dynamic light scattering (DLS) instrument (Nano ZS, Malvern Instruments, UK). Afterward, samples were placed in an electrophoretic cell and zeta potential was determined.

Surface morphology

Scanning electron microscopy (SEM, Philips XL 30, Philips, The Netherlands) was used to determine the shape and surface morphology of the produced NPs. NPs were coated with gold under vacuum before scanning electron microscopy.

FT-IR analysis

To examine the conjugation was done correctly IR analysis. To perform this procedure we prepared a uniform mixture of lyophilized PLGA and PLGA-HSA NPs (separately) and KBr.

Differential scanning calorimetry (DSC)

Different ratio of physical mixture of raw materials included PLGA, HSA, PTX and also PLGA NPs and PLGA-HSA NPs were weighted equivalently (7 mg) and then sealed in standard aluminum pans. The experiment carried out using

Table 1 Particle size, zeta potential, encapsulation, and loading of NPs before and after conjugation

NPs	Size (nm)	Zeta (mV)	Encapsulation %	Loading
PLGA	187.0 ± 10.0	-6.7 ± 1.5	80.1 ± 11.0	10.7 ± 2.6
PLGA-HSA	207.0 ± 5.2	-13.6 ± 1.4	75.4 ± 12.0	8.2 ± 1.3

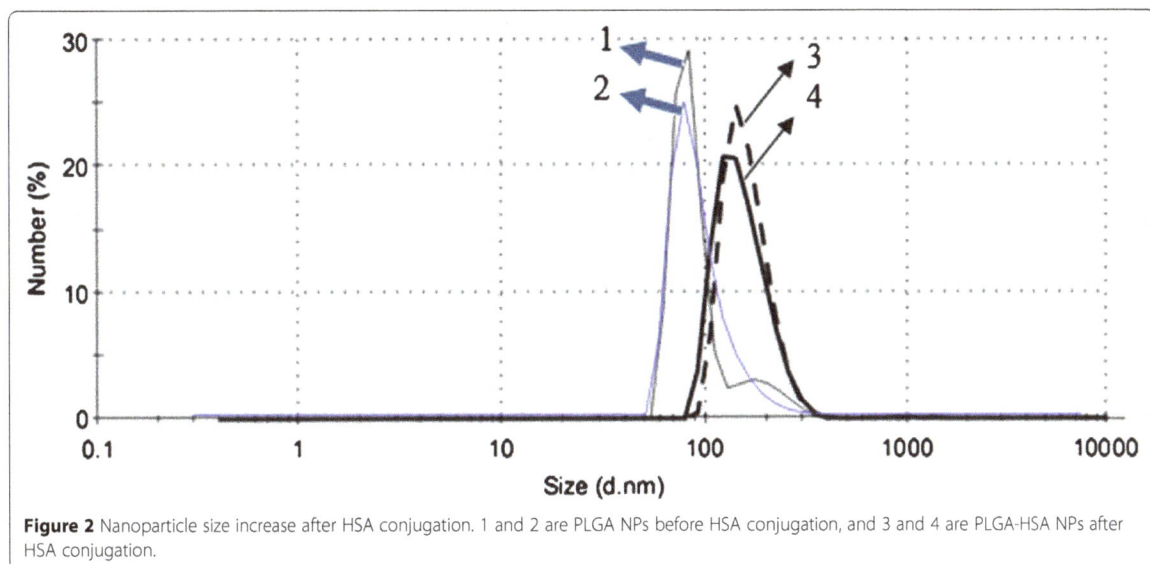

Figure 2 Nanoparticle size increase after HSA conjugation. 1 and 2 are PLGA NPs before HSA conjugation, and 3 and 4 are PLGA-HSA NPs after HSA conjugation.

(Mettler Toledo, GmbH, Switzerland) in ascending mode (10°C min/min) started from 40°C to 600°C.

Drug loading and encapsulation efficiency

To determine the drug loading and encapsulation efficiency, PTX entrapped in the NPs was measured by HPLC (Agilent LC1100, Agilent, Tokyo, Japan) at room temperature. The column was C18 column (25 cm × 0.46 cm internal diameter, pore size 5 μm; Teknokroma, Barcelona, Spain). The mobile phase consisted of acetonitrile/water (1/1 v/v). Lyophilized NPs (2.5 mg) were dissolved in acetonitrile (1 ml) (a common solvent for PLGA and drug) and shaken lightly followed by sonication for 6 min. Then, 2 ml of methanol was added to precipitate the polymer. The sample was filtered and drug quantity in filterant was determined by HPLC analysis.

$$Drug\ Loading\ \% = \left(\frac{weight\ of\ drug\ in\ NPs}{weight\ of\ NPs}\right) \times 100$$

$$Encapsulation\ Efficiency\ \% = \left(\frac{weight\ of\ drug\ in\ NPs}{weight\ of\ feed\ NPs}\right) \times 100$$

In vitro drug release

In order to evaluate in vitro release profile of PTX from PLGA and PLGA-HSA NPs, 2.5 mg of lyophilized samples were dispersed in 5 ml phosphate buffer saline solution (PBS, 0.01 M) containing 5% w/v of sodium dodecyl sulphate (SDS) with different pH (5 and 7.4) [21]. Afterward, suspensions poured into dialysis bags (cut off molecular weight 12000 g/mol) and immersed into the 50 ml of PBS with similar pH to the PBS in the bags. Subsequently, beakers placed on a shaker pre-set its temperature on 37°C

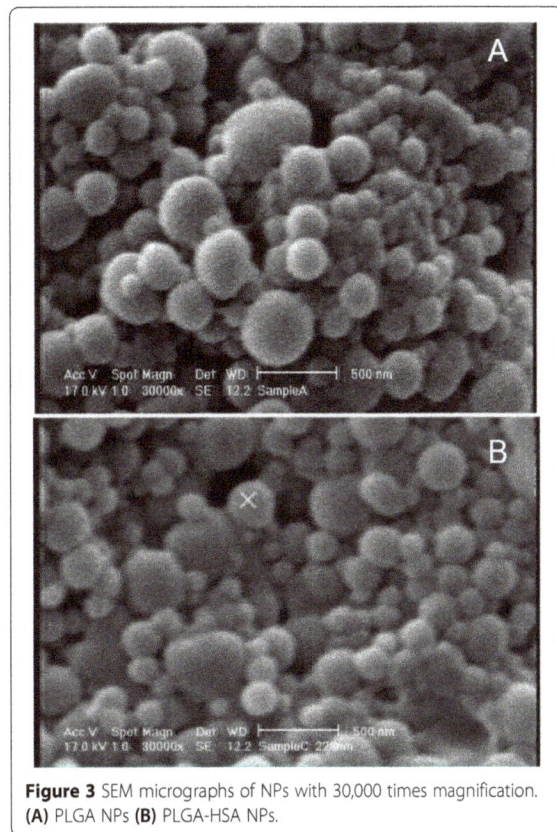

Figure 3 SEM micrographs of NPs with 30,000 times magnification. **(A)** PLGA NPs **(B)** PLGA-HSA NPs.

and 100 cycles per minute for during 33 days because of slow degradation proses of PLGA. For further assessments, all 50 ml of media (PBS) replaced with a same amount of new PBS at predetermined time intervals. The amount of released PTX was determined by HPLC in wavelength of 228 nm.

In vitro cell viability

MTT test was used to study the in vitro cytotoxicity of the subsequent PTX formulations on cell line of T47D: PTX loaded PLGA-HSA NPs, PTX loaded PLGA NPs, free PTX, and unloaded NPs.

T47D cells were seeded at the density of 1×10^4 viable cells/well in 96-well plates (Costar, Chicago, IL) and it is also incubated for 24 hours to providing enough time for cell attachments. Then the formulation (100 µL, 1–200 nM, and 48 h) was used to substitute the medium. A stock solution made in dimethyl sulfoxide (1 mg/ml PTX) for PTX. The concentration of dimethyl sulfoxide kept under 0.5% since at this concentration it has no effect on proliferation of cells and RPMI-1640 culture medium was used as diluents for preparing the working solution of free PTX drug and NPs. 20 µl MTT (5 mg/ml in phosphate-buffered saline) was added at specified periods of time to each well, and after 3 – 4 hours the culture medium containing MTT solution was eliminated. Then, micro plate reader (570 nm)

used to read it after dissolve of formazan crystals in dimethyl sulfoxide (100 µL). At last following equation used to evaluate cell viability:

$$\text{Cell viability } (\%) = (\text{Ints}/\text{Intcontrol}) \times 100$$

In this equation Ints equal to the colorimetric intensity of cells which is incubated with the samples, and Intcontrol is the colorimetric intensity of cells that incubated with the phosphate-buffered saline only as positive control.

Results and discussion
Synthesis of polymer

PLGA functionalized with maleimide group was synthesized and characterized. 1H-NMR and FT-IR analysis was used for confirmation of the primary chemical structure of PMBH–PLGA.

There was overlapping doublets at 1.6 ppm which are a confirmation for the methyl groups of the lactic acid. The multiples peaks at 4.8 ppm and 5.2 ppm correspond to the $-CH_2$ of glycolic acid and -CH of lactic acid, respectively. The high complexity of the peaks at 4.8 ppm and 5.2 ppm resulting from different sequences of glycolic acid and lactic in the backbone of polymer. There are also some detectable proton signals from maleimide and phenyl groups. Peaks which were present the hydrogens of linker are very weak compered to peaks present

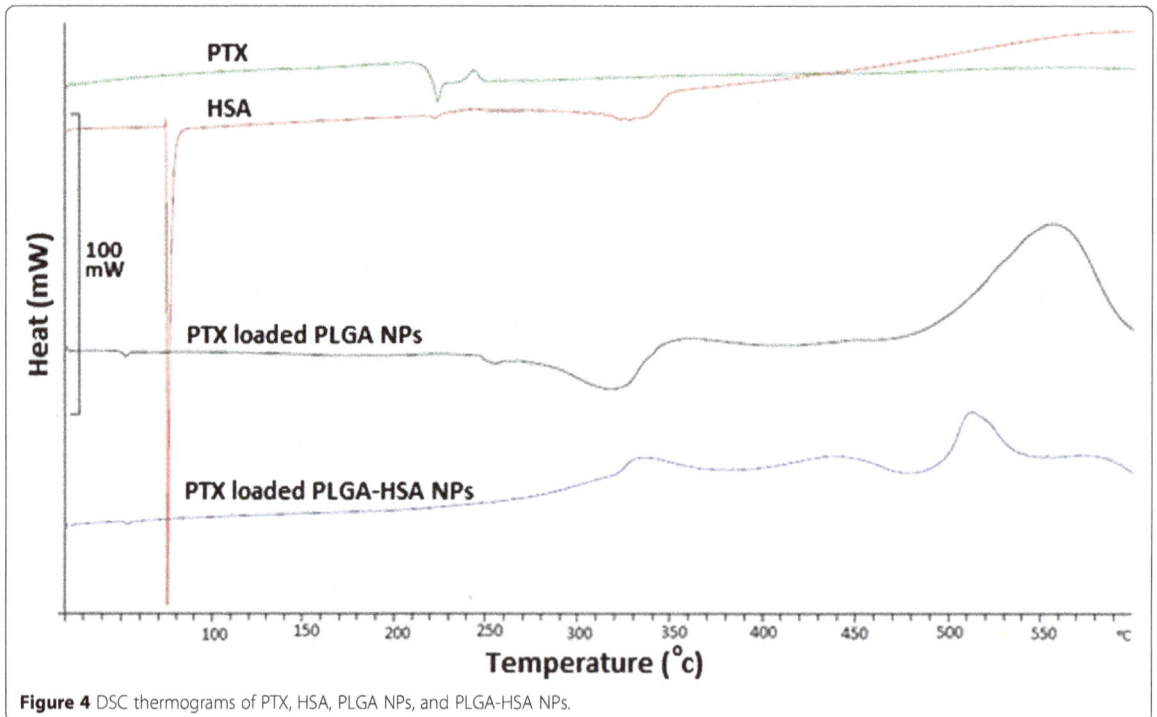

Figure 4 DSC thermograms of PTX, HSA, PLGA NPs, and PLGA-HSA NPs.

PLGA hydrogens because of the small ratio of linker to PLGA. A triplet peak on 7.2- 7.4 can be interoperating as benzoic hydrogens and a small peak found on 6.6 ppm shows the maleimide's hydrogens [22].

Conjugation of PLGA-PMBH was shown by FT-IR assessment (Figure 1). Formation of amide bonds are one of the most important reactions in synthesis of PLGA-PMBH. FTIR spectrum of synthesised polymer verified the amide group formation by some peaks, more specifically; the weak bands at 1620 cm^{-1} were assigned to amide bonds. These results verified the formation of PLGA-PMBH was done successfully.

Nanoparticles characterization

In the current study the modified nanoprecipitation method was chosen for NPs preparation. Several parameters in NPs preparation such as surfactant concentration, ratio of organic to aqueous, ratio of drug to polymer, and applied external energy have crucial effects on the eventual size of NPs and drug loading, so all of these parameters effects were assessed and the optimized formulations were used to prepare NPs to obtain optimized size [23]. Zeta potential, drug loading, and size of NPs were assessed using DLS and HPLC, respectively (Table 1). The evaluation of NPs size by DLS instrument revealed that the mean particle size of NPs was 190 ± 10 nm and when it was conjugated with HSA it increased about 20–30 nm and reached the mean size of 210 ± 10 nm. Theoretically if HSA with axial ratio of 2.66 nm and hydrodynamic radius of 3.7 nm conjugates in high amount around the surface of NPs, it should increase the size of each NPs roughly 19.7 nm and DLS assessment shows the predicted growth in dimension of each NPs (Figure 2). This phenomenon is clearly observed in SEM pictures that are shown in Figure 3. SEM pictures evaluation shows that NPs have spherical shape and mostly have monodispersed size distribution. The nanoparticle's zeta potential assessed by DLS display that PLGA NPs have negative charge (-6 mV) and the zeta potential reaches to -13 mV after HSA conjugation in PLGA-HSA NPs. HSA is also is a negative protein and conjugation will reduce the NPs charge [24].

DSC thermograms of pure PTX, pure HSA, and PTX loaded PLGA NPs and PTX loaded PLGA-HSA NPs demonstrated in Figure 4. In the drug diagram an endothermic peak observed around 220°C and the absence of that in NPs calorimetric curves proposes the lack of crystallinity after NPs preparation; this suggests that during NPs formation polymer hinders crystallization of PTX and the drug exist in the amorphous state. Other verifications, the differences between PLGA NPs and PLGA-HSA NPs peaks show the conjugation of HSA because of the faster degradation of HSA in PLGA-HSA NPs compared to PLGA NPs [25].

HSA conjugation

The infrared spectra of PLGA NPs and PLGA-HSA NPs were recorded by using the KBr pellet method (Figure 1). A very sharp peak at 1650 cm^{-1} in PLGA-HSA NPs that obviously point towards amide bonds existed in amino acids in HSA proved the conjugation take place correctly. FT-IR spectrum, faster degradation of HSA in DSC characterization, increasing the size of NPs, and decreasing the zeta potential are reasons which were proved the conjugation of HSA to PLGA-PMBH.

Drug release profile

In vitro drug release was evaluated in PBS with 2 different pH including 5.5 and 7.4 to assess how the different pH may affect the release profile. Acidic pH was chosen to simulate drug release behavior in the cancer cells. It also was examined before and after conjugation of HSA. In all NPs, 80% of loaded PTX released continuously in a sustained manner during 33 days when assessed in pH of 5.5 and about 70% drug released when experiment was carried out in neutral medium. This phenomena

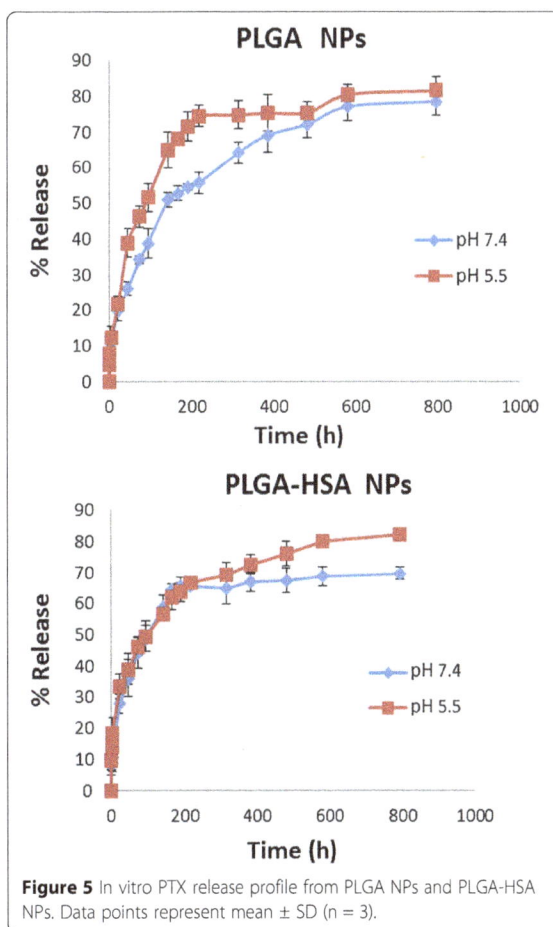

Figure 5 In vitro PTX release profile from PLGA NPs and PLGA-HSA NPs. Data points represent mean ± SD (n = 3).

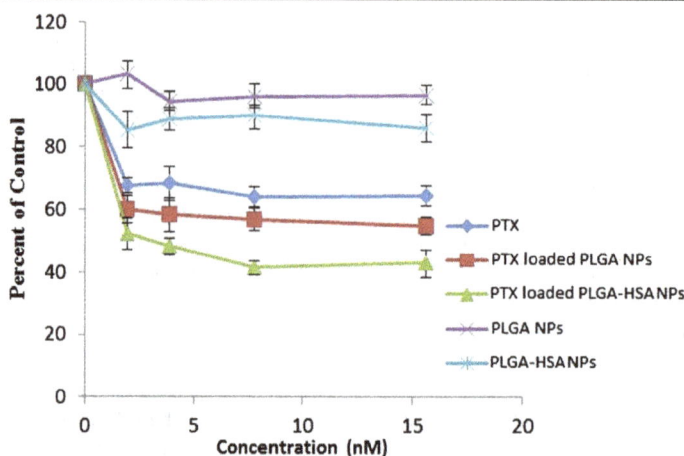

Figure 6 The in vitro cytotoxicity of free PTX, PTX loaded PLGA NPs, and PTX loaded PLGA-HSA NPs with different amount of PTX on T47D breast cancer cells. Data points represent mean ± SD (n = 3).

shows that drug disperse uniformly inside particles and it comes out of it by diffusion. Figure 5 shows that the drug release in acidic environment is faster than neutral ones for all NPs. Hence, this carrier can release drug faster in acidic surroundings of tumors. Acidic pH enhances hydrolization of ester linkage in PLGA and help encapsulated drug to release in control and sustain manner [24-27].

In vitro cytotoxicity

Figure 6 shows the in vitro cytotoxicity of free PTX, PTX loaded PLGA NPs, and PTX loaded PLGA-HSA NPs with different amount of PTX on breast cancer cells (T47D). Figure 6 illustrate that the cytotoxicity of PTX loaded PLGA-HSA NPs was significantly higher than the free PTX and PTX loaded PLGA NPs. Moreover, PTX loaded PLGA NPs have significantly more cytotoxic effect than free PTX. The percent viability of free PTX, PTX loaded PLGA NPs, and PTX loaded PLGA-HSA NPs were 64%, 54%, and 43% in 15 nM concentration, respectively. The enhancement of antitumor activity of PLGA-HSA NPs may be caused by gp60 (albondin) receptor and caveolar transport which both help these particles to increased transendothelial cell transportation of HSA [23,24]. First, HSA molecules bind to gp60 receptors and this binding activates caveolin. After caveolin configuration, HSA and other plasma constituents transfer transversely the endothelial cell to the interstitial space. Improved intratumor delivery of PTX may also other reason for the increased antitumor activity of PLGA-HSA NPs. Activated gp60 receptors which are specific for HSA help transportation of this molecule into tumor tissues by bypassing blood vessel wall barriers [25]. Unloaded NPs tested to evaluate the effect of polymerization and conjugation on cell viability

and statistical analysis proved that these parameters do not affect cell viability.

Conclusions

Preparation of the PTX loaded PLGA NPs were done by modified nanoprecipitation method. The hydrophobic PLGA NPs were decorated by hydrophilic HSA as novel anticancer delivery system. The PMBH was used as linker for the conjugation of HSA on the surface of PLGA NPs. The drug loading and encapsulation efficiency were 13% and 80%, respectively. Our results demonstrated that by using PMBH as linker and this method of nanoprecipitation, HSA conjugated NPs would be obtained with desired size, morphological, and drug loading properties. The in vitro cytotoxicity also showed that the HSA decorated NPs are more cytotoxic when compared with plain NPs and free anticancer agent, so these NPs can be used successfully in drug delivery of anticancer agents.

Competing interests
The authors declare that they have no competing interests.

Authors' contributions
MEM conceived the study and drafted the manuscript. SHM carried out the experiments and assisted in preparation of the manuscript. RFM and MNK supervised the synthesis and characterization of nanoparticles. NSR reviewed and revised the manuscript, MA supervised the synthesis and characterization of nanoparticles, BD helped with the characterization tests. SNO supervised the cell culture study, FA co-supervised the study, and RD supervised and coordinated the study and is the corresponding author of the manuscript. All authors read and approved the final manuscript.

Authors' information
Mehdi Esfandyari-Manesh and Seyed Hossein Mostafavi are considered as first author with equal responsibility and rights.

Author details
[1]Nanotechnology Research Centre, Faculty of Pharmacy, Tehran University of Medical Sciences, Tehran, Iran. [2]Novel Drug Delivery Lab, Department of Pharmaceutics, Faculty of Pharmacy, Tehran University of Medical Sciences,

Tehran, Iran. [3]Department of Bioengineering, University of California, Riverside, CA, USA. [4]Medical Nanotechnology Department, School of Advanced Technologies in Medicine, Tehran University of Medical Sciences, Tehran, Iran. [5]Department of Medicinal Chemistry, Faculty of Pharmacy, Tehran University of Medical Sciences, Tehran, Iran. [6]Department of Toxicology and Pharmacology, Faculty of Pharmacy, Tehran University of Medical Science, Tehran, Iran.

References

1. Soppimath KS, Aminabhavi TM, Kulkarni AR, Rudzinski WE. Biodegradable polymeric nanoparticles as drug delivery devices. J Control Release. 2001;70:1–20.
2. Langer R. Drug delivery and targeting. Nature. 1998;392:5–10.
3. Koopaei MN, Khoshayand MR, Mostafavi SH, Amini M, Khorramizadeh MR, Jeddi Tehrani M, et al. Docetaxel loaded PEG-PLGA nanoparticles: optimized drug loading, in-vitro Cytotoxicity and in-vivo Antitumor Effect. Iran J Pharm Res. 2014;13:819–33.
4. Koo OM, Rubinstein I, Onyuksel H. Role of nanotechnology in targeted drug delivery and imaging: a concise review. Nanomed Nanotechnol, Biol Med. 2005;1:193–212.
5. Koopaei MN, Maghazei MS, Mostafavi SH, Jamalifar H, Samadi N, Amini M, et al. Enhanced antibacterial activity of roxithromycin loaded pegylated poly lactide-co-glycolide nanoparticles. Daru. 2012;20:92–9.
6. Sourabhan S, Kaladhar K, Chandra PS. Method to enhance the encapsulation of biologically active molecules in PLGA nanoparticles. Trends Biomater Artif Organs. 2009;22:211–5.
7. Mostafavi SH, Aghajani M, Amani A, Darvishi B, Noori Koopaei M, Pashazadeh AM, et al. Optimization of paclitaxel-loaded poly (D, l-lactide-co-glycolide-N-p-maleimido benzoic hydrazide) nanoparticles size using artificial neural networks. Pharm Dev Technol. 2014;1:1–9.
8. Danhier F, Feron O, Preat V. To exploit the tumor microenvironment: passive and active tumor targeting of nanocarriers for anti-cancer drug delivery. J Control Release. 2012;148:135–46.
9. Park K. Questions on the role of the EPR effect in tumor targeting. J Control Release. 2013;172:391.
10. Fang J, Sawa T, Maeda H. Factors and mechanism of "EPR" effect and the enhanced antitumor effects of macromolecular drugs including SMANCS. Adv Exp Med Biol. 2003;519:29–49.
11. Maeda H, Sawa T, Konno T. Mechanism of tumor-targeted delivery of macromolecular drugs, including the EPR effect in solid tumor and clinical overview of the prototype polymeric drug SMANCS. J Control Release. 2001;74:47–61.
12. Hirsjarvi S, Passirani C, Benoit JP. Passive and active tumour targeting with nanocarriers. Curr Drug Discov Technol. 2011;8:188–96.
13. Okamura Y, Fujie T, Maruyama H, Handa M, Ikeda Y, Takeoka S. Prolonged hemostatic ability of polyethylene glycol-modified polymerized albumin particles carrying fibrinogen gamma-chain dodecapeptide. Transfusion. 2007;47:1254–62.
14. Moghimi SM, Hunter AC, Murray JC. Long-circulating and target-specific nanoparticles: theory to practice. Pharmacol Rev. 2001;53:283–318.
15. He X, Ma J, Mercado AE, Xu W, Jabbari E. Cytotoxicity of Paclitaxel in biodegradable self-assembled core-shell poly (lactide-co-glycolide ethylene oxide fumarate) nanoparticles. Pharm Res. 2008;25:1552–62.
16. Marcucci F, Lefoulon FO. Active targeting with particulate drug carriers in tumor therapy: fundamentals and recent progress. Drug Discov Today. 2004;9:219–28.
17. Stylianopoulos T. EPR-effect: utilizing size-dependent nanoparticle delivery to solid tumors. Ther Deliv. 2013;4:421–3.
18. Manjappa AS, Chaudhari KR, Venkataraju MP, Dantuluri P, Nanda B, Sidda C, et al. Antibody derivatization and conjugation strategies: application in preparation of stealth immunoliposome to target chemotherapeutics to tumor. J Control Release. 2010;150:2–22.
19. Weber C, Reiss S, Langer K. Preparation of surface modified protein nanoparticles by introduction of sulfhydryl groups. Int J Pharm. 2000;211:67–78.
20. Fonseca C, Simões S, Gaspar R. Paclitaxel-loaded PLGA nanoparticles: preparation, physicochemical characterization and in vitro anti-tumoral activity. J Control Release. 2002;83:273–86.
21. Wang YM, Sato H, Adachi I, Horikoshi I. Preparation and characterization of poly (lactic-co-glycolic acid) microspheres for targeted delivery of a novel anticancer agent, Taxol. Chem Pharm Bull. 1996;44:1935–40.
22. Fessi H, Puisieux F, Devissaguet JP, Ammoury N, Benita S. Nanocapsule formation by interfacial polymer deposition following solvent displacement. Int J Pharm. 1989;55:R1–4.
23. Liu J, Meisner D, Kwong E, Wu XY, Johnston MR. A novel trans-lymphatic drug delivery system: Implantable gelatin sponge impregnated with PLGA "paclitaxel microspheres. Biomaterials. 2007;28:3236–44.
24. Tessmar J, Mikos A, Gopferich A. The use of poly (ethylene glycol)-block-poly (lactic acid) derived copolymers for the rapid creation of biomimetic surfaces. Biomaterials. 2003;24:4475–86.
25. Manchanda R, Fernandez-Fernandez A, Nagesetti A, McGoron AJ. Preparation and characterization of a polymeric (PLGA) nanoparticulate drug delivery system with simultaneous incorporation of chemotherapeutic and thermo-optical agents. Colloids Surf B: Biointerfaces. 2009;75:260–7.
26. Musumeci T, Ventura CA, Giannone I, Ruozi B, Montenegro L, Pignatello R, et al. PLA/PLGA nanoparticles for sustained release of docetaxel. Int J Pharm. 2006;325:172–9.
27. Gindy ME, Ji S, Hoye TR, Panagiotopoulos AZ, Prud'homme RK. Preparation of poly (ethylene glycol) protected nanoparticles with variable bioconjugate ligand density. Biomacromolecules. 2008;9:2705–11.

Preliminary investigation of the effects of topical mixture of *Lawsonia inermis* L. and *Ricinus communis* L. leaves extract in treatment of osteoarthritis using MIA model in rats

Atousa Ziaei[1], Shamim Sahranavard[1], Mohammad Javad Gharagozlou[2] and Mehrdad Faizi[3*]

Abstract

Background: Many plants have been introduced in Iranian traditional medicine for treatment of different joint problems including knee pain. Topical application of the mixture of *Lawsonia inermis* L. leaves (Henna) with aqueous extract of *Ricinus communis* L. leaves have been mentioned to have significant effects on reducing knee pain. The present study was designed to evaluate the analgesic and anti-inflammatory effects of the mixture of these two herbs in male rats.

Methods: We induced knee osteoarthritis as a model of chronic pain by intra-articular injection of mono sodium iodoacetate (MIA). Mechanical allodynia, hotplate latency test, spontaneous movements and gait analysis were used for the evaluation of analgesic activity. Anti-inflammatory activity was evaluated by measuring the diameter and the volume of the injected paw compared to contralateral paw. These tests were monitored at days 1, 3, 7, 14 and 21 of MIA administration. Histopathological evaluations were also used to assess the efficacy of the treatment on inflammation and lesions in knee tissue. In all tests, diclofenac topical gel was used as a positive control. The herbal extracts, their mixture, and vehicle or diclofenac gel were administered daily for 14 days by topical route.

Results: The mixture of these two extracts significantly reduced the knee joint width and volume of the injected paws and also improved foot prints in gait analysis after 3 days of MIA injection. Analysis of mechanical allodynia (after 21 days), hotplate latency test (after 10 days), spontaneous movements (after 7 days) and in positive control group (after 3 days in all tests and in mechanical allodynia after 14 days) compared to the vehicle group, showed significant effects. Topical usage of the selected formulation made significant histopathological changes on the knee of the rats. Compared to the vehicle group, the tests and diclofenac groups showed less reactions characterized by negligible edema and a few scattered inflammatory lymphoid cells.

Conclusion: The present findings showed that the present formulation not only was able to mitigate pain and inflammation in the paws but also made significant histopathological changes on the knee of the rats. Further studies are necessary to confirm the effect of the formulation.

Keywords: *Lawsonia inermis* L, Leaves, MIA, Osteoarthritis, Rats, *Ricinus communis* L

* Correspondence: m.faizi@sbmu.ac.ir
[3]Department of Pharmacology and Toxicology, School of Pharmacy, Shahid Beheshti University of Medical Sciences, Tehran, Iran
Full list of author information is available at the end of the article

Background

Pain is a major symptom in many medical conditions and it is the most common reason for medical consultation. Approximately half of all licensed drugs that had been registered worldwide in a 25 years period prior to 2007 were natural products or synthetic derivatives of natural products [1]. For thousands of years, natural products derived from plants, animals and microorganisms have been used as treatments for human diseases. Knowledge of the medical use of natural products has been transmitted from generation to generation over the years [2]. It seems that drugs, especially those which have plant origin and have been used in the Iranian traditional medicine (ITM) could be an appropriate initiative in research projects aiming at development of new analgesic drugs.

A formula containing the mixture of *Lawsonia inermis* L. and *Ricinus communis* L. was chosen for evaluation of knee pain reduction from the Iranian traditional medicine books such as: *Makhzan-ol Advieh* [3], *Gharabadin-e-kabir* [4] and *Tohfat al-mu'minin* [5]. In these books, the mixture of mentioned plants has been recommended for knee pain treatment.

Osteoarthritis (OA) is a degenerative joint disease characterized by joint pain and progressive loss of articular cartilage [6]. Mono sodium iodoacetate (MIA) is a chemical substance that induced OA as a model of knee pain. This model is used for the study of pain and analgesic drug effects because it is reproducible and mimics the pathological changes and the pain of osteoarthritis in humans [7]. Injection of MIA, an inhibitor of glycolysis, into the femorotibial joint of rodents, promotes loss of articular cartilage similar to that observed in human OA [6]. The joint problem induced in this way, is called induced MIA hereafter.

Lawsonia inermis L. (Lythraceae) is used in the treatment of diseases such as leprosy and headache and has cosmetic purposes like accelerating the growth and dying hair and nails [8] and has also been reported to have anti-inflammatory, antinociceptive and antipyretic effects [9]. The natural constituents of *L.inermis* are Lawsone (2-hydroxy-1,4-naphthoquinone), mucilage, essential oils, tannic acid, gallic acid, fats, glucose, mannitol, and resin [10].

Ricinus communis L. (Euphorbiaceae) is used for the treatment of swelling, gout and skin diseases [11]. Polyphenols and flavonoids are the major compounds found in this plant and have anti-inflammatory and antioxidant activities [11, 12].

The present study was designed to evaluate the analgesic and anti-inflammatory effects of the mixture of topical extracts of *L.inermis* and *R.communis* according to the Iranian traditional manuscripts. The efficacy of the used formulation in reducing knee pain was evaluated by inducing osteoarthritis. All of the pharmacological experiments were also performed to determine the effects of *L.inermis* or *R.communis* extract separately.

Methods
Preparation of the extracts

Dry leaves of *Lawsonia inermis* L. were gathered from Yazd, Iran and identified and authenticated by a plant taxonomist at the herbarium of School of Traditional Medicine, Shahid Beheshti University of Medical Sciences, Tehran, Iran. The voucher specimen was deposited with number of HMS 331 in the herbarium. The dried leaves were powdered coarsely with a mechanical grinder (Desktop mill, 8300, Iran). The powder was passed through sieve No.40 and stored in an airtight container for further use. The powdered leaves were macerated in ethanol and water (80:20) and allowed to shake for 24 h and then were filtered through a filter paper (Whatman filter paper No.1). The maceration process was repeated 3 times. The filtered extract was concentrated in a rotary evaporator (Heidolph, HB digital, Germany) at 40 °C and then used freeze drier (Benchtop, SLC Virtis, USA) to remove water (the herbal extract ratio was 19 %). The dry extract was stored in cool place until used.

Fresh leaves of *Ricinus communis* were gathered from Tehran, Iran and identified and authenticated and deposited similar to *L.inermis* with voucher number of 3577. Subsequently, leaves were dried in shade and powdered by a mechanical grinder. The powdered leaves were macerated in water and allowed to shake for 24 h, same as described for *L.inermis* (the herbal extract ratio was 22 %). The herbal extracts were added at the same concentrations as mentioned in ITM references [3–5] and we did not perform comparative evaluation of different doses of the extracts.

Drug administration

The dry extracts were mixed with the same percentage, suspended in water (0.2 g/0.3 ml). This is the maximum amount of the mixture of extracts that solved in the lowest amount of the vehicle and cover all of the animal 's knee and administered topically on the left hind paw of the animal in all groups, from day 1 to 14 (once a day dosing) respectively. The control group (Vehicle) received the same volume of vehicle (water) by the same route. 0.4 g of diclofenac 1 % gel (Razak Pharmaceutical Company) was used topically in the positive control group [13].

Animals and experimental groups

Wistar male rats (160–180 g body weight) were purchased from the Pasteur Institute of Iran. They were housed in standard polypropylene rat cages and kept in a room with controlled condition (temperature 25 ± 2 °C and relative humidity 40–50 %) in a 12 h light-dark cycle. The rats were given a standard laboratory diet and have free access to food and water. Each rat was only used once. All procedures for the treatment of animals were approved by the Research Committee of Shahid Beheshti University of Medical Sciences and institutional animal care and use committee with approval code SBMU.REC.1392.343.

For induction of OA, rats were anesthetized with ketamine-xylazine (100 and 10 mg/kg) intra-peritoneally [14, 15]. Osteoarthritis was induced by an injection of mono sodium iodoacetate (MIA, Sigma-Aldrich, USA) at a dose of 3 mg/50 μL normal saline to intra articular space of the left hind limb [16–18].

In this study, 36 adult male wistar rats were used. They were randomly divided in to 6 groups including sham group (S; $n = 6$) that received saline instead of MIA, negative control group (N; $n = 6$) with OA induction and treating by vehicle, combination group (T; $n = 6$) with OA induction and treating by topical mixture of the plant extracts, L.inermis group (L; $n = 6$), R.communis group (R; $n = 6$) and positive control group (P; $n = 6$) with OA induction and treating by diclofenac topical gel. On day 21, after performing behavioral tests, rats of all groups were sacrificed by overdosing ether [19]. To evaluate the histological changes, rats were sacrificed on day 14 after 3 h of the formulation or diclofenac gel administration and left knee was collected for histological examination.

Behavioral tests
Mechanical allodynia (Von Frey test)
Von Frey filaments (North Coast Medical, Inc. CA, USA) have been used to assess the mechanical sensitivity of the hind paw of the animals with knee joint arthritis. Typically, paw withdrawal threshold (PWT) is measured in response to increasing pressure stimuli applied to the plantar surface by von Frey filaments. Rats were removed from their home cages and placed in a Plexiglass cage with a wire mesh bottom [20]. The rats were allowed to acclimate for 15 min (or until exploratory and grooming behavior declined to a level compatible with behavioral testing). Von Frey monofilaments were applied at a 90° to the mid-plantar of the left hind paw of the rats (ipsilateral side of MIA injection) with a series of monofilaments that ranged from 0.6 to 26 g in stiffness. Filaments were held in place and then removed; they were applied at the same location; 5 times for 1.5 s with inter stimulus intervals of 1 min. Rats were tested using the up-down method. A positive response was defined as a rapid withdrawal of the left hind paw or licking of the paw (three out of five were considered positive). The first day of the testing provided a baseline measure of tactile sensitivity. Rats in each group

were then tested with von Frey monofilaments on post-injection days 1, 3, 7, 10, 14 and 21.

Spontaneous locomotor activity (Open field test)
This method has been used to evaluate the locomotor activity of rodents [21]. The test was performed in a Plexi glass box of $40 \times 40 \times 40$ cm with transparent walls and black floor (in contrast with the color of the rat). Each rat was initially placed in the center of the box and its activity was recorded by a video camera for 10 min (at the same temperature and light conditions). Locomotor activity was measured in the square arena. The behavior was recorded by a video camera mounted on the ceiling, relayed to a monitor and total distance moved of the rat was analyzed by tracking software (EthoVision, Noldus, The Netherlands). Spontaneous locomotion was assessed on six consecutive days. On each day, each rat was placed in the center of the arena and allowed to explore it for 10 min. In this period, the rat's movements were recorded with a video camera. The computer software calculated the distance that the rat moved and the total distance during 10 min period was measured. At the end of each test, the box was removed and the entire test chamber was cleaned with a damp cloth and subsequently dried [22].

Gait analysis test (Footprint)
Analyzing the walking patterns of the rat by recording its footprints is a well-established and widely employed method for the assessment of motor nerve recovery after nerve injury [23]. We used the software image J to analyze the rat's footprints. Analysis footprints by image J 1.37 software is extremely useful and reduces intervention results such as operator subjectivity which can limit the statistical significance of the numerical data generated.

Tracking tunnels are basically rectangular, designed to allow the target animal to walk through unhindered. A tracking paper made of an absorbent white paper was used. Rats were stained with the ink-foot stump then each animal attracted into the tunnel after walking across the ink leaves footprints on the absorbent paper. The ink is absorbed into the paper leaving tracks which can be analyzed by the software image J [24].

Hotplate test
The analgesic response was the latency observed from the time the rat was placed on the heated surface until the first overt behavioral sign of nociception such as (a) the rat licking a hind paw, (b) vocalization or (c) an escape response [25].

Animals were placed individually on a hotplate with the temperature adjusted to 52 °C (UgoBasile, Varese, Italy). Exposure to heat continued until a nociceptive reaction in either of the hind paws occurred. The latency of the withdrawal response of each of the hind paws was determined at 1, 3, 7, 10, 14 and 21 days after injection of MIA. The heat source was maintained at constant intensity, which produced a stable withdrawal latency of approximately 8–10s in vehicle group. The animals were tested in only one series of measurements and the typical responses were hind paw shaking and/or lifting and the rat was immediately removed from the hotplate after the response was observed. The latency to the response was recorded manually with a chronometer and the maximum permanence permitted on the hot surface was 60s. The experiments were performed in a sound-attenuated and air-conditioned (25–30 °C) laboratory.

Inflammatory tests
Measuring paw diameter
The paw diameter was measured at intervals of 1, 3, 7, 10, 14 and 21 days after the injection of MIA using Colis (Helios, Germany) after MIA injection. The difference between inflamed and right knee's joint width at 6 time points was calculated (indicating the degree of inflammation) and was compared to the amount for vehicle group (N) [26].

Measuring paw edema using mercury
This method was done by the method previously reported by Fereidoni and his colleagues [27]. A cylinder filled with mercury was placed on a sensitive digital balance. The values on the digital balance were recorded. According to the gravity of mercury, the expected measures were calculated and compared with the observed value. The formula used for this measurement is $V = W/p$, in which V stands for volume, W for weight and p for gravity [27]. Measurements of the inflamed paw were continued for 21 days after MIA injection and performed five times on each rat and the average of middle three values was calculated.

Histological evaluation
Histological studies were performed to ensure the responses obtained from the pharmacological experiments. On MIA post day 14, rats were sacrificed and MIA or saline injected knee joints (including distal femur and proximal tibia) were fixed in 10 % buffered formaldehyde solution, decalcified using formic acid-sodium citrate method [28]. This method is superior to other decalcification techniques, since preserves the histological and staining properties of tissues very well. The formalin-fixed specimens were washed properly by distilled water to remove the residues of formaldehyde from the tissues. Then, the specimens were transferred into a jar containing sufficient volume of formic acid–sodium citrate solution, prepared as follows [28].

Solution A: 50 g of sodium citrate was dissolved in 250 ml of distilled water.
Solution B: 125 ml of 90 % formic acid were added to 125 ml of distilled water.
To make a working solution, equal volumes of the solutions A and B were mixed before use. Due to higher volume of the bone tissue of the specimens, the decalcifying solution was changed every single day until decalcification was completed. The decalcified specimens were washed very well with distilled water in order to remove decalcified residues.
A longitudinal section was made at the extensor site in such a manner that divided the specimen into two equal pieces. The tissue samples were processed in a tissue processor, paraffin blocks were made and 5–6 μm thick sections were made with a microtome. Sections were stained with the Harris haematoxylin and eosin method [28]. The histology was evaluated through double-blind observations following the method described previously.
Scoring of the severity of the articular or periarticular tissue lesions including acute or chronic inflammatory lesions in the tissue sections stained with Harris haematoxylin and eosine method was done by using a magnification of X100-X400 as follows:

0: **Negative;** Normal tissue architecture.
1: **Mild;** A very mild tissue edema accompanied by a few scattered mononuclear cells including lymphocytes.
2: **Moderate;** Many mononuclear or polymorphonuclear leukocytes accompanied by hyperemia and edema or beginning of granulation tissue formation.
3: **Severe;** Marked acute or chronic inflammation characterized by fibrinopurulent exudates or granulation tissue formation accompanied by mononuclear infiltration with or without tendinal adhesions to the adjacent tissues.
4: **Very severe;** Marked severe acute or chronic inflammation accompanied by tissue necrosis and tendinal adhesions.

The number of pathology sections that were used: three sections in the Sham group, four sections in rats, a day after they were injected with MIA(Inflammation peak), four sections in group (P), four sections in group (T), five sections in group (N) with no treatment.

Histological studies were done on five groups: 1-Sham injected by Saline (group S). 2- One day after injection of MIA that substantial inflammation of the synovial joints was observed in the model. Some days later, the inflammatory response in the synovium subsides, necrotic cartilage collapse, and chondrocytes are lost [29, 30]. 3- Diclofenac gel or group (P) as positive group 4-Mixture of the extracts or group (T) 5- Vehicle or no treatment or group (N).

Statistical analysis

The obtained data were analyzed by the statistical program Prism 5. Results launched by Average ± SEM. Due to the two interventions (different groups on different days), we used two-way ANOVA to determine the differences between the experimental groups and the mean obtained in the presence of interference interaction between groups. To evaluate the significant differences between the groups, the post hoc Bonferroni test was used. Amounts of $p < 0.05$ were considered as the minimum level of significance. Asterisks indicate a statistically difference from group (N); * $p <0.05$, **$p <0.01$, ***$p <0.001$.

Results

Mechanical allodynia

Results are expressed as pain threshold measurements with von Frey filament stimulation of the area. A decrease in pain threshold compared to group (N) was demonstrated in all of the groups on the ipsilateral side (Fig. 1).

Treatment was initiated 1 day after the MIA injection and pain was assessed on the days 1, 3, 7, 10, 14 and 21. Paw withdrawal threshold significantly increased (indicating less pain) in the test group and the diclofenac gel group compared with vehicle and sham groups. The pain threshold specifically increased in group (P) after 10 days and in group (T) after 21 days compared to group (N) ($p < 0.05$) (Fig. 1).

Spontaneous locomotor activity

Total distance traveled in the arena during 10 min showed a significant effect after 7 days compared to group (N). Topical administration of diclofenac gel also

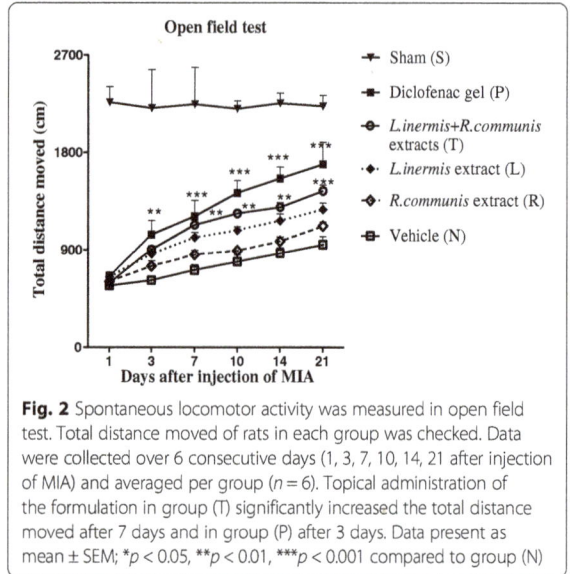

Fig. 2 Spontaneous locomotor activity was measured in open field test. Total distance moved of rats in each group was checked. Data were collected over 6 consecutive days (1, 3, 7, 10, 14, 21 after injection of MIA) and averaged per group ($n = 6$). Topical administration of the formulation in group (T) significantly increased the total distance moved after 7 days and in group (P) after 3 days. Data present as mean ± SEM; *$p < 0.05$, **$p < 0.01$, ***$p < 0.001$ compared to group (N)

significantly increased the total distance moved after 3 days (Fig. 2).

Footprint

Images of footprint patterns enabled the observation of abnormalities in the foot placing (Fig. 3). The rats in group MIA presented measurable foot placing for 21 days. These animals loaded their weight on the medial part of their affected foot. In group sham, no changes were developed. Significant changes were seen in group (T) and group (P) after 3 days compared to group (N). They were measured both in the affected and in the non affected hind legs (Fig. 4).

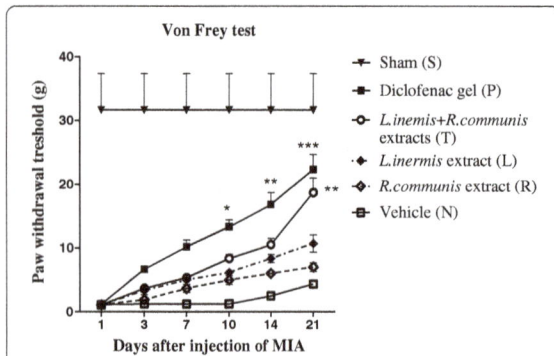

Fig. 1 Paw withdrawal threshold (PWT) was measured by von Frey monofilaments. At days 1, 3, 7, 10, 14, 21 after injection of MIA ($n = 6$), von Frey testing on the inflamed paw showed significant effect compared to group (N); after 21 days in test group (T) and after 10 days in positive control or group (P) of MIA injection. Data present mean ± SEM; *$p < 0.05$, **$p <0.01$, ***$p <0.001$ compared to group (N)

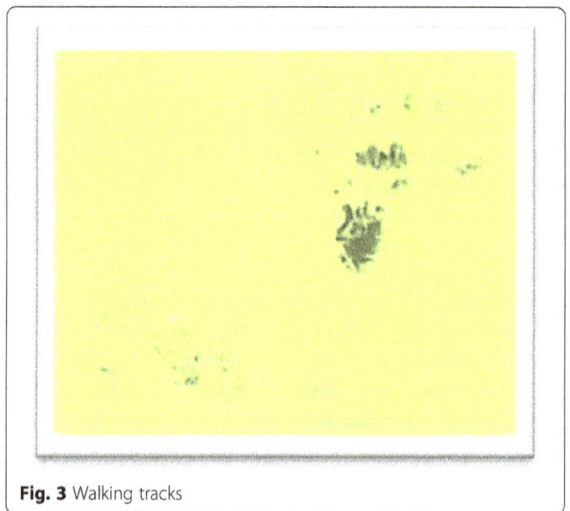

Fig. 3 Walking tracks

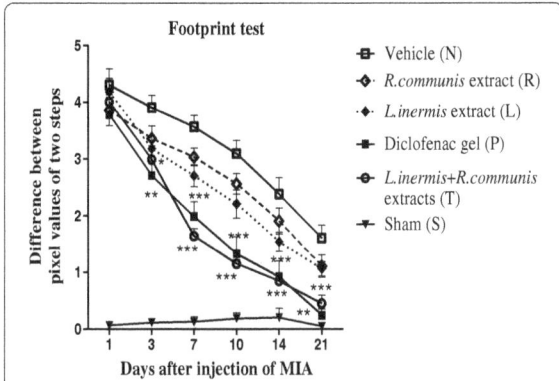

Fig. 4 MIA injection affected weight bearing of the paws during locomotion. Comparing the differences between pixel values of right and left hind paw tracks on the paper which obtained by image J software in different days. Significant reduction between pixel values of two steps were seen in group (T) and group (P) after 3 days compared to group (N). Data presented as mean ± SEM; *$p < 0.05$, **$p < 0.01$, ***$p < 0.001$ compared to group (N)

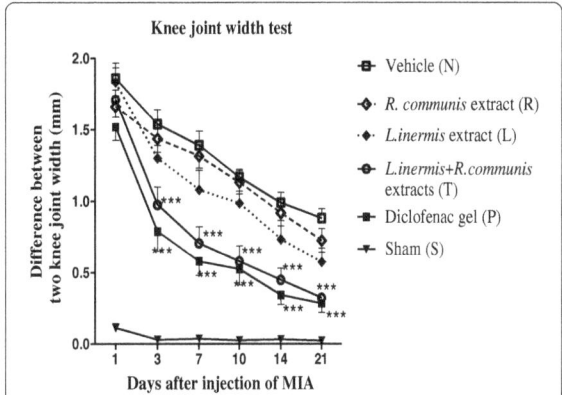

Fig. 6 Comparison the differences between the inflamed and right knee's joint width. The knee's joint width was measured by colis in different days 1, 3, 7, 10, 14, 21 for each group. Treatments were continued for 14 days. Compared to group (N), differences between two knee joint widths were significantly reduced in group (T) and group (P) after 3 days. Data are expressed as mean ± SEM; *$p < 0.05$, **$p < 0.01$, ***$p < 0.001$

Hotplate

As illustrated in Fig. 5, the Intra- articular injection into the left hind paw of the rats caused a reduction in the latency of the withdrawal response to heat stimulation compared to sham group (S). The latency values as compared to group (N), was increased after 10 days and in group (P) after 3 days compared to group (N) (Fig. 5).

Measuring paw diameter

In Fig. 6, Data of anti-inflammatory activity of the extracts in MIA induced paw edema are shown. The left paw diameter after different day s intervals was used as criteria for evaluation of inflammation. Generally, data indicated that the extracts possessed anti-inflammatory

activity compared to the vehicle group and it showed after 3 days significant effect as compared to group (N) can be seen and it was as the same as the effect of group (P) (Fig. 6).

Measuring paw volume

Chronic pain suffering rats were given daily topical administration of extracts, diclofenac and vehicle for 14 days. The volume of the left hind paw was measured with mercury column in different days. The effect was observed after 3 days as the same as diclofenac gel and the paw volume was reduced compared to the vehicle group (Fig. 7).

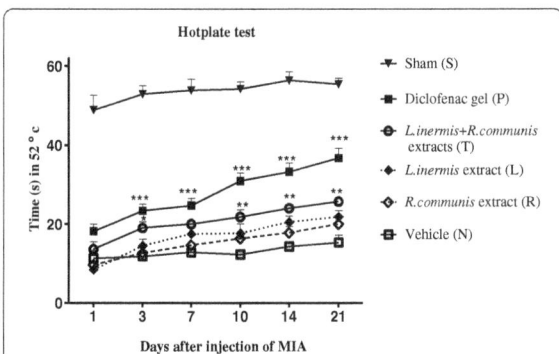

Fig. 5 The response latency time of the paws to heat stimulation in hotplate test. The response latency time of the paws was measured at 1, 3, 7, 10, 14, 21 days after injection MIA compared to group (N) in each group. The latency values were increased after 10 days in group (T) and after 3 days in group (P). Data are expressed as mean ± SEM; *$p < 0.05$, **$p < 0.01$, ***$p < 0.001$ compared to group (N)

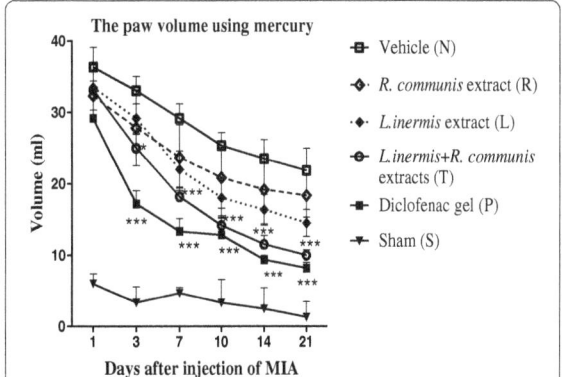

Fig. 7 The volume of the inflamed paw was measured with mercury coloumn in different days. The paw volume significantly reduced after 3 days in group (T) and group (P) compared to group (N). Data are showed as mean ± SEM of edema volume induced by MIA; *$p < 0.05$, **$p < 0.01$, ***$p < 0.001$ compared to group (N)

Topically using *L.inermis* (henna) extract on each paw was effective in reducing the OA pain and inflammation, compare to vehicle but p value was not less than the accepted level of significance ($p > 0.05$) therefore it did not achieve complete pain remission. Topically using *R. communis* was not effective as *L. inermis* and showed little antinociceptive and anti-inflammatory activities in pharmacological tests.

Histology

The results of the pathological findings and scoring of the lesions are depicted in Table 1. As seen in Table 1, the Sham group received saline and was euthanized 14 days later. The articular tissue structures including synovium, synovial tissue, adjacent ligaments, tendons and tendinal sheath and subcutaneous tissues and muscles had normal tissue architecture and were intact (score0) (Fig. 8).

Rats that received MIA and were euthanized 24 h later showed severe acute fibrinopurulent inflammatory reaction. Fibrinopurulent exudates were affected synovial tissues, ligaments, tendons, tendinal sheath, muscles and subcutaneous tissues (score 4) (Fig. 9).

In those groups treated by diclofenac gel group (P) or group (T) that received the mixture of the extracts remedy and euthanized 14 days later the same results were obtained. A very mild edema and presence of a few scattered lymphocytes were observed. Articular tissue structure, including synovium, ligament, tendons and subcutaneous tissue were histologically normal (score1) (Fig. 10).

In the vehicle group that only received MIA and euthanized 14 days later, chronic inflammatory reactions accompanied by tendinal adhesion were noticed. Formation of granulation tissue with neovascularization, edema, infiltration of mononuclear leucocytes including lymphocytes and adhesion of tendons to its tendinal sheath were observed (score 3) (Fig. 11).

According to the obtained data, topical use of the mixture extracts showed anti-inflammatory and analgesic effects on osteoarthritis induced by MIA.

Discussion

Previous studies have shown that lawsone, isoplumbagin and lawsaritol isolated from *Lawsonia inermis* exhibit anti-inflammatory and analgesic effects in rats [8, 31]. Besides, experiments showed that methanolic extract of *Ricinus communis* leaves, contain flavonoids: rutin, quercetin, epicatechin and polyphenols and gentisic acid have anti-inflammatory activity in rats when administered orally [12] but the topical usage of their combination has not yet been investigated.

Studies showed that intra- articular injection of MIA in rats produces chronic osteoarthritis pain, pharmacological tests were performed in the early (up to 1 week after MIA) versus late (between 2 and 4 weeks after MIA) phase of the rat MIA model [32]. In the present study, six time points 1, 3, 7, 10, 14 and 21 days were taken for determining pain and inflammation to see the effect of the formulation on both acute and chronic phases.

In this study mixture of *Lawsonia inermis* L. and *Ricinus communis* L. extracts were used as a topical medication to relief induced joint pain and diclofenac gel which has analgesic and anti-inflammatory effects and has been shown to be effective in the treatment of a variety of acute and chronic pains and inflammatory conditions such as osteoarthritis [33], was used as positive control.

The mixture of extracts showed analgesic effect by reducing mechanical allodynia measured by von Frey filaments increased from a baseline of 0.6 g to 26 g. Comparing the rats of group (N), the significant effect was seen in group (T) after 21 days and in group (P) after 10 days. The responses after day 10, 21 showed that the formulation affected the late inflammatory reactions to painful mechanical stimuli.

Table 1 Comparison of the histological effects of different groups and their scores

Groups	Pathological finding	Score
Sham or group (S)	The articular tissue structures including synovium, synovial tissue, adjacent ligaments, tendons and tendinal sheath and subcutaneous tissues and muscles had normal tissue architecture.	0
A day after injected MIA (Inflammation peak day)	Severe acute fibrinopurulent inflammatory reaction. Fibrinopurulent exudates were affected synovial tissues, ligaments, tendons, tendons sheath, muscles and subcutaneous tissues.	4 sharp
Diclofenac gel or group (P)	A very mild edema and presence of a few scattered lymphocytes. Articular tissue structure, including synovium, ligament, tendons, subcutaneous tissue were histologically normal	1
The mixture of extracts or group (T)	As the same as diclofenac.	1
No treatment or group (N)	Chronic inflammatory reactions accompanied by tendinal adhesion were noticed. Formation of granulation tissue with neo vascularization, edema, infiltration of mononuclear leucocytes including lymphocytes and adhesion of tendons to its tendinal sheath were observed.	3

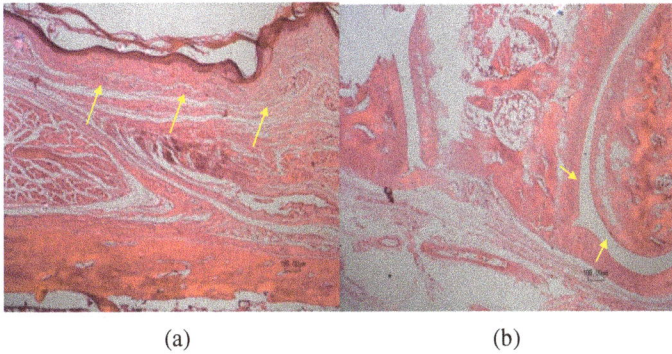

Fig. 8 A section of articular tissue from group (S) or sham. The H&E stained paraffin tissue sections of covering skin tissues (*large arrows*) and articular (*small arrows*) from saline injected group can be seen. The skin (**a**) and articular tissue (**b**) have normal tissue architecture. Scale bar = 100 μm (**a,b**)

We further examined the effects of the mixture using the hot-plate test. The present study has demonstrated the analgesic effect of topical mixture of extracts (0.2 g/0.3 ml) significantly increased the response latency time to heat stimulation after 10 days. This could be the possible explanation for its central analgesic activity observed in hotplate test.

We examined our hypothesis also by using the open field test to exclude false positives in nociceptive tests. The open field test is commonly used for pharmacological selection of drugs that act on the locomotor activities [19]. Rats treated with the mixture of extracts displayed significantly better locomotor recovery at the late stages of the treatment when compared to group (N) after 7 days of MIA injection.

We utilized the differential in weight bearing between the left (osteoarthritic) and right (contralateral control) limbs as an indication of joint discomfort by analysis the rat paw prints. The number and intensity of pixel values of left compared to contralateral paw decreased after 3 days of injection of MIA, same as in group (P).

The acute inflammatory response in the MIA model lasts approximately during the first weak, but afterward inflammation plays a minor role in pain and it is more likely caused by biomechanical forces affecting articular cartilage and subchondral bone [34].

The study showed that topical usage of the mixture of the extracts was useful in the treatment of the inflammation induced by MIA. The effect of reducing inflammation was initiated after 3 days. It showed that the formulation has an effect on acute inflammatory response same as diclofenac gel.

Gross morphological observations and histological evaluation of the knee joints were performed to evaluate the protective effect of the mixture of extracts on cartilage and articular tissue structures. The results of the pathological findings and scoring of the lesions showed that topical usage of the selected formula made

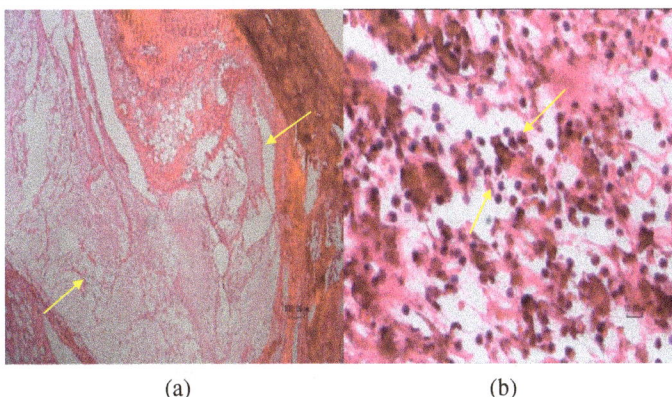

Fig. 9 Pathological findings one day after MIA injection. Severe fibrinopurulent exudates (*arrows*) can be seen within articular and adjacent tissues (**a&b**). Scale bar =100 μm (**a**), Scale bar =10 μm (**b**)

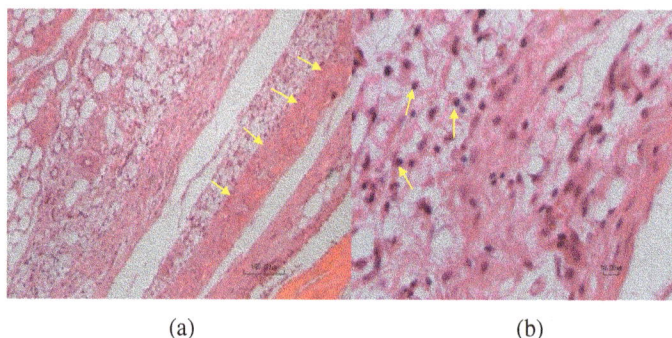

(a)   (b)

Fig. 10 A section of articular tissue from group (P). A very mild reaction including a few scattered lymphoid cells (*arrows*) can be seen. The same tissue reaction was seen in group (T). Scale bar =100 μm (left handed Fig.) and Scale bar =10 μm (right handed Fig.)

significant changes on the knee of the rats histologically. Compared to vehicle group, in which granulation, tissue formation, tendinal adhesion and mixed inflammatory cell infiltration were seen fourteen days after MIA administration, test and diclofenac groups showed only very mild reactions characterized by negligible edema and a few scattered inflammatory lymphoid cells.

According to the pharmacological responses of each herb extract, it could be concluded that the main effect of the formulation related to *L.inermis* extract efficacy.

Although because of the different active compounds in the extracts, the mechanism of action is unknown but the comparable effect on the inhibition of inflammation and pain compared to diclofenac makes the suggestion that they work through the same pathways.

In conclusion, the present study provided clues for further studies on pharmacological methods to analyze the anti-inflammatory and analgesic activities of topical drugs. The results demonstrated that topical preparation of *L.inermis* and *R.communis* was not only be able to mitigate pain and inflammation but also inhibit MIA-induced histological changes on the knee of the rats. Therefore, this formula could be a good candidate for further studies as a new efficient treatment in patients with osteoarthritis.

Conclusion

This study demonstrated that based on the different anti-inflammatory and analgesic evaluations, the pain and inflammation induced by intra-articular injection of MIA in rats were reduced with topical application of a mixture of *Lawsonia inermis* and *Ricinus communis* extracts. Further clinical studies are required to evaluate the safety and efficacy issues of the extracts mixture.

Ethic approval

This research was approved by the Research Committee of Shahid Beheshti University of Medical Sciences and institutional ethics committee with approval code SBMU.REC.1392.343.

Competing interests
The authors declare that they have no competing interests.

Authors' contributions
AZ, MF, MG and SS conceived and designed the experiments. AZ performed experimental procedures. MG produced all histological figures and datas. AZ, MF analyzed the data. MF, MG, AZ contributed materials/analysis tools. AZ, MF, SS and MG wrote the paper. All authors read and approved the final version of the manuscript.

Acknowledgements
This study was the result of a PhD thesis of Atousa Ziaei (no:141) and financial support was provided by a grant (N-128) from Department of Traditional Pharmacy, School of Traditional Medicine, Shahid Beheshti University of Medical Sciences, Tehran, Iran. The authors wish to thank the

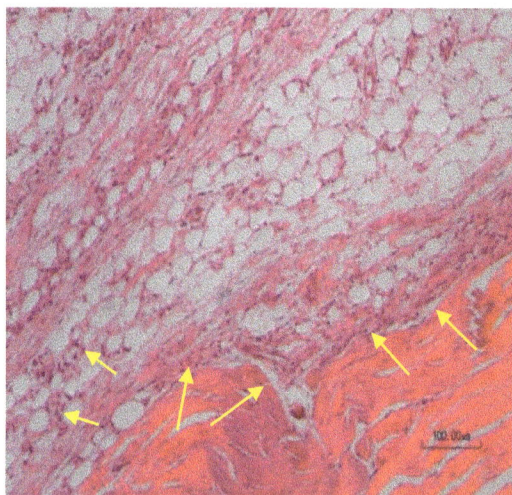

Fig. 11 A section of articular tissue from group (N). 14 days after MIA injection, a mixed inflammatory cell infiltration (*small arrows*) and tendinal adhesion to the adjacent tissue (*large arrows*) are evident. Scale bar =100 μm

Department of Pathology, Faculty of Veterinary Medicine, University of Tehran, for performing the histological tests and their technical assistance.

Author details
[1]Traditional Medicine and Material Medical Research Center; Department of Traditional Pharmacy, School of Traditional Medicine, Shahid Beheshti University of Medical Sciences, Tehran, Iran. [2]Department of Pathology, Faculty of Veterinary Medicine, University of Tehran, Tehran, Iran. [3]Department of Pharmacology and Toxicology, School of Pharmacy, Shahid Beheshti University of Medical Sciences, Tehran, Iran.

References

1. Kennedy DO, Wightman EL. Herbal extracts and phytochemicals: plant secondary metabolites and the enhancement of human brain function. Adv Nutr. 2011;2:32–50. doi:10.3945/an.110.000117.

2. Soares-Bezerra RJ, Calheiros AS, Da Silva Ferreira NC, Da Silva FV, Alves LA. Natural products as a source for new anti-inflammatory and analgesic compounds through the inhibition of puringic p2x receptors. Pharmaceuticals. 2013;6:650–8.

3. Aghili Khorasani MH. Makhzanol Advieh. 1th ed. Research Institute for Islamic and Complementary Medicine, Iran University of Medical Sciences. Tehran, Iran: Bavardaran Press; 2001. p. 243–55.

4. Aghili Khorasani MH. Gharabadin Kabir. 2nd ed. Tehran: Tehran medical university; 2005. p. 899–901.

5. Tonkaboni MM (1699). Tohfeh al-momenin. In: Rahimi R, Ardekani MS. Farjadmand F, editors. Tehran: Shahid beheshti university of medical sciences; 2007. p.166

6. Guzman RE, Evans MG, Bove S, Morenko B, Kilgore K. Mono-iodoacetate-induced histologic changes in subchondral bone and articular cartilage of rat femorotibial joints: An animal model of osteoarthritis. Toxicol Pathol. 2003;31:619–24.

7. Neugebauer V, Han JS, Adwanikar H. Techniques for assessing knee joint pain in arthritis. Mol Pain. 2007;3:30–42.

8. Alia B, Bashir A. Anti-inflammatory, antipyretic and analgesic effects of Lawsonia inermis L. (henna) in rats. Pharmacol. 1995;51:356–63.

9. Nithya V. Anti-inflammatory activity of Lawsonia ulba Linn., in wistar albino rats. Asian J Sci Tech. 2011;4:001–3.

10. Chaudhary G, Goyal S, Poonia P. Lawsonia inermis Linnaeus: a phytopharmacological review. Int J Pharm Sci Drug Res. 2010;2:91–8.

11. Darmanin S, Wismayer PS, Camilleri Podesta MT, Micallef MJ, Buhagiar JA. An extract from Ricinus communis L. Leaves possesses cytotoxic properties and induces apoptosis in sk-mel-28 human melanoma cells. Nat Prod Res. 2009;23:561–71.

12. Nemudzivhadi V, Masoko P. In vitro assessment of cytotoxicity, antioxidant, and anti-inflammatory activities of Ricinus communis (Euphorbiaceae) leaf extracts. Evid Based Complement Alternat Med. 2014;2014:625961. doi:10.1155/2014/625961.

13. Sengupta S, Velpandian T, Kabir SR, Gupta SK. Analgesic efficacy and pharmacokinetics of topical nimesulide gel in healthy human volunteers: double-blind comparison with piroxicam, diclofenac and placebo. Eur J Clin Pharmacol. 1998;54:541–7.

14. Xu Q, Ming Z, Dart AM, Du XJ. Optimizing dosage of ketamine and xylazine in murine echo cardiography. Clin Exp Pharmacol Physiol. 2007;34:499–507.

15. Horváth A, Tékus V, Boros M, Pozsgai G, Botz B, Borbély E, Szolcsányi J. Transient receptor potential ankyrin 1 (TRPA1) receptor is involved in chronic arthritis: in vivo study using TRPA1-deficient mice. Arthritis Res Ther. 2016;18:6. doi:10.1186/s13075-015-0904-y.

16. Lee Y, Pai M, Brederson JD, Wilcox D, Hsieh G, Jarvis MF, Bitner RS. Monosodium iodoacetate-induced joint pain is associated with increased phosphorylation of mitogen activated protein kinases in the rat spinal cord. Mol Pain. 2011;7:39. doi:10.1186/1744-8069-7-39.

17. Bove SE, Calcaterra SL, Brooker RM, Huber CM, Guzman RE. Weight bearing as a measure of disease progression and efficacy of anti-inflammatory compounds in a model of monosodium iodoacetate-induced osteoarthritis. Osteoarthr Cartilage. 2003;11:821–30.

18. Schuelert N, McDougall JJ. Grading of monosodium iodoacetate-induced osteo- arthritis reveals a concentration-dependent sensitization of

19. nociceptors in the knee joint of the rat. Neurosci Lett. 2009;465:184–8. doi:10.1016/j.neulet.2009.08.063.

19. Rainsford KD, Velo GP, editors. Side-effects of anti-inflammatory drugs, part two studies in major organ systems. Lancaster: MTP press limited; 1987. p. 114.

20. Beyreuther B, Callizot N, Stohr T. Antinociceptive efficacy of lacosamide in the monosodium iodoacetate rat model for osteoarthritis pain. Arthritis Res Ther. 2007;9:R14.

21. Archer J. Tests for emotionality in rats and mice: a review. Anim Behav. 1973;21:205–35. doi:10.1016/S0003-3472(73)80065-X.

22. Lacroix L, Broersen L, Weiner I, Feldon J. The effects of excitotoxic lesion of the medial prefrontal cortex on latent inhibition, prepulse inhibition, food hoarding, elevated plus maze, active avoidance and locomotor activity in the rat. Neurosci. 1998;84:431–42.

23. Dijkstra JR, Meek MF, Robinson PH, Gramsberge A. Methods to evaluate functional nerve recovery in adult rats: Walking track analysis, video analysis and the withdrawal reflex. J Neurosci Meth. 2000;96:89–96.

24. Hasler N, Klette R, Agnew W. In: Pariman D, North H, Mcneill S, editors. Footprint recognition of rodents and insects. New Zealand: Landcare Reasearch Ltd; 2004. p. 167–73.

25. South SM, Smith MT. Apparent insensitivity of the hotplate latency test for detection of antinociception following intraperitoneal, intravenous or intracerebroventricular M6G administration to rats. J Pharmacol Exp Ther. 2002;286:1326–32.

26. Hajarolasvadi N, Zamani MJ, Sarkhail P, Khorasani R, Mohajer M, Amin G, Shafiee A, Sharifzadeh M, Abdollahi M. Comparison of antinociceptive effects of total, water, ethyl acetate, Ether and N-Butanol extracts of Phlomis anisodonta boiss and indomethacin in mice. Int J Pharmacol. 2006;2:209–12.

27. Fereidoni M, Ahmadiani A, Semnanian S, Javan M. An accurate and simple method for measurement of paw edema. J Pharmacol Toxicol Methods. 2000;43:11–4.

28. Luna LG. Manual of histologic staining methods of the armed forces institute of pathology. 3rd ed. New York: The Blakiston Division, Mc Graw Hill Book Company; 1960. p. 8–9. 38–39.

29. Woong Park C, Wan Ma K, Woo Jang S, Son M, Joo KM. Comparison of Piroxicam Pharmacokinetics and anti-inflammatory effect in rats after Intra-articular and intramuscular administration. Biomol Ther (Seoul). 2014; 22:260–6. doi:10.4062/biomolther.2014.037.

30. B.McMahon S, Koltzenburg M, Tracey I, Turk D. Wall & Melzack's textbook of Pain. Sixth ed. Philadelphia, PA, USA: Elsevier/Churchill Livingstone; 2013.

31. Makhija IK, Dhananjaya DR, Kumar VS, Devkar R, Khamar D, Manglani N, Chandrakar S. Lawsonia inermis-from traditional use to scientific assessment. Afr J Pharm Sci Pharm. 2011;2:145–65.

32. Rashid MH, Theberge Y, Elmes SJ, Perkins MN, McIntosh F. Pharmacological validation of early and late phase of rat mono-iodoacetate model using the Tekscan system. Eur J Pain. 2013;17:210–22. doi:10.1002/j.1532-2149.2012.00176.x.

33. Eidman DS, Benedito MA, Leite JR. Daily changes in pentylenetetrazol-induced convulsions and open-field behavior in rats. Physiol Behav. 1990;47:853–6.

34. Kumari RR, More AS, Gupta G, Lingaraju MC, Balaganur V, Kumar P. Effect of alcoholic extract of Entada pursaetha DC on monosodium iodoacetate-induced osteoarthritis pain in rats. Indian J Med Res. 2015;141:454–62. doi:10.4103/0971-5916.159296.

Permissions

All chapters in this book were first published in JPS, by BioMed Central; hereby published with permission under the Creative Commons Attribution License or equivalent. Every chapter published in this book has been scrutinized by our experts. Their significance has been extensively debated. The topics covered herein carry significant findings which will fuel the growth of the discipline. They may even be implemented as practical applications or may be referred to as a beginning point for another development.

The contributors of this book come from diverse backgrounds, making this book a truly international effort. This book will bring forth new frontiers with its revolutionizing research information and detailed analysis of the nascent developments around the world.

We would like to thank all the contributing authors for lending their expertise to make the book truly unique. They have played a crucial role in the development of this book. Without their invaluable contributions this book wouldn't have been possible. They have made vital efforts to compile up to date information on the varied aspects of this subject to make this book a valuable addition to the collection of many professionals and students.

This book was conceptualized with the vision of imparting up-to-date information and advanced data in this field. To ensure the same, a matchless editorial board was set up. Every individual on the board went through rigorous rounds of assessment to prove their worth. After which they invested a large part of their time researching and compiling the most relevant data for our readers.

The editorial board has been involved in producing this book since its inception. They have spent rigorous hours researching and exploring the diverse topics which have resulted in the successful publishing of this book. They have passed on their knowledge of decades through this book. To expedite this challenging task, the publisher supported the team at every step. A small team of assistant editors was also appointed to further simplify the editing procedure and attain best results for the readers.

Apart from the editorial board, the designing team has also invested a significant amount of their time in understanding the subject and creating the most relevant covers. They scrutinized every image to scout for the most suitable representation of the subject and create an appropriate cover for the book.

The publishing team has been an ardent support to the editorial, designing and production team. Their endless efforts to recruit the best for this project, has resulted in the accomplishment of this book. They are a veteran in the field of academics and their pool of knowledge is as vast as their experience in printing. Their expertise and guidance has proved useful at every step. Their uncompromising quality standards have made this book an exceptional effort. Their encouragement from time to time has been an inspiration for everyone.

The publisher and the editorial board hope that this book will prove to be a valuable piece of knowledge for researchers, students, practitioners and scholars across the globe.

List of Contributors

Ketan Patel, Vidur Sarma and Pradeep Vavia
Sciences and Technology, Institute of Chemical Technology, University under Section 3 of UGC Act 1956, Elite Status and Center of Excellence – Govt. of Maharashtra, TEQIP Phase II Funded, N. P. Marg, Matunga (E), Mumbai 400 019, India

Rasool Haddadi
Student Research Committee, Tabriz University of Medical Sciences, Tabriz, Iran
Department of Pharmacology and Toxicology, Faculty of Pharmacy, Tabriz University of Medical Sciences, Tabriz, Iran

Safar Farajniya and Shahla Eyvari Brooshghalan
Drug Applied Research Center, Tabriz University of Medical Sciences, Tabriz, Iran
Alireza

Mohajjel Nayebi
Drug Applied Research Center, Tabriz University of Medical Sciences, Tabriz, Iran
Department of Pharmacology and Toxicology, Faculty of Pharmacy, Tabriz University of Medical Sciences, Tabriz, Iran

Hamdolah Sharifi
Urmia University of Medical Science, Urmia, Iran

Mohammad Hossein Boskabady, Azadeh Feizpour, Milad Hashemzahi, Lila Gholami, Farzaneh Vafaee Bagheri and Esmaeil Khodaei
Neurogenic Inflammation Research Centre and Department of Physiology, School of Medicine, Mashhad University of Medical Sciences, Mashhad 9177948564, Iran

Ahmad Ghorbani
Pharmacological Research Center of Medicinal Plants, School of Medicine, Mashhad University of Medical Sciences, Mashhad, Iran

Mahmoud Hosseini
Neurocognitive Research Center and Department of Physiology, School of Medicine, Mashhad University of Medical Sciences, Mashhad, Iran

Mohammad Soukhtanloo
Department of Clinical Biochemistry, School of Medicine, Mashhad University of Medical Sciences, Mashhad, Iran

Nema Mohammadian Roshan
Department of Pathology, School of Medicine, Mashhad University of Medical Sciences, Mashhad, Iran

Alireza Vatanara and Abdolhossein Rouholamini Najafabadi
Department of Pharmaceutics, Faculty of Pharmacy, Tehran University of Medical Sciences, Tehran, Iran

Mohammad Ali Shokrgozar
National Cell Bank of Iran, Pasteur Institute of Iran, Tehran, Iran

Vahid Ramezani
Department of Pharmaceutics, Faculty of Pharmacy, Tehran University of Medical Sciences, Tehran, Iran
Department of Pharmaceutics, Faculty of Pharmacy, Shahid Sadoughi University of Medical Sciences, Yazd, Iran

Alireza Khabiri
Department of Mycology, Pasteur Institute of Iran, Tehran, Iran

Mohammad Seyedabadi
Department of Molecular Imaging, The Persian Gulf Biomedical Sciences Research Institute, Bushehr University of Medical Sciences, Bushehr, Iran

Hosein Shabaninejad and Ahmad Baratimarnani
Department of Health Services Management, School of Health Management and Information Sciences, Iran University of Medical Sciences, Rashidiasemi st, Valiasr st, Vanak sq., P.O.Box: 1995614111, Tehran, Iran

Hamid Reza Rasekh and Gholamhossein Mehralian
Department of Pharmacoeconomics and Pharma Management, School of Pharmacy, Shahid
Beheshti University of Medical Sciences, Tehran, Iran

Arash Rashidian
Department of Health Management and Economics, School of Public Health & Knowledge
Utilization Research Center, Tehran University of Medical Sciences, Tehran, Iran

Mohammad Hossein Yazdi, Neda Setayesh, Mohammad Esfandyar and Ahmad Reza Shahverdi
Department of Pharmaceutical Biotechnology, Faculty of Pharmacy and Biotechnology Research Center, Tehran University of Medical Sciences, Tehran, Iran

Mehdi Mahdavi
Department of virology, Pasteur Institute of Iran, Tehran, Iran

Elham Akhtari, Mansoor Keshavarz and Soodabeh Bioos
Department of Traditional Medicine, School of Medicine, Tehran University of Medical Sciences, Tehran, Iran

Firoozeh Raisi
Psychiatry, Fellow of the European Committee of Sexual Medicine (FECSM), Roozbeh Psychiatric Hospital, Psychiatric and Clinical Psychology, Research Center, Tehran University of Medical Sciences, South Kargar Street, Tehran 13337, Iran

Hamed Hosseini
School of Public Health, Tehran University of Medical Sciences, Tehran, Iran
Clinical Trial Center, Tehran University of Medical Sciences, Tehran, Iran

Farnaz Sohrabvand
Department of Gynecology and Infertility, Imam Khomeini Hospital, Tehran University of
Medical Sciences, Tehran, Iran

Mohammad Kamalinejad
Department of Pharmacognosy, School of Pharmacy, Shaheed Beheshti University of Medical Sciences, Tehran, Iran

Ali Ghobadi
Department of Traditional Medicine, School of Traditional Pharmacology, Tehran University of Medical Sciences, Tehran, Iran

Parisa Sarkhail and Pantea Sarkheil
Pharmaceutical Sciences Research Center, Tehran University of Medical Sciences, Tehran, Iran

Marjan Nikan
Medicinal Plants Research Center, Faculty of Pharmacy, Tehran University of Medical Sciences, Tehran, Iran

Soodabeh Saeidnia and Ahmad R Gohari
Medicinal Plants Research Center, Faculty of Pharmacy, Tehran University of Medical Sciences, Tehran, Iran
Division of Pharmacy, College of Pharmacy and Nutrition, University of Saskatchewan, Saskatoon, Canada

Yousef Ajani
Institute of Medicinal Plants (IMP), Iranian Academic Centre for Education, Culture and Research (ACECR), Karaj, Iran

Rohollah Hosseini
Department of Toxicology and Pharmacology, Faculty of Pharmacy, Tehran University of Medical Sciences, Tehran 1417614411, Iran

Abbass Hadjiakhoondi
Medicinal Plants Research Center, Faculty of Pharmacy, Tehran University of Medical Sciences, Tehran, Iran
Department of Pharmacognosy, Faculty of Pharmacy, Tehran University of Medical Sciences, Tehran 1417614411, Iran

Mehrdad Rafati-Rahimzadeh
Department of Nursing, Babol University of Medical Sciences, Babol, Iran

Mehravar Rafati-Rahimzadeh
Department of Medical Physics, Kashan University of Medical Sciences, Kashan, Iran

Sohrab Kazemi
Department of Pharmacology, Faculty of Medicine, Babol University of Medical Sciences, Babol, Iran

Ali Akbar Moghadamnia
Department of Pharmacology, Faculty of Medicine, Babol University of Medical Sciences, Babol, Iran
Cellular and Molecular Research Center, Babol University of Medical Sciences, Babol, Iran

Mohammad Hossein Karimi, Salimeh Ebrahimnezhad and Mandana Namayandeh
Transplant Research Center, Shiraz University of Medical Sciences, Shiraz, Iran

Zahra Amirghofran
Department of Immunology, Autoimmune Disease Research Center and Medicinal and Natural Products Chemistry Research Center, Shiraz University of Medical Sciences, Shiraz, Iran

Saeedeh Noushini and Eskandar Alipour
Department of Chemistry, Islamic Azad University, Tehran-North Branch, Zafar St, Tehran, Iran

Saeed Emami
Department of Medicinal Chemistry and Pharmaceutical Sciences Research Center, Faculty of Pharmacy, Mazandaran University of Medical Sciences, Sari, Iran

Maliheh Safavi and Sussan Kabudanian Ardestani
Institute of Biochemistry and Biophysics, University of Tehran, Tehran, Iran

Ahmad Reza Gohari
Medicinal Plants Research Center, Tehran University of Medical Sciences, Tehran, Iran

Alireza Foroumadi
Medicinal Plants Research Center, Tehran University of Medical Sciences, Tehran, Iran
Department of Medicinal Chemistry, Faculty of Pharmacy and Pharmaceutical Sciences Research Center, Tehran University of Medical Sciences, Tehran, Iran

Abbas Shafiee
Department of Medicinal Chemistry, Faculty of Pharmacy and Pharmaceutical Sciences Research Center, Tehran University of Medical Sciences, Tehran, Iran

Hamid Soraya and Peyman Mikaili
Department of Pharmacology, Faculty of Pharmacy, Urmia University of Medical Sciences, Urmia, Iran

Milad Moloudizargari, Shahin Aghajanshakeri and Soheil Javaherypour
Student of Veterinary Medicine, Faculty of Veterinary Medicine, Urmia University, Urmia, Iran

Aram Mokarizadeh
Department of Immunology, Faculty of Medicine, and Cellular & Molecular Research Center, Kurdistan University of Medical Sciences, Sanandaj, Iran

Sanaz Hamedeyazdan
Department of Pharmacognosy, Faculty of Pharmacy, Tabriz University of Medical Sciences, Tabriz, Iran

Hadi Esmaeli Gouvarchin Ghaleh
Department of Microbiology, Faculty of Veterinary Medicine, Urmia University, Urmia, Iran

Alireza Garjani
Department of Pharmacology & Toxicology, Faculty of Pharmacy, Tabriz University of Medical Sciences, Tabriz, Iran

Zahra Hami
Department of Medical Nanotechnology, School of Advanced Technologies in Medicine, Tehran University of Medical Sciences, Tehran, Iran

Mohsen Amini
Department of Medicinal Chemistry, Faculty of Pharmacy and Drug Design & Development Research Center, Tehran University of Medical Sciences, Tehran, Iran

Mahmoud Ghazi-Khansari
Department of Pharmacology, School of Medicine, Tehran University of Medical Sciences, Tehran, Iran

Seyed Mehdi Rezayat
Department of Medical Nanotechnology, School of Advanced Technologies in Medicine, Tehran University of Medical Sciences, Tehran, Iran
Department of Pharmacology, School of Medicine, Tehran University of Medical Sciences, Tehran, Iran
Department of Toxicology & Pharmacology, Faculty of Pharmacy, Pharmaceutical Sciences Branch, Islamic Azad University (IAUPS), Tehran, Iran

Kambiz Gilani
Aerosol Research Laboratory, Department of Pharmaceutics, School of Pharmacy, Tehran University of Medical Sciences, Tehran, Iran

Roshanak Salari and Zahra Khashyarmanesh
Department of Drug and Food Control, School of Pharmacy, Mashhad University of Medical Sciences, Mashhad, Iran

BiBi Sedigheh Fazly Bazzaz
Department of Drug and Food Control, School of Pharmacy, Mashhad University of Medical Sciences, Mashhad, Iran
Biotechnology Research Centre, School of Pharmacy, Mashhad University of Medical Sciences, Mashhad, Iran

Omid Rajabi
Department of Drug and Food Control, School of Pharmacy, Mashhad University of Medical Sciences, Mashhad, Iran
Targetted Drug Delivery Research Centre, School of Pharmacy, Mashhad University of Medical Sciences, Mashhad, Iran

Christina Woodward, Ali Pourmand and Maryann Mazer-Amirshahi
Department of Emergency Medicine, George Washington University, Washington, DC 20037, USA

Fereshteh Haghighi, Fatemeh B Rassouli and Azadeh Haghighitalab
Department of Biology, Faculty of Science, Ferdowsi University of Mashhad, Mashhad, Iran

Maryam M Matin and Ahmad Reza Bahrami
Department of Biology, Faculty of Science, Ferdowsi University of Mashhad, Mashhad, Iran Cell and Molecular Biotechnology Research Group, Institute of Biotechnology, Ferdowsi University of Mashhad, Mashhad, Iran

Mehrdad Iranshahi
Biotechnology Research Center and School of Pharmacy, Mashhad University of Medical Sciences, Mashhad, Iran

Monireh Afzali, Maliheh Parsa, Hamed Montazeri, Mohammad Hossein Ghahremani and Seyed Nasser Ostad
Department Toxicology & Pharmacology, Faculty of Pharmacy, Toxicology & Poisoning Research Center, Tehran University of Medical Sciences, 14155/ 6451 Tehran, Iran

Padideh Ghaeli
Department Clinical Pharmacy, Faculty of Pharmacy & Rational Drug Use Research Center, Tehran University of Medical Sciences, 14155/6451 Tehran, Iran

Mahnaz Khanavi
Department Pharmacognosy, Faculty of Pharmacy, Tehran University of Medical Sciences, 14155/6451 Tehran, Iran

Sabrina Giacoppo, Maria Galuppo, Placido Bramanti and Emanuela Mazzon
IRCCS Centro Neurolesi "Bonino-Pulejo", Via Provinciale Palermo, contrada Casazza, 98124 Messina, Italy

Federica Pollastro
Dipartimento di Scienze del Farmaco, Università del Piemonte Orientale, Largo Donegani 2, 28100 Novara, Italy

Gianpaolo Grassi
Consiglio per le Ricerca e la sperimentazione in Agricoltura – Centro di Ricerca per le Colture Industriali (CRA-CIN), Viale G. Amendola 82, 45100 Rovigo, Italy

Somayeh Rajabi and Tahereh Naji
Cell and Molecular Biology Departments, Pharmaceutical Sciences Branch, Islamic Azad University, Tehran, Iran

Ali Ramazani
Cell and Molecular Biology Departments, Pharmaceutical Sciences Branch, Islamic Azad University, Tehran, Iran
Biotechnology Departments, School ofPharmacy, Zanjan University of Medical Sciences, Zanjan, Iran

Mehrdad Hamidi
Zanjan Pharmaceutical Nanotechnology Research Center, Zanjan University of Medical Sciences, Zanjan, Iran

Raju Dash, Md Firoz Hossen, Mohammad Mohiuddin and Md Rashadul Alam
Department of Pha rmacy, BGC Trust University Bangladesh, Chittagong 4000, Bangladesh

Talha Bin Emran
Department of Pha rmacy, BGC Trust University Bangladesh, Chittagong 4000, Bangladesh
Department of Biochemistry and Molecular Biology, University of Chittagong, Chittagong 4331, Bangladesh

Md Atiar Rahman
Department of Biochemistry and Molecular Biology, University of Chittagong, Chittagong 4331, Bangladesh

Mir Muhammad Nasir Uddin
Department of Pharmacy, University of Chittagong, Chittagong 4331, Bangladesh

Muhammad Faheem Akhtar, Nazar Muhammad Ranjha and Muhammad Hanif
Faculty of Pharmacy, Bahauddin Zakariya University, P.O.Box: 60800, Multan, Pakistan

Saeed Abbasi
Anesthesiology and Critical Care Research Center, Isfahan University of Medical Sciences, Isfahan, Iran

Shadi Farsaei
Department of Clinical Pharmacy and Pharmacy Practice, Isfahan University of Medical Sciences, Isfahan, Iran

Kamran Fazel
Department of Anesthesia and Critical Care Medicine, Bagiatalla University of Medical Sciences, Tehran, Iran

Samad EJ Golzari
Medical Education Research Center, Tabriz University of Medical Sciences, Tabriz, Iran

Ata Mahmoodpoor
Cardiovascular Research Center, Tabriz University of Medical Sciences, Tabriz, Iran

Vivek K. Bajpai, Gyeong-Jun Nam, Rajib Majumder, Irfan A. Rather and Yong-Ha Park
Department of Applied Microbiology and Biotechnology, Microbiome Laboratory, Yeungnam University, Gyeongsan, Gyeongbuk 712-749, Republic of Korea

Chanseo Park, Jeongheui Lim, Woon Kee Paek and Jeong-Ho Han
National Science Museum, Ministry of Science, ICT and Future Planning, Daejeon 32143, Republic of Korea

Mehdi Esfandyari-Manesh, Nazanin Shabani Ravari, Fatemeh Atyabi and Rassoul Dinarvand
Nanotechnology Research Centre, Faculty of Pharmacy, Tehran University of Medical Sciences, Tehran, Iran
Novel Drug Delivery Lab, Department of Pharmaceutics, Faculty of Pharmacy, Tehran University of Medical Sciences, Tehran, Iran

Mona Noori Koopaei
Novel Drug Delivery Lab, Department of Pharmaceutics, Faculty of Pharmacy, Tehran University of Medical Sciences, Tehran, Iran
Seyed Hossein Mostafavi
Novel Drug Delivery Lab, Department of Pharmaceutics, Faculty of Pharmacy, Tehran University of Medical Sciences, Tehran, Iran
Department of Bioengineering, University of California, Riverside, CA, USA
Medical Nanotechnology Department, School of Advanced Technologies in Medicine, Tehran University of Medical Sciences, Tehran, Iran

Reza Faridi Majidi
Medical Nanotechnology Department, School of Advanced Technologies in Medicine, Tehran University of Medical Sciences, Tehran, Iran

Behrad Darvishi
Nanotechnology Research Centre, Faculty of Pharmacy, Tehran University of Medical Sciences, Tehran, Iran
Medical Nanotechnology Department, School of Advanced Technologies in Medicine, Tehran University of Medical Sciences, Tehran, Iran

Mohsen Amini
Department of Medicinal Chemistry, Faculty of Pharmacy, Tehran University of Medical Sciences, Tehran, Iran

Seyed Nasser Ostad
Department of Toxicology and Pharmacology, Faculty of Pharmacy, Tehran University of Medical Science, Tehran, Iran

Atousa Ziaei and Shamim Sahranavard
Traditional Medicine and Material Medical Research Center; Department of Traditional Pharmacy, School of Traditional Medicine, Shahid Beheshti University of Medical Sciences, Tehran, Iran

Mohammad Javad Gharagozlou
Department of Pathology, Faculty of Veterinary Medicine, University of Tehran, Tehran, Iran

Mehrdad Faizi
Department of Pharmacology and Toxicology, School of Pharmacy, Shahid Beheshti University of Medical Sciences, Tehran, Iran

Index

A

Acrylic Acid-polyvinyl Alcohol Hydrogel, 174, 176
Albumin Surface Modification, 204-205, 207, 209, 211
Angiogenic Effect, 97, 99, 101-103
Anti-tyrosinase Activity, 192, 202
Antimalarial Molecule, 1
Artemia Salina, 160-161, 163, 165
Autoimmune Encephalomyelitis (eae), 143

B

Bacopa Monnieri L, 166
Beta Cyclodextrin, 32-33
Beta-blocker, 120, 123
Bladder Cancer, 125, 130-132

C

Calcium Channel Blocker, 120-121, 123
Cancer Chemotherapy, 87
Cannabidiol (cbd), 143-144, 158
Cannabis Sativa L, 143-145
Cell Culture, 32, 34, 46, 48-49, 51, 54, 81, 126, 142, 160-161, 164, 210
Cell Cycle Arrest, 125-126, 130, 132-133
Cell Viability, 32, 35, 37, 95, 110, 127, 160-162, 208, 210
Chelating Agents, 70, 75-77
Chroman-4-one, 87
Chronic Obstructive Pulmonary Disease (copd), 20
Cichorium Intybus, 80-81, 83, 85-86
Competitiveness, 39-45
Cynodon Dactylon, 97, 99, 101-104
Cytotoxic Activity, 87-88, 92-95, 110

D

Dendritic Cells, 80-81, 83, 85-86
Difficult Weaning, 184
Donepezil, 184-191
Doxorubicin-conjugated, 105-107, 109, 111
Dynamic Swelling, 174, 177, 179

E

Emphysema, 20-21, 23, 25-27, 29-31, 72
Endothelial Cells, 21, 97-98, 100-101, 104, 183
Ethylene Glycol Dimethacrylate, 174-175, 177, 179, 181, 183

F

Fish Microbiota, 192, 198-199

G

Genotoxicity, 135-136, 141-142
Glutaraldehyde, 174-175
Gold Nanoparticles, 70, 74, 79
Granulation Tissue, 97, 99-102, 104, 215, 218

H

Hemi-parkisonian Rats, 13, 15, 17
High Dose Insulin Therapy, 120-121, 123
Human Capital, 39, 41, 43, 45
Hydroxypropyl Beta Cyclodextrin, 32

I

Immune Responses, 46-47, 49, 51, 53-54, 80-81, 84, 158, 203
Immunomodulatory Agents, 47
Inhibition Studies, 166-167, 169, 171, 173
Ionic Complex, 2-3, 5, 7, 9

L

Lactic Acid Bacteria, 46, 192, 194-195, 202-203
Liver Metastasis, 46, 52-53

M

Malondialdehyde, 13, 17, 20, 27
Mercury Poisoning, 70-71, 73-75, 77-79
Microencapsulation, 118-119
Molecular Docking, 166-167, 169-171, 173
Monoclonal Antibodies, 35
Multiple Sclerosis, 143-144, 158

N

Nanoscience, 160

Natural Biologic Scavengers, 70
Neuroinflammation, 11-12, 16, 18-19, 144, 155-158
Noscapine, 135-138, 140-142

O
Opium Alkaloids, 135, 137, 139, 141
Osteoarthritis, 84, 86, 212-214, 218, 220-221
Oxidative Stress, 11, 15-18, 20-21, 23, 25, 27, 29-31, 72, 76, 78-80, 104, 111, 133, 143, 156, 165

P
Pharmaceutical Industry, 39-45
Phlomis (lamiaceae), 61
Pla-peg-folate, 107, 109-111
Polymeric Micelle, 107, 109, 111
Poor Aqueous Solubility, 1-2

Q
Quantification, 36, 61-63, 65, 67, 69

R
Reticuloendothelial System (res), 204
Ricinus Communis L, 212-213, 221

S
Saccharomyces Cerevisiae Yeast Cells, 112, 115-117
Selenium Enriched L. Brevis, 46
Self Nanoemulsifying, 1-3, 5-7, 9
Sexual Dysfunction, 55, 57, 59-60
Silymarin, 11-13, 15-19
Spray Drying, 32-33, 35-37
Staphylococcus Aureus, 166-167, 170, 173, 193-194
Stromal Cells, 20-31

T
T Cell Responses, 80
Therapeutic Options, 167
Tlc Scanner, 61, 64, 67-68
Traditional Medicine, 55-56, 60, 80, 104, 212-213, 220-221
Trastuzumab, 32-38
Tribulus Terrestris, 55-57, 59-60
Tumor-targeted Delivery, 211

V
Verbascoside, 61-69